SECOND EDITION

INTRODUCTION TO
EVIDENCE-BASED PRACTICE
in Nursing and Health Care

Edited by

Kathy·Malloch, PhD, MBA, RN, FAAN
President
Kathy Malloch Leadership Systems, LLC

Clinical Professor
College of Nursing and Healthcare Innovation
Arizona State University

Tim Porter-O'Grady, PhD, EdD, RN, FAAN
Senior Partner
Tim Porter-O'Grady Associates, Inc.

Associate Professor
College of Nursing and Healthcare Innovation
Arizona State University

JONES AND BARTLETT PUBLISHERS
Sudbury, Massachusetts
BOSTON   TORONTO   LONDON   SINGAPORE

World Headquarters

Jones and Bartlett Publishers
40 Tall Pine Drive
Sudbury, MA 01776
978-443-5000
info@jbpub.com
www.jbpub.com

Jones and Bartlett Publishers
Canada
6339 Ormindale Way
Mississauga, Ontario L5V 1J2
Canada

Jones and Bartlett Publishers
International
Barb House, Barb Mews
London W6 7PA
United Kingdom

Jones and Bartlett's books and products are available through most bookstores and online booksellers. To contact Jones and Bartlett Publishers directly, call 800-832-0034, fax 978-443-8000, or visit our website, www.jbpub.com.

Substantial discounts on bulk quantities of Jones and Bartlett's publications are available to corporations, professional associations, and other qualified organizations. For details and specific discount information, contact the special sales department at Jones and Bartlett via the above contact information or send an email to specialsales@jbpub.com.

The authors, editor, and publisher have made every effort to provide accurate information. However, they are not responsible for errors, omissions, or for any outcomes related to the use of the contents of this book and take no responsibility for the use of the products and procedures described. Treatments and side effects described in this book may not be applicable to all people; likewise, some people may require a dose or experience a side effect that is not described herein. Drugs and medical devices are discussed that may have limited availability controlled by the Food and Drug Administration (FDA) for use only in a research study or clinical trial. Research, clinical practice, and government regulations often change the accepted standard in this field. When consideration is being given to use of any drug in the clinical setting, the healthcare provider or reader is responsible for determining FDA status of the drug, reading the package insert, and reviewing prescribing information for the most up-to-date recommendations on dose, precautions, and contraindications, and determining the appropriate usage for the product. This is especially important in the case of drugs that are new or seldom used.

Production Credits

Publisher: Kevin Sullivan
Acquisitions Editor: Emily Ekle
Acquisitions Editor: Amy Sibley
Associate Editor: Patricia Donnelly
Editorial Assistant: Rachel Shuster
Associate Production Editor: Katie Spiegel
Marketing Manager: Rebecca Wasley

V.P., Manufacturing and Inventory Control: Therese Connell
Composition: Spoke & Wheel/Jason Miranda
Cover Design: Scott Moden
Cover Image: © WebStudio24h/Shutterstock, Inc.
Printing and Binding: Malloy, Inc.
Cover Printing: Malloy, Inc.

Library of Congress Cataloging-in-Publication Data

Introduction to evidence-based practice in nursing and health care / [edited by] Kathy Malloch and Tim Porter-O'Grady.—2nd ed.
    p. ; cm.
  Includes bibliographical references and index.
  ISBN 978-0-7637-6542-2
  1. Evidence-based nursing. 2. Evidence-based medicine. I. Malloch, Kathy. II. Porter-O'Grady, Timothy.
  [DNLM: 1. Evidence-Based Nursing. 2. Nursing Process. WY 100 I61 2010]
  RT42.I584 2010
  610.73—dc22

                              2009010260

6048
Printed in the United States of America
13 12 11 10   10 9 8 7 6 5 4 3 2

Contents

Preface

The second edition of *Introduction to Evidence-Based Practice in Nursing and Health Care* provides new and updated information in nearly every chapter—new insights, new evidence, and new references for the evolving work. Two new chapters—Chapter 11, "Evidence-Based Regulation: Emerging Knowledge Management to Inform Policy" by Joey Ridenour, and Chapter 12, "Evidence-Based Leadership: Solid Foundations for Management Practices" by Tim Porter-O'Grady and Kathy Malloch—provide a framework for evidence-based management that further add to the richness of this reference book.

In a perfect world, the expenditure of energy, time, and money would result in corresponding value that is clearly evident to both the giver and the receiver of the energy, time, and money. Evidence of the relationship between the expenditure of resources and the value to the recipient is readily apparent and appreciated. In recent years, however, the new world focusing on the value of information has seriously challenged the allocation of resources and the basis from which future decisions are made. Consumers are not content to expend resources for undefined and unpredictable results; they want proof that they are getting their money's worth. Clear evidence linking expenditures to outcomes that provide value given limited human, physical, and financial resources is essential for survival and sustainability.

Interestingly, expectations that outcome value will be linked to resource expenditures have not been a priority or an expectation in health care in the past. Instead, the marketplace has largely focused on providing ready access to health care and financial coverage for citizens, without attempting to link that effort to value-based outcomes. Healthcare workers—particularly nurses—have yet to fully identify and articulate the value consumers receive for the time and energy that nurses expend, the fiscal support provided by the marketplace for those services, and the specific relationships between the resources expended and the value received.

Nurses, as both providers and consumers of healthcare services, are well positioned not only to improve the economic status of healthcare organizations, but also to advance the science of evidence-based resource allocation through the advancement of evidence-based practice in nursing. The continuing evolution of world complexity in today's "age of technology" presents new challenges and expectations for the profession of nursing. In fact, producing evidence of value in practice cannot be achieved without using a level of digital technology that simply has not as yet been fully adopted by the healthcare system. Increasing consumer involvement in healthcare services and the expectation that healthcare organization will provide hard evidence that value does, indeed, result from the fiscal resources expended on health care is the reality now faced by all providers. Never before have the challenges been so motivating for nursing and the potential so significant for the explication of its value.

During the last 10 years, nursing has embraced and begun to integrate the gold standard of health care—evidence-based practice (EBP)—to advance the profession of nursing. Never in the history of nursing has there been a better time for the nursing professional to be recognized for the differences he or she makes in the healthcare system and in the outcomes associated with individual patient services. Creating evidence will serve to validate and document the value of nursing practice, and doing so is also a call to celebrate the incredible value and efficacy of nursing. This compelling opportunity is much more than a mere invitation: It is a mandate for the profession to continue the journey initiated by Florence Nightingale.

To be sure, the journey is not only transformational, but also requires the involvement of all forces affecting the world of nursing practice. This book provides an overview of the world of evidence for nursing practice and highlights the application of EBP principles presented from differing perspectives, thereby combining theoretical underpinnings and real-world experience from experts with practical application to the practice of nursing. Specifically, the governance structure, organizational vision and values, goals, allocation of resources, implications for technology, educational processes, support for staff nurse clinical excellence, management of errors through application of high reliability theory, workload management systems embedded in the reality of the marketplace, and evaluation for excellence using the Magnet framework are covered in this book to provide a broad overview of the far-reaching implications when evidence is emphasized within an integrated, highly interconnected healthcare system. In addition, barriers to the integration of an evidentiary approach to nursing are discussed as well as strategies to overcome those barriers.

Closing the gap between evidence and practice requires knowledge, commitment, resilience, and a belief that this is the right course to explicate the essence of nursing and to further embed the value of nursing in the marketplace. As always, this work is a journey, not a destination. Your comments and suggestions to further enhance this work are encouraged and welcomed.

Kathy Malloch and Tim Porter-O'Grady

Acknowledgments

The collective wisdom of the contributing authors of this text not only illuminates the essence of evidence-based practice—that is, the best research available, the expertise of the practitioners, and the values of those involved—but also raises many thought-provoking and innovative challenges intended to enhance the journey of nursing practice along its evidence-based pathway. We are deeply grateful for the collective expertise of the contributors to this work, which represents a single source collecting information on the 12 critical areas of nursing practice that affect a large majority of the United States' 2.8 million nurses.

Each chapter author provides significant insight into nursing practice area and provides a welcome depth of discussion; each also amply demonstrates his or her passion for the topic. Our colleagues have shared their wisdom, their passion, and their very precious time in the preparation of these chapters. We have learned much from each of the chapters, and we continue to marvel at the incredible knowledge and willingness of each author to contribute his or her special expertise to this evidence-based practice knowledge reference book for other nurses. To be sure, no one nurse can know it all; it is only through collective generosity that the profession of nursing evolves and advances its science.

Thank you to our authors:

- To Dolly Sanares, Dr. Diane Heliker, and Dr. Phyllis Waters, for their willingness to share their updated model of disciplined clinical inquiry (DCI). This model represents the ultimate application of evidence-based practice principles in the practice setting and was developed in collaboration with the University of Texas Medical Branch at Galveston.

- To Dr. Bob Geibert, for his creative and thorough review of the literature specific to technology and the electronic health record. The new insights he has added in his chapter will be essential for those seeking to advance electronic media into healthcare mainstream work. Dr. Geibert's insight and ability to present the complex issues and challenges of the management of computerized information is a gift for those of us who struggle with the challenge of integrating the work of nursing into the world of technology.

- To Dr. Marie Farrell, for her wisdom and rich overview of the challenges of information synthesis. Her global perspective continues to offer a new lens for analysis and integration of the science of nursing into practice.

- To Dr. Amy Steinbinder and Elaine Scherer, for taking the risk to go above and beyond the norm in the development of the chapter on evidence for Magnet accreditation. While their assessment of Magnet leaders found in the first edition of this book was outstanding, their updated interview data continue to build the evidence base supporting the necessity of Magnet designation.

- To Dr. Kathy Scott, for her willingness to share her recent dissertation findings and evolving expertise in the area of patient safety and high-reliability organizations. Her work is essential reading in this time of great emphasis on patient safety.

- To Roz Cama, nationally recognized architect for creating healing spaces. She has brought this body of knowledge to a new level in documenting the link between physical space design, color, light, and nature and the processes of healing, as well as the creation of space that supports the work of nursing in a safe and ergonomically sound manner. The updates to this chapter will further assist healthcare professionals in the creation of evidence-based healing environments.

- To Drs. Marcia Flesner, Louise Miller, Roxanne McDaniel, and Marilyn Rantz, educators and innovators who continually push the walls of learning and practice advancement. Their insights into the need for and encouragement of evidence-based practices in learning and leading in clinical practice challenge us to think deeply and differently about the future of learning.

- Ginna Betts and her colleagues Susan Cooper, Karen Butler, and Jill Gentry, who work tirelessly to meet the needs of the health of the community and challenge their nursing and other healthcare colleagues to demonstrate a commitment to advocacy, meeting the needs of the marginalized, and making sure that we are actually improving the health of those we serve.

- Joey Ridenour, a national expert in nursing regulation, who has provided a new and important chapter on the evidence paradigm—namely, evidence-based nursing regulation. This chapter provides a historical overview of nursing regulation, offers examples of successful initiatives based on evidence, and presents the continuing challenges in and strategies needed to advance an evidence-based regulatory model.

Tim Porter-O'Grady and I also added a new chapter to this edition; it is designed to help leaders work from an evidence-based model while cultivating similar values among managers and knowledge workers. This information will greatly assist leaders, managers, and knowledge workers in advancing the infrastructure to support the most effective patient care work.

Finally, our own work on governance, workload management, and building preferred health models for the future is designed to provide new and innovative strategies for understanding current challenges, evaluating available evidence, and continuing to develop new skills in asking better questions about our work that will open the doors to new models and structures for evidence-based practice.

Kathy Malloch and Tim Porter-O'Grady

Contributors

Virginia Trotter Betts, MSN, JD, RN, FAAN
Commissioner for Policy
Tennessee Department of Mental Health and Developmental Disability
Nashville, Tennessee

Karen Butler, MSN, RN
Lecturer and Clinical Instructor
College of Nursing
University of Kentucky
Lexington, Kentucky

Rosalyn Cama, FASID
President
CAMA, Inc.
New Haven, Connecticut
Chair of the Board
The Center for Health Design
Concord, California

Susan R. Cooper, MSN, RN
Assistant Dean of Faculty Practice
Assistant Professor
Vanderbilt University School of Nursing
Nashville, Tennessee

Marie P. Farrell, MPH, RN, FAAN
Doctoral Faculty
School of Human and Organizational Development
Fielding University
Santa Barbara, California

Marcia K. Flesner, PhD, RN
Clinical Educator
Sinclair School of Nursing
University of Missouri–Columbia
Columbia, Missouri

Robert C. Geibert, EdD, RN
Senior Management Consultant
ACS Healthcare Services
Staff Nurse II, Pediatrics, Infusion Center, and GI Lab
Kaiser Permanente Medical Center
San Rafael, California
Consultant to the Vietnam Nurse Project
University of San Francisco School of Nursing and the Bach Mai Medical Nursing School
Hanoi, Vietnam

Jill Gentry
Special Assistant to the Commissioner
Tennessee Department of Mental Health and Developmental Disability
Nashville, Tennessee

Diane Heliker, PhD, RN
Professor
School of Nursing
University of Texas Medical Branch
Galveston, Texas

Roxanne McDaniel, PhD, RN
Associate Dean
Sinclair School of Nursing
University of Missouri–Columbia
Columbia, Missouri

Louise Miller, PhD, RN
Assistant Professor of Clinical Nursing
Sinclair School of Nursing
University of Missouri–Columbia
Columbia, Missouri

Marilyn Rantz, PhD, RN, FAAN
Professor
Sinclair School of Nursing
University of Missouri–Columbia
Columbia, Missouri

Joey Ridenour, MSN, RN, FAAN
Executive Director
Arizona State Board of Nursing
Phoenix, Arizona

Dolora (Dolly) C. Sanares-Carreon, MPA, RN
Program Manager, Evidence-Based
   Practice
Nursing Program Development,
   Hospitals and Clinics
University of Texas Medical Branch
Galveston, Texas

Elaine Scherer, MA, RN
Director
Mountain Area Health Education Center
Asheville, North Carolina

Kathy A. Scott, PhD, RN
Regional Vice President
Clinical Services
Banner Health
Phoenix, Arizona

Amy Steinbinder, PhD, RN, CNA
Managing Partner
Thunderbird Consulting
Phoenix, Arizona

Phyllis J. Waters, PhD, RN
Director, Nursing Practice &
   Professional Advancement
University of Texas Medical Branch
Galveston, Texas

Many practitioners are concerned about evidence-based practice, often describing it as "cookie cutter" or "cookbook" clinical practice. Nothing could be further from the truth. Evidence-based practice is generated from the practice setting, is guided by practitioners, and represents the aggregation and integration of actual applied clinical experience in the generation of objective data through practice-based processes and methodologies (Breslin & Lucas, 2003). At the same time, evidence-based practice respects—and, indeed, includes— the vagaries of individual human circumstances and applications that frequently call for adjustment and change in practice. Introduction of human variability becomes one of the elements of evidence requiring accommodation as a part of the value of applying evidence-based practice within specific clinical settings. This match between external and objective clinical data and applied subjective clinical judgment is one of the critical clinical values for an evidence-based practice. Operating out of this framework ensures that specific clinical practice is not only relevant and based on the best available knowledge, but also adaptive, reflecting the particular needs of individual patients as reflected in good clinical decision making.

At the same time, it is important to recognize that the evidentiary process is currently in its infancy. As the database with regard to clinical practices expands and the technology for recording, integrating, and reporting practices becomes more seamless, relevant, and accurate, evidence-based practice will be more strongly incorporated into ongoing practice (Laurie, Draus, & Klem, 2009).

Clinical practitioners frequently suggest that evidence-based practice is used as a means for justifying cost-cutting and resource-reduction measures. Some believe that widespread adoption of evidence-based practice would simply aid the nonclinical money managers in reducing resources so that clinical efficacy can be sacrificed on the altar of profitability. Furthermore, many clinical practitioners fear that these financial regulators will hold them hostage to specific clinical practices that tend to favor cost reduction rather than quality performance, thereby leading to a failure to act in the best interests of the patient. Of course, any such policy would be a profound misuse of the processes of evidence-based practice—as well as wholly unethical and clinically inappropriate. One of the major characteristics of evidence-based practice is the continual change in clinical practice to reflect the most current and relevant evidence. Any attempt at ritualizing and permanently formalizing a clinical practice simply to obtain economic advantage

> Evidence-based practice does not comprise a cookbook or cookie-cutter approach to developing or managing clinical practice. It requires a degree of flexibility and fluidity based on firm scientific and clinical evidence validating appropriate and sustainable clinical practice.

defeats the purpose of evidence-based methodologies. In fact, such unilateral cost-based initiatives undermine the effectiveness and value of evidence-based practice and ultimately eliminate any potential for cost saving that might be discovered in efficient and effective practice approaches.

Evidence-based practice provides a framework for a specific clinical way of life. It involves developing structures, methodologies, and clinical practice approaches that reflect a specific way of doing business. It requires a commitment to tracking down and applying the best available knowledge related to any clinical process that specifically meets patient needs and answers the critical questions related to best practices *in real time*. Within this paradigm, the practitioner is determined to ensure the most accurate diagnosis and treatment, and can apply the best possible information to clinical judgments related to that treatment. Evidence-based practice engages the whole range of research approaches, from randomized to the most structured, as a way of both gathering data and establishing an information base upon which to advance sound clinical decision making (McGill, 2002).

An analogy that demonstrates the new contextual framework for the use of evidence relates to the question, "Why do physicians and nurses kill more people than airline pilots?" The answer is complex: Pilots are required to have sufficient time off and complete every check in duplicate. The systems in which they work have sufficient checks and balances as well as redundancy; pilots follow specific and validated protocols for action; and, if they commit a serious error, they are required to die with their passengers. Some have suggested that if the same rules applied to physicians, nurses, and other practitioners, there would be fewer errors and better practice in health care. Evidence-based practice begins to address this disparity, as it provides a dependable frame of reference upon which nurses, physicians, and other practitioners can depend for assessing the efficacy and effectiveness of practice and its influence on clinical outcomes (Friedland, 1998).

Currently, healthcare literature is impossibly diverse, with a database that is unmanageably large. Furthermore, it is disorganized, uncoordinated, unwieldy, and often filled with bias. Also, many clinical research studies are so poorly designed that the validity of their results is readily subject to question. In fact, much clinical activity is based on previous experience or clinical research that is not sufficiently accurate; it does not have a rigorous scientific design or validity to be applied to specific clinical circumstances (Bakken, Crimino, & Hripcsak, 2004). The feasibility of obtaining trustworthy evidence related to the large range of clinical decisions remains open to question, especially given the ongoing issues related to number of test subjects and the timing of testing, intervention, and treatment. Furthermore, the implications of personal mythology, sociology, psychology, and cultural concerns are frequently missing from the array of information related to appropriate and evidentiary clinical practices. All of these factors influence the clinical process and the healing dynamic, and require further explication to more fully understand their value and applicability.

Often, current clinical guidelines are not sufficient and do not provide the right kind of answers that clinical professionals are hoping to use as basis for clinical action and decision making. As currently devised, such recommendations are slow to develop, require a great deal of resources whose generalizability is often questionable, and are often surprisingly anecdotal. Taken together, these factors make the current state-of-the-art with regard to clinical practice highly controversial and subject to broad variability. In this circumstance, the work of evidence-based practice is a complex, yet vital undertaking that begins to more rigorously and systematically codify evidence, link experience, and create more valid and sustainable foundations for effective clinical decision making and applied practice (Cadmus et al., 2008).

BEGINNING WITH CRITICAL THINKING AND CLINICAL SYNTHESIS

Over the years, much has been written about reflective and critical thinking processes, especially as applied to clinical practice (Kozier, Erb, Berman, & Snyder, 2003). Critical thinking is simply the ability to deconstruct events and apply reasoning to determine the origins of situations (Brookfield, 1987). Essentially, critical thinking is a format or a methodology of problem solving that requires reflection and disciplined process. Critical thinking builds on particular standards, practices, protocols, values, and ideals. It is goal directed and specifically intended to inform effective decision making. Specific characteristics unique to critical thinking include inductive and deductive reasoning; application of knowledge; translation and interpretation of research; validation and implementation of experience; innovation and creativity; and the evaluation of impact and/or outcomes. Critical thinkers are generally systematic, organized, informed, and purposeful, such that their activities lead to defined and expected results (Oermann, 1991; Vacek, 2009).

The critical thinker is able to reflect concomitantly on both information and situation. Reflected in good critical thinking are a facility at priority setting; balancing and competing priorities; making judgments about specific risks and benefits; and determining how those factors might influence decision making. The good critical thinker makes effective decisions about specific interventions, their timing, and subsequent decisions and their impact; such an individual also effectively communicates process, decisions, and impact to other providers and to the patient.

Critical thinkers adhere to rigorous intellectual and academic standards. As a part of this adherence, the critical thinker commits to using appropriate and referenced research information, validated and accepted data sources, and accurate sources for clinical decision making. The critical thinker is always working to remain precise, clear, complete, and accurate in all decision making and in communication. Because evidence-based practice requires the same level of rigor, there is a necessary goodness of fit between the demands of good critical thinking and the process expectations for evidence-based practice (**Figure 1-2**).

Critical reasoning, in common with the processes associated with evidence-based practice, involves the process of effective problem solving. The critical thinker enters into the process of identifying problems and issues, and tying them as best as possible to the structure and elements of good thinking. As in the evidence-based process, the critical thinker attempts to delineate the problem; understand its indications; define the elements and components of the problem; develop the frames of reference related to the problem; and, ultimately, define the direction that needs to be pursued to appropriately address the problem. Clearly delineating the facts related to the issue and all elements that constitute the issue helps develop a deep understanding of the basic components of the problem and drives the critical thinker toward the elements of solution seeking. The same process forms the foundation for evidence-based practice. Problem formation is the foundation for both critical thinking and the mechanics of evidence-based applications.

Evidence-based practice is purposeful and so is critical thinking. Evidence-based practice and critical thinking hold the following elements in common:

- A problem exists that requires exploration.
- A purpose or goal needs to be addressed.
- A frame of reference is constructed that looks at all of the elements of the problem.

Figure 1-2   From process to synthesis.

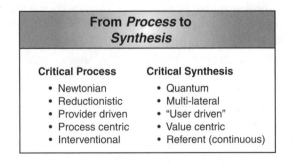

From *Process* to *Synthesis*	
Critical Process	**Critical Synthesis**
• Newtonian	• Quantum
• Reductionistic	• Multi-lateral
• Provider driven	• "User driven"
• Process centric	• Value centric
• Interventional	• Referent (continuous)

- Assumptions about the problem, its characteristics, and elements are drawn from an assessment of the problem.
- Some central concepts, themes, and indicators emerge as a result of clarifying the problem.
- Evidence, data, information, and sources are accessed to better inform, explain, or expand the problem.
- Interpretations, evidence, applications, and protocols are informed by the aggregation of information as applied to a specific problem or situation.
- Reasoning, planning, processing, defining, and documenting lead to a format or process that will guide subsequent action in addressing the problem.
- Action consistent with the protocols and parameters is undertaken, all the while assessing process, impact, and effect.
- Mechanisms for evaluating, making judgments, adjusting, generalizing, and applying to a broader set of like problems indicate the effectiveness and utility of the critical problem-solving process (Paul, 1990).

The essential personal attributes of critical thinking and the external objective attributes of evidence-based practice combine to create the essential requisites and conditions for providing an evidence base to clinical activity. Both require an element of discipline, rigor, and objectivity within the deliberative process. Both are complementary and reflect an approach to clinical practice, the goal of which is to ensure a clear and rational basis upon which practice decisions are made and clinical activities are undertaken.

Like critical thinking, evidence-based practice requires clinical decision makers to use the best available evidence, including both clinical expertise and specific patient circumstances and preferences. To effectively carry out evidence-based practice, sufficient exploration, research, and evidence gathering must have been generated with regard to the specific clinical issue or case. Furthermore, the clinician must have sufficient and appropriate skills, and apply those skills during the critical process and analysis, to be able to read the research, understand its implications, translate it into the language of practice, and, finally, apply it within specific patient circumstances (Dawes, 1999).

Finally, the clinician must be able to make sound decisions based on the evidence, implement the requisite practice, and ultimately change that practice as the evidence indicates a need for change. This fluidity and flexibility between the discipline of process and the practice, as well as the requirements for a good outcome, are cornerstones of evidence-based practice. This continual confluence between the foundations of practice and the ability to change when the need for a modification of practice is articulated establish a foundation upon which all practice parameters must be based. The challenge to historic clinical practice is found in the contradiction between the fluidity, flexibility, and commitment to changing practice when the demand for it occurs, as opposed to rigid and formal policies, procedures, and practices that do not lend themselves to fluid, flexible, and immediate changes.

The processes associated with formalizing the clinical process create a challenging, yet important demand for fundamental shifts in practice. To clearly identify an issue or problem, this analysis must be based on an accurate assessment of the current knowledge base, research data, and practice. Included in that effort must be the ability and the facility to search for relevant information in the literature to glean the data upon which clear decision-making processes can rely. In addition, the skills necessary to evaluate the research or data generated using clearly defined criteria regarding its merit and applicability are now a fundamental aspect of clinical practice (Pape, 2003). Interventions will be chosen and will be effective to the extent that the skills necessary to undertake this process are in place in the individual practitioner and within the context of collective practice standards.

CLINICAL SYNTHESIS: EXTENDING THE NURSING PROCESS

The nursing process has been a foundation for nursing practice action for the last three decades. It simply comprises the nursing format for the critical thinking process. The nursing process provides a clinical overlay that is specific and unique to nursing-based activities and to achieving anticipated nursing care outcomes.

As applied to the clinical process, critical thinking has been transformed to include the elements of activity and of care. This caring component provides an overlay that is unique to the nursing experience and includes elements of interaction, relationship, communication, and satisfaction. Using formative, summative, and confirmative strategies, the critical thinking processes are transformed into nursing actions that influence the patient's clinical process. These formative processes help the nurse develop understanding and create a feedback loop related specifically to personal knowledge, current applications, and the need for further learning and application of clinical care (Martin, 2002).

In the summative process, competency and the application of care become the critical centerpieces in ensuring that the right choices are undertaken in the application of nursing activities. These elements draw upon the nurse's critical translation skills as he or she begins to apply assessment and thought into clinical action. It is at this point that all of the critical information related to clinical action is correlated with the specific circumstances and conditions of the patient to both inform and guide critical clinical action.

The confirmative component of the critical process relates to the integration between thinking, acting, and reflecting on currency, applicability, and value of the clinical action in relationship to expectations and to clinical outcomes. Confirmation ensures that a solid relationship exists between the process chosen, the action undertaken, and any outcomes achieved. At this stage, the intent is to make sure that there has been a goodness of fit and that the expectation actually leads to changing conditions in a way that benefits the patient (O'Connell & Landers, 2008; Oermann, 1999).

While each of these elements is important to the active practice and application of nursing, there is a need for a shift in emphasis to reflect the characteristics of evidence construction and contemporary clinical practice. Evidence-based approaches require a heavy emphasis on the linkage and integration of information in a systematic and organized way that ultimately influences both the choice and the delivery of patient care. This notion of combining significant sources of data with appropriate decision-making processes and subsequent clinical activity changes the dynamic and emphasis in clinical process. Specifically, this shift alters the fundamentals of the nursing process and of practice as the driving force for choice making, such that subsequent action based on decisions relates to the quality and integration of the data available for good clinical decision making.

In an era where evidence is now an essential component of validating action, becoming critical to the foundations upon which this action is taken requires that the evidence is substantial enough to justify the action and sustain it. Historically, the intensity of this relationship in clinical practice has been rather tenuous. While critical thinking and clinical process have been perceived as valuable in terms of learning and process application for nurses and other providers, what has been missing is an ability to draw on a large enough database in a way that validates the clinical choices that are subsequently made and to do so in real time. In the old model of thinking, knowledge was viewed as a capacity—that is, as something that someone has and subsequently expresses, ultimately translating it into action. The flaw in this approach is the assumption that sufficient and valid knowledge is present, upon which subsequent action is taken. Indeed, precious little evidence supports the truth of this approach.

While practitioners judiciously and dutifully identify the elements of competence and build competency in clinical approaches, little hard evidence supports the notion that competence is present. Ensuring competency assumes the foundations for action are clear, precise, understood, and held in common. In reality, this state is rarely achieved. The only measure for adequate clinical performance that has provided any veracity is experience. Nurses and other clinicians draw heavily on the value of experience in terms of clinical activity.

The problem with this approach, however, is that experience is based on past practice. The question related to past practice thus becomes, "What are the legitimate, clear, accurate, and valid foundations upon which this experience is based?" Much of clinical experience is not validated by any truly objective and sustainable methodology, other than the aggregation of the number of clinical processes, procedures, and clinical interventions. Without a firmer foundation bolstered by a continuous and dynamic access to objective and validated clinical performance, experience is just that—experience. There is no evidence, no clarity, and no validity as to whether the experience has real meaning and value. This concept is especially difficult to grasp in contemporary nursing, because so many nurses claim competency through valuing their own experience without recognizing that, in an evidence-based framework, such claims are more an indictment than a source of value.

Missing most often in this scenario are the structural elements of synthesis. These components include the ability to link and integrate all of the elements, sources, and databases necessary in a dynamic way to best inform *real-time* decisions and action (Figure 1-2). This notion of critical clinical synthesis is now the centerpiece for clinical process in an evidence-based framework. Synthesis simply means having access to both the hardware and the software processes that are essential to make the most appropriate clinical decision under any given set of circumstances (O'Neil, Dluhy, Fortier, & Michel, 2004).

Just a brief word about policy and procedure: In an evidentiary dynamic, predescribed and foundational policy and procedure are anathema to good practice. Yet, almost all clinical practices in healthcare institutions are based on, reflect, or extend clinical processes that include policy and procedure as the driving element. In a truly evidence-based dynamic, the notion of policy and procedure does not hold sway. Perhaps the greatest "noise" in health care today is the almost absolute dependence on policy and procedure as the driving foundation for legitimacy in practice. Such a frame for practice is no longer consonance with all of the characteristics of an evidentiary practice dynamic. Indeed, evidence-based practice is embedded in the quantum reality and requisite of constant change. The evidence-driven practitioner is committed to the constancy of the fluidity of clinical practice. Within this framework, the need to change practice is expressed continuously, reflecting the applications of the most current and relevant evidence, which itself serves as the driving foundation upon which the veracity of practice is based. Static, process-oriented, predescribed, and fixed notions of practice foundations (such as policies and procedures) stand in direct contradiction to the prevailing reality of the evidentiary dynamic. Evidence-based practice will be successful as both a framework and a dynamic for clinical practice only when the structures, infrastructure, format, and processes of policy and procedure are eliminated from healthcare institutions and no longer serve as a rationale or justification for clinical practice.

ACCESS AND CLINICAL SYNTHESIS

For evidence-based practice to be sustainable, access to a digital information framework is essential to its success. This notion of access becomes critical to the clinical process in today's framework for evidence-based practice. Access simply means the availability and ability to obtain and use information in a way that will inform practice and guide the action (Wulff & Nixon, 2004). For nurses and other clinical providers, it is the essential cornerstone of critical clinical synthesis.

This notion of clinical access skills is a fundamental concept for developing both attitude and facility in evidence-based processes. An "access" clinician is one who has both facility and means to obtain real-time information in the act of clinical processing, in such a way that the information can be assessed, translated, applied, and evaluated within the context of the clinical circumstance. Essentially, this means that the access-enabled nurse or clinician is able to utilize real-time technology in the course of clinical decision making and acting as a part of the clinical process (Podichetty & Penn, 2004). This essential real-time approach calls for access to digital equipment and hardware as well as facility in the real-time use of software in the course of undertaking clinical work.

The establishment of an evidence-based context that is fundamentally necessary for evidence-based practice to operate effectively over time depends upon the information and infrastructure, as well as its goodness of fit with the clinical process. This real-time clinical process requires portability, fluidity, and mobility of both the hardware and the software of information services in a way that increases its utility in present-time clinical decision making and action (Hougaard, 2004). If evidence-based practice is to become a real experience for the first-line practitioner, an ongoing availability, facility, and utility of the interface between technology and clinical decision making must become a way of life for practitioners. Without this seamless integration of data and decision, evidence-based practice remains at considerable distance from reality in the lives of the majority of practitioners.

Access skill development within an evidence-based conceptual framework calls for a different approach to both basic education in clinical practice and ongoing performance expectations in the clinical environment. The education of nurses and clinicians must include higher levels of expectation with regard to development of access skills. Furthermore, it must incorporate an understanding of the fluidity of knowledge and the development of competency in knowledge management rather than knowledge capacity (synthesis). Perhaps the greatest impediment to effective knowledge management is the prevailing notion that enough knowledge capacity is available to affirm competence. Of course, competency is not what one has; instead, it is what one does and the efficacy of that action. Competency is not an outcome measure, but rather a process value. Furthermore, competency is dynamic. It is not static, nor is it a condition that one achieves and then retains forever. Competency is fluid, reflecting currency, appropriateness, and applicability. The competency of today can become the error of tomorrow if it does not reflect the latest reality in terms of measures of effectiveness (Lucia & Lepsinger, 1999; Tanner, 2006).

In addition, competency must reflect the changing dynamic of technology, information, and a state-of-the-art (or science). This fluidity of prevailing clinical reality affects the notion of competence to the extent that it cannot be contained or owned. Competency is simply a reflection of relevance, with relevance being defined as the confluence between the latest known information and evidence and its relevance and relationship to the practice that reflects it (Dubois, 1993; Williams, 2008). That goodness of fit is the highest indication of competence and the best reflection of effective evidence-based practice.

Evidence-based practice calls upon our clinical disciplines to adopt an entirely new approach to education for practice. Producing the competent practitioner now requires creating a skilled practitioner who is facile in computer information technology management, has sufficient translation skills to apply that knowledge to the clinical situation, and possesses a high level of real-time application and evaluation techniques that are able to both validate clinical practice and feed the outcomes of that practice back into the information loop (Horak, Welton, & Shortell, 2004). Skilled practitioners recognize the continuous, dynamic connection between the action of practice and return of information into the scientific network, so that it both informs and is informed by the action taken by individual practitioners (Eysenbach, Powell, Rizo, & Stern, 2004). This continuing dynamic between the practitioner and the virtual reality is now a fundamental element of the practice itself. Access to information, use of that information, evaluation of that information after it is applied, and feedback of that information into the database system is a fundamental subset of the present-day nursing process. It represents one component of the dynamic of critical synthesis.

Evidence-based practice can be accurately and dynamically informed over time and in real time only to the extent that information can be accessed quickly, documented effectively, aggregated appropriately, and reaccessed in a continuous loop of data management, access, and application. If the nodes and networks are sufficiently complex and integrated, this dynamic can occur at the point of service, within clinical services, across organizational networks, and, conceivably, across a national database (Scavuzzo & Gamba, 2004). If best practices are ever to be truly obtained and utilized, this kind of node and network framework will necessarily become a foundation of managing clinical care nationwide.

Nodes and Networks

In evidence-based practice and in clinical synthesis, understanding the nodes and networks is critical to sustainability. Networks consist of nodes that are generally connected together by links. Networks are frequently depicted graphically using dots or circles to represent specific nodes, and straight and curved lines between nodes to represent linkages (**Figure 1-3**). The critical element here is the understanding that the network is defined by its nodes and not by its links. Links are simply the points, lines, and processes that operate between the nodes. Nodes and networks represent real system processes and form the theoretical framework that ultimately ensures the effective management of networks and aggregates of information. While network theory, analysis, and synthesis are a field of study onto themselves, it is important to recognize the impact of the network's knowledge on evidence-based practice (Moorehead & Delaney, 1998; Paley, 2007).

Figure 1-3   Nodes and networks.

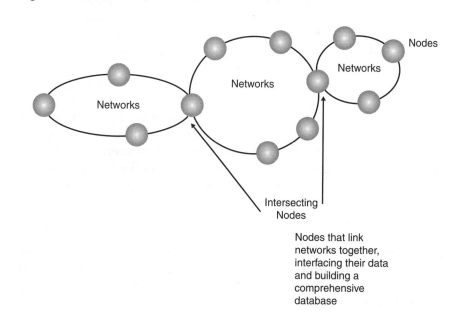

Network management and an awareness of the network's impact on clinical decision making are important factors necessary to understand current time management in terms of evidence-based practice. Issues of degrees exist—for example, the number of direct connections to nodes indicates the kinds of connectors and hubs in the network. Elements of "betweenness"—such as the number of direct connections in a network—help determine the degree of integration between either elements or members of the network. The degree of closeness of the nodes and the short distance between the connectors determine the level of immediacy and intensity that elements (or individuals) have in relation to one another. Those nodes that act as integrators and boundary spanners link aggregates of elements (or people) with other large data points (or groups). These major points often serve as entry or access points to one another, and to nodes and clusters, thereby facilitating connection in creating the use of access to a wide radius of information. Complexity or decentralization of the network and the accommodations of the links and connections that reflect those relationships are critical influences on access and action. All of these network elements are important to the future development and management of evidence-based processes.

Understanding and applying systems management are important when constructing an infrastructure to manipulate evidence-based processes so as to make evidence-based practice a way of life in organizations. This endeavor calls for more than simply incremental approaches to evidence-based activities. In fact, the ability to create truly sustainable evidence-based processes requires the creation of a continuous, dynamic evidence-based infrastructure that supports, manages, and interfaces the data and practice relationship within the clinical environment, between clinical practitioners, and across specific clinical practice parameters (Saranto & Hovenga, 2004).

Here again, understanding the critical link between the digital capacity to aggregate clinical data in a pool with a huge confluence of related information, and the human ability to manage and access that network, translate it into practice, evaluate its impact, and then feed the results back into the digital network as a cybernetic dynamic, represents the best in critical synthesis. This notion of synthesis is now a fundamental part of critical clinical practice. Nurses and other practitioners must now recognize that the ability to synthesize a broad diversity of information, circumstances, conditions, and patient vagaries in a way that influences critical judgment and subsequent clinical action is the foundation of contemporary practice.

Critical synthesis calls for the practitioner—primarily the nurse—to be able to live at the intersection of these various forces and to recognize that the practitioner is essentially managing the intersection and addressing the confluence of elements and forces operating there, linking them and using them in a way that affects patient care in a positive way (Segal, Dunt, & Day, 2004). Living at this intersection, which mandates skills in managing the variables that define clinical life, making decisions, and undertaking clinical practices, is the focal point of contemporary and future clinical practice. Competency, in this set of circumstances, is reflected in the ability to manage this confluence of factors and forces, integrate them, prioritize them, make decisions, and, finally, act. This is nursing synthesis.

Evidence-based practice draws on an increasing level of understanding related to systems processes and their application to clinical decision making. A systematic, day-to-day scheme for managing information, digital infrastructure, and clinical practice is essential for administrative and management leadership in creating a supportive environment for evidence-based practice. This new environment further requires a shift in the mental model of organizational structure and human systems. The movement from a twentieth-century model of finite institutional structural references is giving way to more fluid, flexible, portable, and mobile notions of structure and organizational format (Porter-O'Grady, Hawkins, & Parker, 1997). Furthermore, healthcare leaders have to reconceptualize the organizational structure of clinical services and practice environments. As the information infrastructure, the Internet, and other digital and fiber-optic infrastructures become a common context for social and clinical life, leaders must reconceive the organization and system structures that support it. Perhaps the greatest impediment to the success of evidence-based practice is the organizational, informational, and interactional infrastructure necessary to support it. Without these structures of support, format, and infrastructure, it will be impossible to sustain an evidence-based frame of reference for ongoing clinical practice in the future (**Figure 1-4**).

Figure 1-4   New model of 21st century practice.

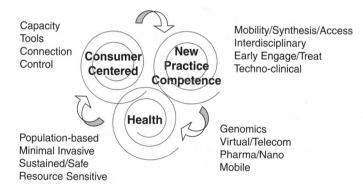

Capacity
Tools
Connection
Control

Consumer Centered

New Practice Competence

Health

Mobility/Synthesis/Access
Interdisciplinary
Early Engage/Treat
Techno-clinical

Population-based
Minimal Invasive
Sustained/Safe
Resource Sensitive

Genomics
Virtual/Telecom
Pharma/Nano
Mobile

BUILDING THE INFORMATION INFRASTRUCTURE FOR EVIDENCE-BASED PRACTICE

If we are to ensure that evidence-based practice does not become yet another fad in health care, we must build a systematic organizational infrastructure that supports this method as a way of delivering care. From the information infrastructure to the interdisciplinary and organizational framework, new approaches to organizing and delivering care are essential.

Creating an Interdisciplinary Frame of Reference

Perhaps the most challenging aspects of contemporary clinical practice within an evidence-based framework are the traditional compartmentalization and fragmentation of disciplinary practice (Coombs & Ersser, 2004). Historically, the various healthcare disciplines, especially nursing and medicine, have developed on parallel but distinct pathways. In an effort to establish independent professional and economic frameworks for practice, nursing and medicine have remained essentially nonaligned. As the complexity of health care has increased and the intensity of clinical practice within disciplines has accelerated, the relationships between the two disciplines have become even more distinct, perhaps even polarized (LeTourneau, 2004). What is unusual about this set of circumstances in an era characterized by clinical and technical integration is that the behavior patterns of independence are no longer relevant to the clinical necessity for integration.

The highly independent practice of medicine and the equally complex interdependent practice of nursing now must intersect in a highly interrelated format if evidence-based practice is to be sustained. Furthermore, this clinical intersection between the two major disciplines must include a concomitant and equally important multidisciplinary intersection between all key disciplines. Such interweaving of nursing and medicine will not happen by accident, of course. Instead, clinical leadership in health care must construct the format for integration and interaction necessary to create the structural and organizational foundations that support interdisciplinary evidence-based practices. Critical among those efforts are the following steps:

- Each discipline must clearly define its specific and unique accountability for clinical decision making, clinical action, and interdisciplinary interaction.
- A mandate and organizational format must require the disciplines to develop clinical protocols and practices in conjunction with each other, such that no discipline unilaterally develops clinical practices that affect other disciplines.
- A structural format must require the decision-making processes of each discipline to act in concert, such that no one discipline can make clinical decisions in isolation of its relationship to other disciplines.

- A clearly defined process, methodology, or mechanism for constructing clinical protocols is ongoing business between the disciplines, and within the process of making decisions that conform to clinical protocols and formats.
- A clinical management structure needs to reflect particular interdisciplinary configurations based on specified organizational formats that support effective interdisciplinary clinical decision making, activities, and evaluation.

Systematic approaches toward organizing and structuring the disciplines are important to systematic delineation and evaluation of care. In fact, evidence-based practice requires an organizing format that essentially forces the disciplines to integrate their clinical activities, reflecting an essential synthesis or confluence of clinical process related to patient care and effective practice. The challenge to creating and sustaining a structural format relates specifically to the past independence and nonaligned practice relationships established by the disciplines independent of each other. Historic disciplinary, gender, knowledge, legal, legislative, and relational issues are clearly components of the first line of dialogue. Many of the cultural and organizational shifts that need to occur are reflected in how these historic issues are resolved, and how subsequent action represents a new set of relationships around these long-held practices.

Getting Past Cultural and Organizational Barriers

Clearly, evidence-based practice has cultural and organizational implications that are vital to its success. Evidence-based practice will remain a marginal or faddish practice if the interdisciplinary interface necessary to advance it does not become a central component of its implementation. When examining organizational mandates, managers and clinical leaders need to realize that the structure for integrated, corollary, and horizontal relationships will be as important as the clinical processes related to establishing evidence in practice. Several priorities must emerge within the manager's table of accountability if the organizational structure supporting evidence-based practice is to operate effectively:

- Create a leadership lexicon that represents the collaborating, correlating, and horizontal relationship between the disciplines and management processes associated with it.
- Create an organizational structure that creates equity, collaboration, dialogue, and distributed decision-making frames of reference for the function and operation of clinically specific services.
- Move away from the organizational delineation of clinical services based on models of medical diagnosis rather than processes of patient care.

- Eliminate turf-based clinical service structures that create discipline-specific clinical alignments and subordinate other disciplines within those alignments, which reflects a change from a pyramidal orientation of authority to more circular clinical relationships and decision making.
- End the "captain of the ship" mental model for organizational and relational interaction between the disciplines, recognizing instead a complexity-based, collaborative decision model for patient care.
- Move to end hierarchy-based pyramidal models of control and decision authority, replacing them with point-of-service oriented clinical decision-making formats driven by patient care professionals.
- Enhance the skills of the management and clinical leadership team to include more facilitative, engaged, and clinically driven decision processes and empowerment strategies so as to more fully engage practitioners in continuous evidence-based practices.

Clearly, new organizational arrangements to create a different set of parameters for practitioners are essential to build the organizational frame necessary to make evidence-based practice a fundamental system of doing business in health care. Managers must understand that the prevailing organizational models of decision making, organizing, and structuring relationships are impediments to engaging practitioners more fully in decisions about effective practice. After years of parental and hierarchical organizational constructs in health care driven by lay business models of organizing work, the evidence is overwhelming: Clinical practice and quality patient care are sacrificed to a high degree in such models. What is important is that sound business principles be applied to clinical service structures. Equally important is that the outcomes of clinical practice not be lost in the effort to maintain financial viability. Loss of focus on the core business end of health care and failure to facilitate cost-effective, outcome-oriented, and sustainable clinical practice ultimately result in the loss of the financial viability of the healthcare organization.

If evidence-based principles are to be applied effectively in the clinical framework of the healthcare system, they must be applied equally effectively in the management and organizational framework. Evidence-based practice does not mean solely clinical activity. To the contrary, the mental model for evidence must permeate the organization and every level of its structure. Clinical efficacy and effectiveness simply should be the results of structural integrity, good financial stewardship, and excellent patient care. The interaction between these forces is as important as the effectiveness of any one of them. Evidence-based practice in the clinical frame of reference is no more sustainable than it would be if operated only in the financial constructs of the organization. Indeed, the true viability of evidence-based practice is found in the intersection of all of the organizational, systematic, and clinical variables affecting the delivery of high-quality patient care. The measurement of each of these components in relationship to the others is the best example of an evidence-based practice framework for clinical services. As a result, in the interface between structural, business, and clinical activities, leaders must recognize the continuing and intersecting dynamics essential for maintaining focus on the core business and for sustaining excellence at all levels of measurement (**Figure 1-5**).

Just as necessary in the information infrastructure, the organizational structure must sacrifice the traditional addiction to hierarchical control, replacing it with a commitment to a highly effective and strongly delineated valuing of horizontal relationships, accountability, individual and collective performance, and evidence of sustainable levels of measurable, quality clinical service (Coombs, 2003). Equally important is that management's demands for accountability, performance-based decision making, professional and individual evaluation, and clinical expectations and outcomes are correlated in a way that demonstrates a confluence of these factors focused on maintaining high levels of patient care and organizational excellence. Here again, the interface between the information infrastructure, performance measurement, and quality patient care is critical. Evidence-based outcomes cannot be obtained simply through the definition of clinical protocols and the clarification of clinical expectations. Without clearly defined relationships between competence, performance, expectations, and outcomes, evidence-based practices would be built on, at best, a superficial and slippery foundation.

Figure 1-5   Building clinical evidence.

Integrating the Elements of Evidence

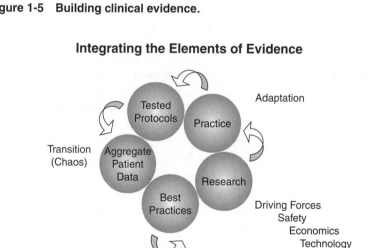

Perhaps the greatest problem with current notions of evidence-based practice is the belief that simply getting at the practices by identifying their relationship to expectations and outcomes will be sufficient to ultimately improve patient care, reduce risk, and advance the practice of medicine. Nothing could be further from the truth. This synthetic and superficial notion of what is necessary to sustain evidence-based practice will surely contribute to its decline. Instead, managers and clinical leaders must reflect on their understanding and recognize, in the design of organizations, the fundamental interface between organizational structure, performance expectations, clinical protocols and practices, and evaluation of clinical care as an outcome of the intersection between all of these variables.

This understanding, of course, should not exclude any discipline. Indeed, the notion of the medical staff as customers of the organization, rather than as partners in practice, is a key impediment to obtaining the kind of medical accountability that is critical to effective evidence-based practice. No disciplines can remain outside the cycle of accountability and expect that practice will be enhanced or improved. Expressing and owning accountability for fiscal, relational, interactional, and disciplinary contributions to defining clinical protocols and practice behavior are essential to success, and must engage all involved disciplines. Neither employment nor partnership is an effective exclusionary consideration.

While most physicians in the U.S. healthcare system are not employed by hospitals, they nevertheless have a history of directing decisions that affect what those who are employed in hospitals and health care systems do. This "closed shop" approach to medical practice is neither viable nor sustainable in today's healthcare environment, especially within the construct of evidence-based practice. The "physician as customer" notion must disappear from the language of administrators and managers in health care, to be replaced by the language of partnership and accountability. Evidence-based practice requires a level of equity and collaborative expectations among all those parties addressed under its rubric. The physician continues to be a key player in this clinical drama. While the complexities of health care and the increased intensity of investment and involvement of all the disciplines have created an interdependence that simply cannot be dissolved, the physician often remains the point of access. No longer can physicians remain outside the circular cycle of relationships necessary to identify protocols, methodologies, practices, and evaluation of the clinical activities that are reflective of the intersections and the intensity of the multiplicity of clinical providers making decisions along the patient's clinical pathway. Just as in the information infrastructure, access to other providers as clinical partners is critical to both the developmental and application elements of evidence-based practice. Access to one another's practice, data, protocols, and clinical behaviors is essential when seeking the normative framework as well as the path to excellence. Mythology and ignorance of one another's actions and contributions to decision making and clinical practice are no longer viable in rendering a clearly delineated and validated level of clinical care (Thomas, Sexton, & Helmreich, 2003).

For clinical leaders and managers, much of the initial effort in building the infrastructure for evidence-based practice lies in reconstructing the formal organizational as well as professional and personal relationships within the clinical service. This endeavor requires thinking and acting in fundamentally different ways with regard to the role of the leader in formatting support systems for evidence-based clinical services. Key components of the leader's armamentarium include the following elements:

- An ability to facilitate interdisciplinary dialogue from the simple to the complex with the intention of establishing the continuing and sustainable mode of communication between disciplines
- Gathering diverse stakeholders together around controversial and "noisy" issues with an ability to achieve an agreeable outcome for all stakeholders
- Helping others delineate clear performance expectations as well as individual and collective accountability for performance, holding each to the commitments and tasks agreed upon
- Developing mechanisms and modalities of organizational and systems support for the clinical decisions and subsequent actions made by the disciplines in advancing patient care
- Addressing crisis, nonperformance, and conflict as a normal part of the managerial function, with the intent of seeking common ground and facilitating sustainable resolution

Leadership is no easy task. This is certainly no less so in an environment that promulgates and facilitates an evidence-based framework for clinical practice. It is vital to the success of evidence-based practice processes that the organization be fully committed to establishing evidence as a frame of reference at all levels of doing business. Consistency and faithfulness to this commitment are essential leadership and administrative criteria upon which the success of evidence-based practice can be predicated. Like most clinical processes, evidence-based practice is sustained on the altar of effective administrative support, continuous organizational encouragement and expectation, and effective application of leadership skills. Concepts such as evidence-based practice rarely fail because the concept is not viable. Rather, they tend to fail because the organization's priorities and leadership skills do not match up well with the expectations and demands for changes in the personal and organizational behavior necessary to support it.

Organizational leadership is often averse to risk and organizational noise. This fear of organizational reaction (especially within the physician community) frequently creates retrenchment and distracts the organization's leadership from the focus that must be maintained through the challenging and high decibel periods of organizational change (Lancaster, 1998). This reality is no less true for evidence-based practice when it is perceived as a systems change. The dramatic shift in locus of control, accountability, expectations, performance, and measurement creates truly significant organizational and systematic noise. A good administrator/manager must anticipate this reaction prior to implementing the changes required for the organization's commitment to effective patient care and evidence-based practices. This anticipation should lead to good preparation, skill development, and careful execution of the supporting and application processes necessary to ensure effective evidence-based practice approaches.

Wise leaders do not enter the arena of evidence-based practice either incrementally or tentatively. Evidence-based practice signifies an entirely new approach to the delivery of high-quality and effective patient care. It incorporates all that is known about what works and what doesn't work. It also begins to utilize, at a high level of intensity, all data that are now available in the digital management of patient care. The leader understands that evidence-based practice reflects the incorporation of a completely new range of processes and elements of data, decision making, and clinical action. He or she sees this interface between the emerging systems of complexity, digital processes, accountability, and expectations for performance and high-quality outcomes as a frame of reference for the future of healthcare practice (Paquette, 2003). Consequently, the leader sees evidence-based practice as the format for a business lifestyle in this contemporary age and for moving healthcare professionals, organizations, patients, and the social system into a twenty-first-century framework for the delivery of healthcare services, which advances the quality of care and raises the level of health.

INFORMATION INFRASTRUCTURE SUPPORTING EVIDENCE-BASED PRACTICE

Evidence-based practice requires a level of information integrity and integration that has not been achieved previously in the practice environment of health care. Although incremental evidence-based activities can certainly rely on a fairly basic array of data steps, establishing a systematic and broad-based approach to building an evidence-based framework requires a much more sophisticated integration between clinical practice and data management.

To build an information foundation and ensure effective clinical data management, the critical factor is access. Widespread availability of basic clinical information is just one element of access assessment, however. A systematic approach to access requires the evidence-based organization to develop an information and operational infrastructure that provides broad-based data access to all available clinical resources in real time, at the point of service to clinical practitioners. This level of sophistication calls for an organizational commitment to building a clinically based information infrastructure that is not yet evident in most healthcare institutions across the United States. The primary fear about relationships in sustainable evidence-based practice today relates to the willingness of clinical organizations to make the financial, resource, and organizational commitments necessary to build a well-designed, practitioner-friendly clinical information management system. To engage in evidence-based practice, organizations must implement a mechanism for integrating existing and historical clinical data, historical and current patient information, and existing clinical practice standards and processes, and then link these individual databases together in a comprehensive, integrated data framework to guide clinical decision making (**Figure 1-6**).

Databases must be able to be accessed simultaneously and in real time. The clinician must have the ability to act on a relatively seamless intersection of data in such a way that judgments can be made and practice actions can be undertaken. Furthermore, the clinician must be able to record instantaneously both the action and the impact of clinical practices based on the data mining that occurred in making the choices for the most appropriate clinical action. Here again, evidence-based practice must be seen as a practice process, not an evaluation mechanism. Evidence-based practice must be designed and developed in an organization as a way of delivering care and a method of doing the clinical business of the organization. For this reason, data management and clinical processing must be directly related such that both are ongoing elements and a subset of the full definition of clinical care (Nada, Keravnou, & Blaz, 1997).

Designing practice within an evidence-based format calls for focus on the following key elements:

- The digital documentation system must include the digital patient records, digital hardware, portability/mobility-based recording and documentation, and software, which facilitates integration of diffuse clinical information.
- Hardware must allow multiple points of access to the same patients and clinical information for a variety of involved healthcare professionals.
- Software must ensure continuous real-time access to the multitude of collateral clinical information provided by any practitioner at every moment in the patient care continuum.

Figure 1-6   Evidence-based clinical system.

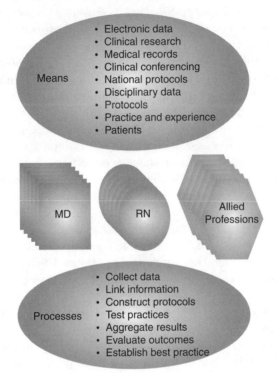

- Implications of specific clinical data in relationship to other elements of clinical data must be highlighted in a way that indicates anomalies or abnormalities in real time and is available to all clinicians.
- Design of the information infrastructure must accommodate the aggregation of evaluative data in ways that automatically enumerate the norms of practice with particular patients, clinical protocols, and/or practices, and subsequently inform standards of patient care.

Constructing this infrastructure calls for a level of understanding of the myriad interfaces that are necessary to ensure an effective data management process. Several levels of construction are important to make the right data infrastructure routinely available within the healthcare facility. Several levels of delineation are important here:

1. Specific clinical protocols are developed with regard to the predominant patient care populations, diagnosis-related groups (DRGs), or specific clinical delineation.
2. Interdisciplinary integration of clinical standards of practice are developed and linked within particular patient care populations, DRGs, or specific clinical delineation.
3. Standards of practice are agreed upon by all the disciplines and become the format for clinical decision-making action as well as clinical and patient evaluation.
4. Adjustments of clinical practice can be made in real time as clinical performance, patient response, and immediate clinical measurement indicate a need for change in specific clinical practice.
5. Individual applications of clinical protocols/standards can be aggregated with the larger consolidated patient database as a mechanism for further validating, refining, adjusting, or validating particular clinical approaches.

Clinical design professionals recognize that two concomitant processes are occurring. The first process relates specifically to the development of clinical protocols and frames of reference for practice to provide the evidence foundation for particular clinical standards and practices. Simultaneously, the evidence-based practice format calls for real-time decisions, applications, and adjustments that are practice-based established protocols, which also reflect adjustments in patient circumstances and conditions. The information infrastructure provides a vehicle to link the developed protocol with the real-time decision making, action, documentation, and evaluation. In addition, clinical adjustments, variances, corrective action, or standards enhancements must be sufficiently available to affect subsequent practices and/or specific populations across the clinical service spectrum. In short, these changes and adjustments, which ultimately result in a shift in the protocol or standard, must be available to all practitioners immediately so that the value of evidence can inform the action of practice. It is this ongoing, living interface between (1) the establishment of sound practice protocols based on the last available data and clinical process and (2) real-time clinical activity and its impact that ensures the effectiveness and ongoing utility of evidence-based practice.

In establishing the foundations of evidence-based practice, ready availability of data becomes critical. Multiple-file indices of discipline-specific scientific journals (especially those on the Internet—that is, e-journals) must be easily and generally accessible. In the past, clinically sound studies that report accurate, meaningful research have been conducted using evidence-based methodologies found using OVID or Medline key word searches. The information structure and the clinical skills necessary to access these resources must be in place to ensure that they are used appropriately to inform evidence-based practice. In fact, many e-guidelines and databases are merging on the Web, thereby providing both data and format guidance to those who are constructing or using evidence-based approaches (Bennett, Casebeer, Kristofco, & Strasser, 2004).

Of course, simply providing access to clinical information is not sufficient to ensure that it is appropriate and utilized correctly in clinical practice. To date, the evidence-based practice approach has failed when it came to the question of adequate translation of best practices into appropriate clinical protocols and with standard practices within the organization. Of course, many behavioral, structural, and organizational reasons explain this observation (Podichetty & Penn, 2004). Perhaps the most significant factor is that much of evidence-based practice remains discipline unilateral and clinically non-aligned. Knowledge is good—but unless it is aggregated, linked, and ultimately translated into continuous behavior, it is not effective.

Clinical interventions that reflect the assessment and management of the potential barriers in multidisciplinary activities can often be more effective than simply addressing the clinical protocols themselves. First, identifying those cross-discipline standards of practice and protocols upon which all disciplines agree can provide a firmer foundation for building evidence-based practice than simply incorporating other disciplines' recommendations and advice into a particular discipline-specific set of standards. Establishing this approach as a principal standard helps inform and define the clinical standards and protocols to which ultimately all practitioners will adhere. Designing the systems infrastructures to incorporate this notion as a principle of design leads to a format for interdisciplinary collaboration and integration that becomes the prevailing characteristic of a systematic evidence-based practice approach.

CREATING A CULTURE OF EVIDENCE

Today, clinical practice faces a new world. As practitioners enter more fully into the digital age, the mechanisms upon which they once depended for clinical decision making, practice application, and documentation are quickly disappearing. The manual and mechanical processes for critical thinking, acting, documenting, and evaluating are no longer valid in an increasingly digital world. This understanding of the virtual implications intersecting the course of human life stands in stark contrast to the process-driven clinical orientation still evident among most practitioners today.

The challenge for clinical leaders in this set of circumstances is to not simply introduce a framework for evidence-based practice. Instead, they must embrace the transformation of the entire approach to healthcare delivery.

A deep understanding that most health care reflects a provider-driven model of clinical decision making and acting that is bereft of ownership and accountability for health is important when contemplating the demand for undertaking major shifts in healthcare delivery. Leadership must be able to see the need for change to support evidence-based practice at three levels of intensity: systems change, disciplinary change, and individual change. This chapter has enumerated some of the fundamental concepts that are essential to implementing those meaningful long-term changes necessary to support evidence-based practice as a way of undertaking clinical work in the twenty-first century. Initiation of evidence-based practice can occur in a number of simple, functional steps that are outlined in a variety of ways in subsequent chapters. Nevertheless, to make evidence-based practice tenable in the context of our digital age, leaders must recognize that a radical transformation in all elements of practice is essential to sustain it and to make a positive difference in the lives of patients.

Even more important to the delivery of effective quality health care is the commitment of every individual practitioner to making evidence-based practice the format and framework for individual decision making and clinical activity. Every practitioner needs to address fundamental and specific conditions to ensure appropriate and effective patient care. Some of these priorities are outlined here:

- An individual critical review of current practice behaviors and dependencies upon which past practice has been based that represent an impediment to the engagement of emerging practice requisites
- Development of a thorough and clear understanding of the elements of evidence-based practice and the implications they have for personal and professional practice, interdisciplinary relationships, and effective patient care
- Full engagement of each practitioner and every discipline to communicate and interact with one another in a common effort to effectively define individual and collective contributions to clinical protocols and practice as an ongoing way of undertaking patient care
- An individual professional commitment to continually evaluate the action of practice, subjecting it to the test of analysis and comparison for the purposes of improving and advancing practice
- A personal, sustaining commitment to a continuously changing practice that is no longer absolutely defined by ritual and routine, which ultimately represents the best response to evidence and outcome
- A commitment on the part of every practicing professional to engage with her or his colleagues in a collective exercise to more clearly define the foundations of practice, joining with other disciplines and with patients to define the foundations of practice, change the elements of practice, advance positive clinical outcomes, and raise the level of social health

In the final analysis, if evidence-based practice is to work and be sustained, it requires commitment at every level of the health system. From government to the private sector, to corporate and community health systems, to professions and providers, to patients and communities—all parties will be required to participate in a fundamental change in the foundations of healthcare delivery. Evidence-based practice provides a format and means for creating effective change in the way health care is delivered and the higher value subsequently obtained from health service providers.

Ultimately, the commitment to improving and changing practice must, at some level, relate to the improvements of the health of society at the individual and collective levels. Reducing errors, establishing practice foundations, and advancing quality are all important elements of effective healthcare delivery systems. Of course, the more important measure of healthcare delivery is the quality of health that the citizens of the community and the nation enjoy. Evidence-based practice must, in the long run, have a definitive impact. At this critical time in U.S. history—indeed, in human history—focusing on the quality of health for all has become increasingly important as we move more inevitably to becoming a global community.

As life expectancy is extended by the miracle of technology and our social constructs continually demand reconfiguration, movement of the healthcare system toward a new frame of reference will be important to its long-term viability. The use of the information infrastructure, including the adoption of emerging digital, nano, and mobility-based technologies, will further refine and increase the level of impact that healthcare therapeutics will have on the future of health. As the importance of portable therapeutics for the delineation and maintenance of health for our aging population grows, the clinical, social, economic, and personal effects of these new care measures will become ever more significant. The age of evidence is truly an age of engagement and validation—a way of explicitly recognizing the value of decisions, actions, and outcomes. Evidence-based practice provides a means, and perhaps a foundation, upon which the health care of the twenty-first century will be built. Recognizing the significance of the work, the depth of the activities associated with building mechanisms for evidence, and the commitment necessary to sustain and advance a new framework for healthcare delivery is the most important clinical work of our time.

REFERENCES

Bakken, S., Crimino, J., & Hripcsak, G. (2004). Promoting patient safety and enabling evidence-based practice through informatics. *Medical Care, 42*(2), 49–56.

Bennett, N., Casebeer, L., Kristofco, R., & Strasser, S. (2004). Positions: Internet information seeking behavior. *Journal of Continuing Education in the Health Professions, 24*(1), 31–38.

Breslin, E., & Lucas, V. (2003). *Women's health nursing: Towards evidence based practice.* Chicago: W. B. Saunders.

Brookfield, S. (1987). *Developing critical thinkers: Challenging adults to explore alternative ways of thinking and acting.* Milton Keynes, UK: Open University Press.

Cadmus, E., Van Wynen, E., Chamberlain, B., Steingall, P., Kilgallen, M., Holly, C., et al. (2008). Nurses at skill level and access to evidence-based practice. *Journal of Nursing Administration, 38*(11), 494–503.

Coombs, M. (2003). Power and conflict in intensive care clinical decision-making. *Intensive & Critical Care Nursing, 19*(3), 125–135.

Coombs, M., & Ersser, S. (2004). Medical hegemony in decision-making: A barrier to interdisciplinary working in intensive care? *Journal of Advanced Nursing, 46*(3), 245–252.

Dawes, M. (1999). *Evidence based practice: A primer for healthcare professionals.* London: Churchill Livingstone.

Dubois, D. (1993). *Competency-based performance improvement: A strategy for organizational change.* Amherst, MA: HRD Press.

Eysenbach, G., Powell, J., Rizo, C., & Stern, A. (2004). Health-related virtual communities and electronic support groups: Systematic review of the effects of online peer-to-peer interactions. *British Medical Journal, 328*(7449), 1166–1176.

Friedland, D. (1998). *Evidence based medicine: A framework for clinical practice.* New York: McGraw-Hill.

Horak, B., Welton, W., & Shortell, S. (2004). Crossing the quality chasm: Implications for health services administration education. *Journal of Health Administration Education, 21*(1), 15–38.

Hougaard, J. (2004). Developing evidence based interdisciplinary care standards and implications for improving patient safety. *International Journal of Medical Informatics, 73*(7/8), 615–624.

Kahn, J. (2009). *Disseminating clinical trial results in critical care* [Conference proceedings No. 37(1) Supplement]. Brussels, Belgium: Critical Care Medicine.

Kozier, B., Erb, G., Berman, A., & Snyder, S. (2003). *Fundamentals of nursing concepts: Process and practice.* New York: Prentice Hall.

Lancaster, J. (1998). *Nursing issues in leading in managing change.* St. Louis, MO: C.V. Mosby.

Laurie, E., Draus, P., & Klem, M. (2009). Description of a Web based educational tool for understanding the PICO framework in evidence-based practice with a citation ranking system. *CIN: Computers, Informatics, Nursing, 27*(1), 44–49.

Law, M. (2002). *Evidence-based rehabilitation: A guide to practice.* New York: Delmar Learning.

LeTourneau, B. (2004). Physicians and nurses: Friends or focus? *Journal of Healthcare Management, 49*(1), 12–15.

Lucia, A., & Lepsinger, R. (1999). *Art and science of competency models: Pinpointing critical success factors in organizations.* San Francisco: Jossey-Bass.

Martin, C. (2002). The theory of critical thinking in nursing. *Nursing Education Perspectives, 23*(6), 243–247.

McGill, S. (2002). *Low back disorders: Evidence-based prevention and rehabilitation.* San Francisco: Human Kinetics.

Melnyk, B.M., & Fineout-Overholt, E. (2004). *Evidence based practice in nursing and healthcare: A guide to best practice.* Philadelphia: Lippincott Williams & Wilkins.

Moorehead, S., & Delaney, C. (1998). *Information systems innovations for nursing: New vision's adventures*. New York: Sage.

Muir, G. (2001). *Evidence based healthcare*. Chicago: W. B. Saunders.

Nada, L., Keravnou, E., & Blaz, Z. (1997). *Intelligent data analysis in medicine and pharmacology*. New York: Kluwer Academic.

O'Connell, E., & Landers, M. (2008). The importance of critical care nurses caring behaviors as perceived by nurses and relatives. *Critical Care Nursing, 24*(6), 349–358.

Oermann, M. (1991). *Professional nursing practice: A conceptual approach*. Philadelphia: Lippincott Williams & Wilkins.

Oermann, M. (1999). Critical thinking, critical practice. *Nursing Management, 30*(4), 40–45.

O'Neil, E., Dluhy, N., Fortier, P., & Michel, H. (2004). Knowledge acquisition, synthesis and validation: A model for decision support systems. *Journal of Advanced Nursing, 47*(2), 134–142.

Paley, J. (2007). Complex adaptive systems and nursing. *Nursing Inquiry, 14*(3), 233–242.

Pape, T. (2003). Evidence based nursing practice: To infinity and beyond. *Journal of Continuing Education in Nursing, 34*(4), 189–190.

Paquette, L. (2003). *Prescription for change: Managing and controlling change in health services*. Hauppauge, NY: Nova Science.

Paul, R. (1990). *Critical thinking: What every person needs to survive in a rapidly changing world*. Rohnert Park, CA: Center for Critical Thinking and Moral Critique.

Podichetty, V., & Penn, D. (2004). The progress of roles of electronic medicine: Benefits, concerns, and costs. *American Journal of the Medical Sciences of the Medical Sciences, 328*(2), 94–109.

Porter-O'Grady, T., Hawkins, M., & Parker, M. (1997). *Whole systems shared governance: Architecture for integration*. Sudbury, MA: Jones and Bartlett Publishers.

Sackett, D., Straus, S., Richardson, S., Rosenberg, W., & Haynes, B. (2000). *Evidence-based medicine: How to practice and teach EBM*. London: Churchill Livingstone.

Saranto, K., & Hovenga, E. (2004). Information literacy: What is it about? Literature review of the concept and the context. *International Journal of Medical Informatics, 73*(6), 503–513.

Scavuzzo, J., & Gamba, N. (2004). Bridging the gap: The virtual chemotherapy unit. *Journal of Pediatric Oncology Nursing, 21*(1), 27–32.

Segal, L., Dunt, D., & Day, S. (2004). Introducing coordinated care: Evaluation of design features and implementation processes implications for preferred health system model. *Health Policy, 69*(2), 215–228.

Tanner, C. (2006). Thinking like a nurse: Research-based model of clinical judgment and nursing. *Journal of Nursing Education, 45*(6), 204–212.

Thomas, E., Sexton, J., & Helmreich, R. (2003). Discrepant attitudes about teamwork among critical care nurses and physicians. *Critical Care Medicine, 31*(3), 956–962.

Vacek, J. (2009). Using a conceptual approach with concept mapping to promote critical thinking. *Journal of Nursing Education, 48*(1), 45–49.

Williams, J. (2008). Competency assessments help strengthen promotion systems, develop staff skills. *Biomedical Instrumentation & Technology, 42*(2), 127–129.

Wulff, J., & Nixon, N. (2004). Quality markers and the use of electronic journals in an academic health sciences library. *Journal of the Medical Library Association, 92*(3), 315–322.

CHAPTER 2

A Framework for Nursing Clinical Inquiry: Pathway Toward Evidence-Based Practice

Dolora Sanares-Carreon, Phyllis J. Waters, and Diane Heliker

Technological and scientific innovations continue to expand the universe of medical interventions, treatments, and approaches to care, ushering in an era rich with the potential for improving the quality of health care (Institute of Medicine [IOM], 2008). The continuous, accelerated pace of knowledge creation that drives these changes and innovation will soon make the status quo a distant memory. Within this environment, only those with appropriate strategies and infrastructure to respond quickly can leverage the promise of innovations (Hagel, Brown, & Davison, 2008). This trend provides nursing with the opportunity to demonstrate its unique value in healthcare services, and evidence-based practice (EBP) provides the framework for realizing this goal. Disciplined clinical inquiry (DCI) is a model that offers a pathway proven effective in integrating EBP into individual and organizational performance.

DCI was inductively developed and fine-tuned through a series of collaborative pilots. This model has proven to be both flexible and useful for all levels of nurses and across all settings. The objectives of this chapter are threefold: (1) to describe EBP in nursing, (2) to delineate the principles and phases of DCI as a proven model to EBP competency development, and (3) to describe organizational development and strategies used by an academic medical center to embed EBP in nursing service philosophy, strategic plans, and essential functions.

EVIDENCE-BASED PRACTICE IN NURSING

Evidence-based practice is a framework for making clinically effective individualized decisions. It employs a reproducible process that focuses on treating the body of evidence relative to a focused question. EBP does not provide the final answer, but rather offers a process for finding the final answer to a clinical question.

In the past, clinical decisions were based on clinical experience, expert opinion, collegial relationships, pathophysiology, common sense, community standards, and published materials. The process of EBP uses the same sources of clinical advice, but passes all of them through the filter of the question, "On what evidence is the advice based?" (Berg, 2000, p. 25). Within the framework of the DCI model, a practice informed by an EBP approach is grounded not on one source of evidence alone, but on the judicious integration of the most relevant, current, available best evidence. Sources of evidence that can best inform nursing practice include research, clinical expertise, the patient's values and perspectives (Sackett, Straus, Richardson, Rosenberg, & Haynes, 2000), and other recognized sources of knowledge (e.g., ethical knowing, sociopolitical knowing, personal experience, and aesthetic ways of knowing) (Carper, 1978; Silva, Sorrell, & Sorrell, 1995; White, 1995).

Research

EBP does not involve conducting a research study. Rather, it involves accessing, examining, and using the research conducted by others in an attempt to answer a focused question. A focused question guides the inquiry to elicit evidence needed for clinical decision making. Clearly, research is a critical source of information in developing the body of evidence for clinical decision making. In particular, two important sources of research-based evidence inform the nurse's clinical decision making: single studies and research summaries.

Single studies are commonly referred to as research or primary studies. Research is the scientific method of discovering new information to contribute to a body of knowledge:

> Best research evidence is clinically relevant research, based on both medical science and patient-centered clinical research. New evidence from clinical research raises questions about previously accepted diagnostic tests and treatments, and recommends interventions that are more powerful, more accurate, more efficacious, and safer (Sackett et al., 2000).

Nursing care is more than a set of investigations and treatment interventions. Clinical nurses draw on a wide range of knowledge sources within and beyond the medical sciences, including the behavioral and social sciences (Craig & Smyth, 2002). Nursing practice is informed by findings from multiple research methodologies both quantitative (e.g., randomized clinical trials) and qualitative (e.g., interpretive phenomenology and participatory action research) (Allen, Benner, & Diekelmann, 1986; Benner, 1994).

The large volume of research flooding the healthcare information super-highway is likely to overwhelm a clinician. To make these research findings easy to access and to use, proponents of EBP advocate a systematic process to bring together a large body of empirical evidence in one single document, known as a research summary/synthesis. Research summaries/synthesis come in several forms, including systematic reviews, meta-analyses, meta-syntheses, and integrative reviews.

"Systematic review is a type of secondary research which provides a summary of all the relevant unbiased studies on a single topic addressing a focused question. A good systematic review incorporates exhaustive searches for evidence, a critical appraisal process, and an explicit process of evidence integration" (Strauss, Richardson, Glasziou, & Haynes, 2005). In other words, systematic review answers the following question: Based on all of the available research-based evidence, what do we know currently about this specific question (Bent, Shojania, & Saint, 2004)?

Meta-analysis is a statistical technique used in systematic reviews to quantitatively combine the results of several separate studies that measure the same outcome into a single pooled or summary estimate. The findings from pooled data that are proven statistically significant may answer questions that cannot be reliably addressed by any single study (Dicenso, Guyatt, & Ciliska, 2005).

Meta-synthesis refers to a family of methodological approaches for integrating the findings from related qualitative studies (Finfgeld, 2003; Thorne et al., 2004).

An integrative review is a research summary method that allows for the simultaneous inclusion of diverse data sources, such as findings from prior quantitative and qualitative research on a particular topic. The potential for systematic bias in integrative reviews can be averted by enhancing the rigor of the data collection and analysis strategies (Whittemore & Knafl, 2005).

Information derived from research is essential for making clinical decisions that lead to best practices. Evidence from research, however, is merely one part of the body of evidence that forms the basis for making and applying nursing practice decisions.

Clinical Expertise

Clinical expertise is the ability to use clinical skills and experience to rapidly identify each patient's unique health state and diagnosis, individual risks and benefits, potential interventions, and personal circumstances and expectations (Strauss, Richardson, Glasziou, & Haynes, 2005). In essence, clinical expertise represents the filter through which research evidence is applied to the individual patient (Porta, 2006).

Individual or consensus opinions of experts are especially important in the absence of research-based studies or in instances of conflicting evidence. These expert opinions may be found on professional Web sites, in conference proceedings, or in peer-reviewed journals. In addition, expert clinicians possess experientially based knowledge that is not available in the literature (Feuerbach & Panniers, 2003). When including individual expertise as a source of evidence for EBP, one must differentiate between clinical experience and clinical expertise. To do so, reported isolated anecdotal experiences must be separated out from a series of grounded and well-documented observations.

A clinical practice guideline (CPG) is an example of a common practice source developed using the consensus opinions of experts. Most credible CPGs use consensual clinical opinions based on a thorough review of relevant evidence. Clinical opinions or consensus is helpful in translating evidence into clinical application recommendations.

Patients' Values and Perspectives

The patient has the greatest stake in his or her own health care and, as such, should be respected as an equal partner. The elevation of the patient to partner is not a ceremonial title bestowed to ensure a "feel good" moment, but rather has significant implications for the quality and safety of care (The Joint Commission, 2008, p. 21). Fully including the patient in decisions about his or her health care means taking into account the individual's views and circumstances when interpreting and applying research evidence. It is expected that patients' willingness and ability to contribute to the decision-making process will vary. Factors influencing the patient's participation may include the patient's health status, the patient's personal characteristics, or the nature of the decision to be made. The process of eliciting preferences begins by assembling an evidence-based summary of the relevant information, linking various options with outcomes, costs, benefits, and complications.

Ask questions. Listen a lot. Continuously examine the patient's changing reactions and responses to treatment plans and perceptions about his or her well-being. Do not forget to acknowledge the perspective of the patient's family and significant others. Indeed, under some circumstances, the patient may rely heavily on the family's input in the decision-making process. The inclusion of the patient's values and perspectives in clinical decision making enhances the probability of applying best evidence in a more effective, humane manner.

Other Sources of Evidence

The pathophysiology data, pharmacokinetics information, and theory found in standard textbooks are essential sources of evidence, but not sufficient bases for making patient care decisions in today's healthcare environment

(Feuerbach & Panniers, 2003). Textbooks may provide a broad overview of knowledge on a subject, but are frequently not fully up-to-date or do not include information at the level of specificity needed. Each text should be critiqued and its contents assessed by comparison with peer-reviewed journal articles and through consultation with experts both from clinical practice and from academe. One approach when considering text references is to form a committee of advanced practice nurses who review acceptable texts on a periodic basis.

Regulatory and professional standards of care that contain statements of minimum expectations for providing safe care are also important sources of evidence. In addition, local evidence generated in the provider's own clinical setting is important to consider when moving toward EBP. These findings might take the form of the results of quality improvement projects, risk management reports, and prevalence surveys, among others.

Integration of Best Evidence

In recent years, a huge amount of attention has been devoted to the synthesis of research-based evidence. The process of integrating the body of best evidence (research, clinical expertise/expert consensus, patients' values, and other sources), however, continues to challenge the proponents and adherents of EBP in nursing. One approach that may offer great promise in this regard is the deliberative process advocated by the Canadian Health Services Research Foundation (CHSRF, 2006). A deliberative process entails a participative approach of eliciting and combining different types of evidence that include representation from experts and stakeholders. It employs a set of criteria and mechanisms for unearthing colloquial evidence while making it subsidiary to the science (CHSRF, 2006). Nursing can also learn a great deal from the processes employed by guideline developers who publish their work in the National Guideline Clearing House.

One of the major challenges for bedside nurses is the use of an EBP approach at the point of care. The DCI approach provides preprocessed evidence in a user-friendly format that the nurse can readily access at the bedside. Examples of these resources include evidence-based practice standards, notes for nurses, and a best evidence digest (a tool currently under development).

THE DISCIPLINED CLINICAL INQUIRY MODEL

DCI is an integrated practice inquiry model that supports the nurse's journey in bringing the best evidence from the workbench to the bedside. In this journey, DCI provides the principles, processes, and tools for an inquiry approach to clinical practice. This model is unique because it was developed inductively by working with a group of practicing clinicians who were part of the research process.

The methodology used, called *participatory action research*, incorporates both quantitative and qualitative approaches that are equally important in understanding the practice of nursing. The theoretical underpinning, *critical theory*, was applied along with the precepts espoused by the following sources:

- Lewin's work (1946), which emphasizes the inclusion of practitioners as local experts on all phases on the inquiry
- Habermas's work (1987), which focuses on critical knowledge based on the principles of collaboration, reflection, and communication
- Freire's work (1970), which underscores the need for an interactive learner-empowered environment (Sanares & Heliker, 2006)

This process allowed the extraction of clinicians' perspectives in designing the inquiry approaches, which then provided a frame of reference and learning pathways that resonated with the clinicians. The learning methods developed for DCI were designed to be congruent with the process of inquiry being taught. Technology that allowed for interactive and self-paced learning was employed so that each step of the learning experience produced meaningful discovery.

The DCI model has five core components. First, DCI clearly delineates the difference between conducting research and engaging nurses in EBP as a process for making clinical decisions. Second, DCI has an interactive online educational component, which consists of five EBP skills sets intended to help individual nurses develop competency. The learning modules are unique in that the nurse produces a measurable outcome demonstrating these skill sets for each step. For example, when the nurse identifies a problem he or she would like to address through an EBP approach, the first skill set required is to formulate a focused question. Upon completing the module, the nurse has a formulated focused question addressing the problem he or she identified. Each skill set moves the nurse closer to having completed the inquiry process of acquiring evidence necessary to answer the stated problem.

The third component consists of the Web-based DCI pathways that offer tools to enhance nurses' skill level in EBP, translate knowledge in accessible format, and engage nurses in inquiry processes. The fourth component of the DCI model consists of a Web site that provides easy access to evidence-based resources. The sources of best evidence are structured online so that accessing them requires the same systematic steps used to access the evidence in the learning module (second component). The fifth component is the application of EBP to essential nursing functions.

In the next section, a more detailed discussion of the components of DCI is seamlessly weaved into coverage of the five phases of the DCI model. This explication of the model is presented from a clinical practice application perspective.

MAINSTREAMING EBP THROUGH USE OF THE DCI MODEL

The five cascading phases of DCI serve as guideposts for turning EBP into a mainstream approach within the clinical practice setting (see **Figure 2-1**):

- Phase 1 focuses on assessing the nurse's knowledge, level of skill, and attitude about EBP, and conducting a scan of the environment in which the nurse practices.
- Phase 2 engages the nurse in learning EBP skill sets and specific pathways.
- Phase 3 confirms the nurse's ability to transfer learning into the practice setting.
- Phase 4 evaluates the patient's receipt of clinically effective, personalized nursing interventions.
- Phase 5 ensures that nurses are engaged in ongoing critiques and evaluation of the process and outcomes of nursing care, making the whole process iterative.

These phases are not linear, but rather cyclical. When indicated, feedback loops are set in motion to facilitate nurse's mastering content in one phase/section prior to moving forward.

Figure 2-1   The DCI model implementation framework.

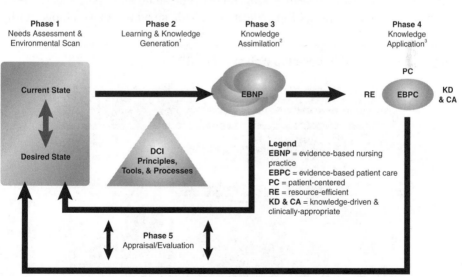

[1]Learning & Knowledge Generation is engagement in the process of aggregating the best evidence relevant to a focused question.
[2]Knowledge Assimilation is engagement in the process of integrating the best evidence within the context of nursing practice.
[3]Knowledge Application is engagement in the process of using evidence-based nursing interventions to an individual patient.

The principles, processes, and tools of the DCI model that are embedded in the various phases are available on a dedicated one-stop Web site (*http://intranet.utmb.edu/dci/*); thus nurses can access them at their leisure. The DCI Web site is currently configured into three centers: (1) the Assessment Center, which contains the need assessment tools and evaluation tools; (2) the Learning Center, which houses the self-directed modules and pathways; and (3) the Knowledge Center, which serves as a repository for nurse's EBP works, such as evidence reviews, summaries, and other resources (see **Figure 2-2**).

Phase 1: Needs Assessment and Environmental Scan

Phase 1 is a diagnostic tool that provides information to map the pathway for successful assimilation of EBP into the clinical setting. This phase is concerned with determining key information about nurses, including their knowledge, attitudes, skills, and perceived learning needs relative to EBP. Equally important, this phase includes an evaluation of the environment in which nurses practice. Phase 1 provides structure and processes to facilitate the DCI model being transported to other settings and used by a wide range of nurses.

Figure 2-3 depicts the key variables that should be considered in determining the current and desired needs of nurses in the organization. Using a structured survey format, nurses are cued to reflect on the context of their practice (professional, institutional, societal) and to become more astute in assessing their current experience, knowledge, learning needs, and areas of interest related to EBP. A five-point Likert-type scale and open-ended questions are used to conduct the assessment. This survey was developed with

---

Figure 2-2   The UTMB one-stop Web site for EBP.

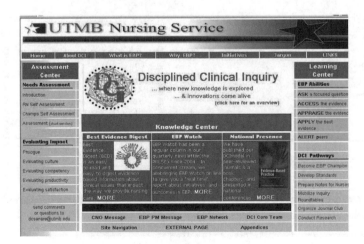

Figure 2-3   Key variables for needs assessment.

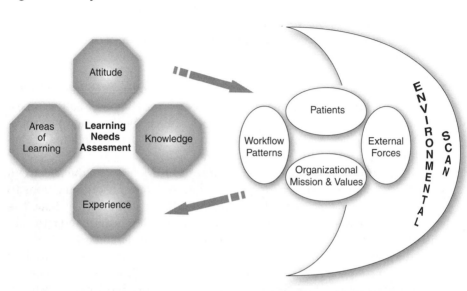

input from clinicians and nurse managers to assure clinical relevance. It may be completed online or in paper-and-pencil format. The assessment results are then compared with the EBP program objectives to determine which knowledge and skill gaps need to be addressed.

Knowledge and skill gaps typically occur to a greater degree among nurses whose basic education did not systematically integrate the principles and utilization of EBP. In recent years, a number of nursing educational programs have begun introducing EBP strategies in their undergraduate curricula. EBP literature and continuing education opportunities also have increased exponentially over the last decade. However, several studies report continuing barriers to nurses' application of EBP (Bostrom, Kajermo, Nordstrom, & Wallin, 2008; Estabrooks et al., 2008; Funk, Tornquist, & Champagne, 1995; McCleary & Brown, 2003; Newman, Papadopoulos, & Sigsworth, 1998; Retsas, 2000). The most notable barriers identified include usage of unfamiliar language, insufficient support, and inadequate knowledge about EBP. The Institute of Medicine reports that support systems that might facilitate nurses in using and accessing the new knowledge and technology at the point of care are not widely available at this time (IOM, 2003, p. 33).

The second segment of Phase 1 involves an environmental scan that takes into account both external and internal factors that influence the environment in which the nurse practices. The individual and environmental components of the assessment are analyzed to identify strengths, weaknesses, opportunities, and threats that may affect the entire practice arena. Processes are identified that may facilitate or disrupt the creation of an ethic of care and a culture (locus or environment of care) that provides the structure, processes, and systems supportive of nurses' efforts to reshape their practice.

Cultures do not turn sharply with the pages of the calendar; rather, they evolve gradually over time. By becoming aware of what is changing today, we determine what we must improve upon tomorrow (Bennis, 2000). Nurses, therefore, must monitor and critique advances in biomedical science, new clinical care technologies, and changes in population socio-demographics and consider their implications for nursing practice.

In its document entitled *Nursing's Agenda for the Future*, the American Nurses Association (2002) recognized that uniting nursing organizations to advance EBP would have significant benefits for the profession as a whole. The landmark 2003 Institute of Medicine publication, which was authored by a multidisciplinary group of nationally recognized professionals, set forth the expectation that healthcare providers would incorporate five competencies into their practice—one of which is to consistently employ EBP. (The other four competencies are to provide patient-centered care, work in an interdisciplinary team, apply quality improvement, and utilize informatics.) The importance placed on the application of EBP by national and international healthcare leaders is already influencing policy and professional trends. Thus these external forces are being incorporated into the streams of change now occurring in health care at the regional and community levels. Nursing leaders and clinicians influenced by these policies and trends are increasingly driving changes within their organizations to support the enculturation of EBP. As the professional and environmental awareness of the nurse is heightened, these resources and directives become both imperative and significant.

A mere statement that EBP is a key strategic initiative to achieve excellence is not sufficient to create organizational change. The first step in ensuring that change is effected is to determine the extent to which EBP principles are embedded in the structure, processes, and outcome patterns within the organization. Using this assessment, nurse leaders and clinicians can then develop plans for systematically implementing EBP throughout the organization. True commitment is manifested in the flow and allocation of resources. Dedicated time for the core EBP team and participating nurses is exceedingly important. Access to major databases (i.e., Cochrane, CINAHL, and Medline/Pub Med) and other Internet-based sources (National Guidelines Clearing House, TRIP, and Joanna Briggs Foundation) is indispensable in this endeavor. If these resources are not currently available in nursing service, special efforts will be required to include these tools in the organizational budget cycle.

Phase 2: Learning, Knowledge Translation, and Systems Development

Phase 2 activities create the conditions necessary to implement EBP successfully. These conditions involve developing nurses' EBP competencies and structuring organizational systems that optimize the application of these competencies. Based on the University of Texas Medical Branch (UTMB) experience, we have learned that development of individual nurses' knowledge and skills should occur in parallel with development of organizational support and structure. We have found that nurses need to take ownership of the EBP initiative to enhance their commitment, fully recognize their accountability, and increase the uptake of evidence-based decision-making processes in the clinical setting.

Principles for Implementation

Traditionally, nursing has implemented educational programs as soon as a gap in knowledge was identified. The DCI approach examines Phase 1 results while at the same time determining how these results are influenced by, or can be influenced by, the other factors in the nursing system environment.

For example, at UTMB the results of Phase 1 informed us that we needed to build our nurses' EBP competencies and structure congruent nursing systems to optimize the application of these competencies. The UTMB Nexus Model for Nursing Practice and Professional Development (Waters, 2003) provides the framework for interweaving all development activities designed for individual nurses with congruent systems development.

At UTMB, two key systems have been restructured to incorporate the process and principles of EBP: the Clinical Advancement Program (CAP) and the Evidence-Based Practice Standards System. A task force composed of nurses in various specialty units led by the EBP Program Manager was commissioned to study how to support and reward nurses' application of EBP competencies. As an outgrowth of its work, a key feature of the current CAP is the designation of EBP as a key domain of nursing practice. To advance to the highest clinician level (expert level), the nurse is expected to demonstrate competency in the five core EBP skills sets specified in the DCI model. The other levels in the CAP entail varying degrees of EBP expectations (see **Figure 2-4**). UTMB's strategies now include outcome and impact indicators that can be regularly evaluated and used to implement course corrections when needed.

As a result of an exploratory study, UTMB's updated nursing policies and standards now subscribe to an Evidence-Based Practice Standard System. Given the explicit expectations specified in the CAP and the Evidence-Based Practice Standard System, nurses are more likely to see investments in learning and knowledge translation as being valuable both to their practice and to the organization (Sanares, Waters, & Marshall, 2007). The goal is for nurses

Figure 2-4   EBP expectations.

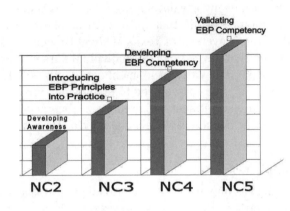

to own the initiative, thereby securing their commitment, accountability, and consequently integration of EBP into the clinical setting.

Three principles emerged from the series of EBP pilot studies conducted at UTMB.

Principle 1: Inquiry is an essential dimension of professional nursing practice.   Nurses are inquiry-based problem solvers as well as co-creators of new knowledge. To be effective, a nurse must have a sense of inquiry and use evidence in problem solving. More than two decades ago, Christman (1987, p. 6) predicted that in the future all nurses would be expected to have clinical investigative ability. According to his prediction, relatively few nurses would be full-time researchers, but application of the scientific method to problems of practice would be commonplace. Today Christman's prediction is being manifested through the EBP movement in nursing. Positive patient outcomes depend on nurses taking on an active role in bringing the best evidence to the bedside. They serve as the front-line staff in providing complex nursing interventions and making hundreds of clinical decisions every day (Swan & Boruch, 2004). The nature of the nursing role places these front-line care providers in a strategic position. It is within these daily face-to-face encounters with patients, their families, and significant others that problems are identified and solved.

Principle 2: Accountability is a prerequisite to achievement.   Accountability is structured at the individual nurse level through performance evaluation tools and clinical advancement criteria that define EBP expectations. At the organizational level, accountability is achieved by structuring evidence-based criteria to assess function and introduce change. These criteria are then evaluated at both individual and organizational levels in terms of their congruence with EBP principles.

To facilitate EBP becoming an integral part of nursing practice, following key points are advocated within the DCI model:

- Clear articulation of the value of EBP as reflected in the nursing services' organizational structure, professional practice model, and strategic plan.
- Appointment of a dedicated EBP expert as a program manager or director to lead the development, planning, implementation, and evaluation of the EBP program of nursing service. The reporting system of the EBP leader should be strategic enough to allow open lines of communication with operational directors and mangers. The EBP program manager/director needs to be master's degree or doctorally prepared, and to have professional experience in research, research utilization, and EBP. He or she should have a sound base in ways of knowing and competency in accessing, critiquing, integrating, and appropriately applying the most current and valid knowledge and technology at the point of care.
- Formalization of the accountability structure for EBP using a network or matrix-type structure that indicates clear lines of communication, areas of cooperation, and resource commitment. The matrix or network structure offers greater flexibility in engaging clinical experts from various nursing specialties who are intensively trained.
- Recruitment and development of clinicians with varying specialties to form the core EBP team. Depending on the size of the nursing organization, specialty-based networks maybe subsequently developed. The Core EBP team will be led and mentored by the EBP Manager/Director.
- Authorization of dedicated time, critical resources, and sufficient autonomy for EBP teams to fulfill their charges.

Principle 3: EBP is a collaborative endeavor. EBP is shaped by those who create it, use it, and evaluate it. The successful adoption of DCI as a framework for EBP requires a shift in thinking. New relationship patterns among all stakeholders must be developed. Nurses in leadership positions and nurses at the bedside need to collaborate as they consciously create a new shared vision of the role of nursing in the organization. Relationships should shift from traditional hierarchical to heterarchial patterns—that is, decision and communication lines should develop in accord with the stakeholders' specialty knowledge rather than through positional authority line designations. Stakeholders will then relate in a circular and interconnected manner to define and achieve desired outcomes (see **Figure 2-5**). These relationships foster a resolve to manifest a shared vision.

If the nursing service is operating under the umbrella of an academic medical center, collegial partnerships with nursing faculty in academe may be established during this phase. Although roles may overlap at times, the following patterns usually emerge: (1) nursing leaders facilitate resource acquisition and utilization; (2) nursing faculty and EBP experts serve as mentors; and (3) front-line staff are recognized as experts of "local" clinical knowledge and co-creators of new knowledge.

The Learning Modules

Learning is an individualized process. While some individuals prefer a structured small-group teaching/learning approach, others prefer a self-paced solitary format. Some learners thrive with Web-based instruction, whereas others maintain that they are best served through traditional learning experiences. DCI offers an e-learning package that is need based, self-directed, and modular, and that provides the opportunity for concurrent learning and knowledge translation. Importantly, this e-learning package can be customized and blended with other learning approaches. This versatility accommodates various levels of engagement in achieving individual and organizational goals for EBP.

The DCI framework is structured so that nurses become actively engaged as inquiry-based problem solvers. They are expected to match the organization's investments in their development by evincing a personal commitment

Figure 2-5   New relationship patterns.

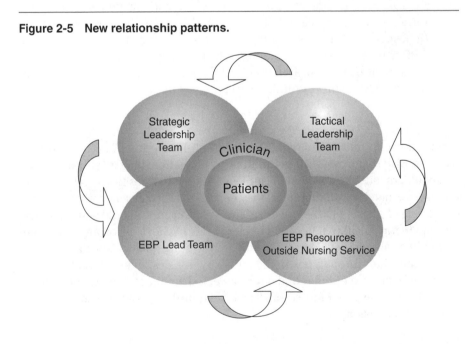

that yields demonstrable results. Interactive exercises provide opportunities for the immediate application of the concepts and principles. As such, as soon as the module is completed, achievement of the targeted outcome becomes a natural outgrowth. Tools and templates that serve as outlines and guides are made available online for ease of access. Each page on the Web site provides easy access to a Webmaster who can respond to questions or facilitate referral to appropriate experts as applicable.

Each of the modules has a specific focus of learning inquiry, as outlined in **Table 2-1**. These learning activities are completed independently and/or with coaching from EBP expert. Several modules offer Type I continuing nursing education credit. The key learning modules focus on the five competencies for EBP, called the "five A's": Asking a focused question, Accessing the evidence, Appraising the evidence, Applying the best evidence, and Alerting peers on the adaptation of new knowledge. These modules provide the foundational knowledge necessary for clinicians to develop EBP competencies.

One DCI online resource that has been found especially useful at the point of care by the other disciplines in the UTMB academic medical center is links. Links is an important tool in the systematic access of best evidence (see **Figure 2-6**).

The DCI Pathways

The DCI pathways are focused applications of EBP skill sets. Nurses may select one or more pathways to demonstrate and further develop their EBP competencies. These pathways are Web based, self-directed, and outcome oriented. Nurses have the option of becoming involved with any of the pathways, or with any combination of pathways, based on their personal interest and capability. Varying degrees of involvement in these pathways are possible, ranging from assuming a leadership role to becoming a member of the team.

Pathway 1: Becoming an EBP-DCI Champion. This pathway is recommended for expert clinicians who were selected/supported by their respective nurse managers and nursing directors based on the following attributes: (1) motivation to become proficient in EBP applications, (2) leadership skills in solving problems and improving practice, and (3) teaching and team building skills or potential. EBP champions are expected to play instrumental roles in developing a critical mass of RNs in EBP initiatives. Put simply, they are expected to serve as coaches and clinical site resources in EBP. Innovation expert Everett Rogers (1995) introduced the notion that the "critical mass occurs at the point at which enough individuals have adopted an innovation so that the innovation's further rate of adoption becomes self-sustain." Use of champions strengthens the EBP infrastructure around "critical connections" and is expected to help

Table 2-1   DCI Learning Inquiry Modules

Learning Modules	Focus of Inquiry
Asking a focused question	Process and tools of developing a searchable focused question
Accessing the evidence	Process and tools of identifying and locating the sources of evidence
Appraising the evidence	Process and principles of critiquing and/or interpreting the body of evidence
Applying the best evidence	Process and principles of synthesizing, interpreting, and translating the body of best evidence in practice
Alerting peers	Process and tools of disseminating the adaptation of new knowledge
Thinking and planning strategically	Values, principles, and process of strategic thinking and action planning.
Becoming a reflective nurse clinician	Values, process, and attributes of reflective nursing practice
Identifying clinical issues and establishing priorities	Process and principles of identifying and prioritizing clinical issues sensitive to nursing interventions
Identifying practice standards and determining priorities	Processes, principles, and tools in identifying priority practice standards
Translating clinical issues into a researchable problem	Process and principles of developing and refining a broad clinical issue into a testable problem statement/question

the nursing service reach the tipping point (moment when something unique becomes common place) in EBP. In addition to influencing nurses, champions have begun to make cross-disciplinary connections. Furthering these intradisciplinary and interdisciplinary connections is considered important in the strategic development of evidence-based clinical practice. This pathway requires at least 100 hours to complete, spread over a three- to four-month period.

Figure 2-6   DCI steps to evidence: Online resources.

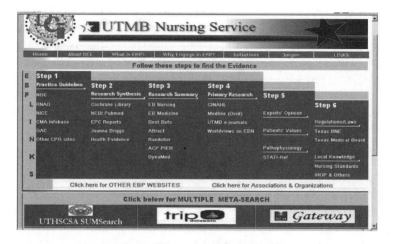

Pathway 2: Developing Evidence-Based Practice Standards. If EBP is to become integral in the healthcare culture, an organized effort to understand organizational influences and to develop an infrastructure that promotes EBP is critical (Foxcroft & Cole, 2004). This goal can be accomplished if the shared vision and experiences of all stakeholders are directly linked with essential nursing functions. "Essential nursing functions" in this context refers to those nursing activities that have been traditionally accepted by both clinicians and management as a component of nursing practice. The most notable of these essential functions are the development of practice standards, provision of patient teaching, and quality improvement projects. If the authoritative statements guiding day-to-day nursing practice are not keeping pace with the most current best evidence, potential adverse effects on patient care may arise.

Despite the significant strides made in clinical practice guideline development at the national level, there is a dearth of systematic studies that apply EBP in the appraisal and development of practice standards at the organizational level. Ensuring that nursing practice standards keep pace with the most current best evidence remains an ongoing challenge. The DCI evidence-based practice standards (EBPS) pathway may be completed in 24–40 hours, spread over a one- to two-month period. The formalized structure and processes facilitate (1) the integration of EBP competencies in the Advancement and Performance Standards and Evaluation criteria appropriate for each level of nursing practice and (2) the incorporation of DCI/EBP structure and processes in the development and update of standards of care.

Pathway 3: Preparing Notes for Nurses. Notes for nurses focuses on practices that address the question, "Why are we doing what we're doing?" Nurses engaged in this pathway use the DCI process to summarize the best evidence derived from the integration of research, expert opinion, pathophysiologic rationale, patient perspectives, and other recognized sources of nursing knowledge. The primary purpose of this pathway is to share with peers the most current, valid, and reliable evidence-based knowledge about nursing practices. New knowledge is presented in a concise one-page summary that nurse clinicians can quickly peruse in the midst of a high-intensity care environment. Some of these summaries have also been presented in posters that were placed on clinical units at UTMB.

Pathway 4: Organizing Journal Clubs. The purpose of a journal club is to review and critique research-based studies related to specific clinical issues. At the end of this pathway, the nurse is expected to facilitate the review and critique of a research study and evaluate its implications and application in practice. If the group decides that the findings of the study should be considered as the basis for making a change in practice, the nurse leading the journal club session is expected to prepare an action plan. This action plan may include finding additional evidence-based information that supports or negates the findings. At the end of the session, the facilitator, in collaboration with the unit-based journal club coordinator, prepares a brief summary using the journal club template link and shares the group's conclusions with those unable to attend the journal club.

Pathway 5: Mobilizing Clinical Inquiry Roundtables. This pathway allows nurses to reflect on actual care provided for a particular patient. The problems encountered and the successes achieved along the care continuum are identified. Evidence-based data are referenced as nurses engage in the inquiry process, exploring the causes and solutions sensitive to nursing interventions. At the end of the session, nurses are expected to acquire better understanding and practice perspectives. Insights gained in the session lead nurses toward the exploration of opportunities for EBP. The inquiry session serves as a reflective lens using one of three structural formats: (1) patient case presentation, (2) multidisciplinary case review and analysis, and (3) multidisciplinary patient care planning.

Pathway 6: Conducting Research. Engaging in the research pathway will help nurses acquire understanding and beginning skills in research methodology, identify resources, and establish partnerships that set the tone for an inquiry-based practice. This pathway focuses on the acquisition of foundational knowledge and skills in preparing a research proposal. The studies are initiated on clinical issues that have little, absence of, or conflicting evidence reported in literature. In this learner-directed pathway, nurses are held personally responsible for tracking their level of research competency and for determining how much coaching is needed to achieve goals. This need is determined by the result of individual self-assessment. The research pathway incorporates intensive mentoring, as nurses are immersed in the acquisition and application of the key elements of the research process.

Phase 3: Knowledge Assimilation

Knowledge assimilation is the process whereby EBP becomes integrated into individual practice patterns and nursing service systems. If EBP abilities and their applications become integral to the nurse's daily practice, he or she will have experienced demonstrable knowledge assimilation. Note that the rate and level of knowledge assimilation are not solely a function of individual nurses' abilities and motivation, but equally a function of the organizational system in which nurses practice.

Individual Practice Patterns

The learning experience is expected to enable the nurses to become reflective and outcome-oriented practitioners, who are open to new possibilities of nursing practice, and who routinely engage in systematic examination of evidence. These patterns of practice lead to the achievement of EBP. The DCI model acknowledges that EBP may be demonstrated in varying degrees based on the level of a nurse's clinical practice. For example, in organizations with a clinical ladder, expert-level nurses are expected to have a higher degree of knowledge and skill in synthesizing and applying the best evidence in particular patient care situations compared to a novice nurse.

> Nurses apply the newly acquired practice patterns in making clinical decisions relative to: (a) intervention effectiveness (e.g., choosing among multiple interventions, which patient will most benefit from the intervention, and the best time to employ particular interventions); (b) communication (e.g., choices relating to ways of delivering and receiving information to and from patients, families, and colleagues); (c) service organization, delivery, and management (e.g., decisions concerning the configuration or processes of service delivery); (d) experience, understanding, and hermeneutics (e.g., relates to the interpretation of cues in the process of care) (Thompson, Cullum, McCaughan, Sheldon, & Raynor, 2004, p. 69).

Nursing Service Practice Systems

If the benefits of EBP are to become widespread in health services, organized efforts to promote EBP are crucial (Foxcroft & Cole, 2004). It is for this reason that DCI advocates forging a link between EBP initiatives and essential nursing functions. This strategy facilitates the creation of an infrastructure for EBP. By the same token, new knowledge does not have any value unless it reaches the intended users. The DCI model provides strategies for transforming new knowledge into an accessible format that nurses can utilize at the point of care. Of course, it is not reasonable to expect all nurses in every situation to access, critique, and integrate best evidence. Instead, DCI offers organized efforts and a medium where sources of best evidence are shared and disseminated.

Phase 4: Knowledge Application

Within the DCI framework, evidence-based nursing practice (EBNP) and evidence-based patient care (EBPC) become two outcomes on a continuum. EBPC is evaluated by the quality of care already received by the patient, where EBPC is defined as the optimal interface of clinically appropriate, resource-efficient, and patient-centered care. A nurse who has acquired EBP competencies is expected to identify and provide unique contributions as a collegial member of the healthcare team. This unique contribution defines the nature of the patient issue that lies within the domain of nursing practice. While interdisciplinary overlapping of functions does occur, nursing—like medicine—has specific domains of practice that are uniquely reflective of the profession.

The study foci and research methodology used to examine practice issues in the two disciplines are also unique to each. For example, when deciding which antibiotic would be most effective for a particular infection, a physician may utilize Cochrane's hierarchy of evidence (**Table 2-2**). In this case, a well-conducted systematic review of randomized controlled trials (RCTs) offers the best evidence. For the patient receiving the prescribed medication, the nurse might go beyond Cochrane's hierarchy to make a series of clinical decisions based on a number of the issues. **Table 2-3** shows the nature of the decisions the nurse has to make and the gold standards for evidence he or she is likely to use.

This example illustrates that a medically prescribed method of hierarchy/ grading system may not be adequate to address real-world nursing practice. Not only are fewer RCTs available to support nursing interventions, but a substantial number of patient issues sensitive to nursing interventions cannot be appropriately or sufficiently validated using RCT. One nursing EBP scholar characterizes this nursing challenge as follows:

> The practice context is complex, people are complex, and clinicians are complex. The best evidence will most probably come in different forms, in different situations, and context… Knowing how to decipher this complexity… and knowing how to match situation and context with appropriate evidence, will perhaps be the most important requirement of the 21st-century practicing nurse (Estabrooks, 1998, p. 30).

Table 2-2   Cochrane's Hierarchy: Levels of Evidence

Level I	Systematic review of well-designed, randomized controlled clinical trials
Level II	Randomized controlled clinical trials
Level III	Nonrandomized clinical trials
Level IV	Well-designed, non-experimental studies
Level V	Opinions of respected authorities based on clinical evidence, reports of expert committees
Level VI	Someone's opinion

Table 2-3   Nursing Decisions

Clinical Issue	Gold Standard
Allergy	Patient's voice
Drug interaction	Randomized controlled trial
IV flush solution	Well-designed nonrandomized study
Site selection	Clinical expertise
Anxiety over a needle stick	Patient
Noncompliance with treatment	Well-designed qualitative study

This perspective reflects the notion that nursing is not prescriptive. The essential components of nursing knowledge—its art and science—are integrated, interdependent, and complementary. They inform and enhance each other, and cannot be easily extrapolated or separated (Bailey, 2004). Nursing practice draws from various sources of knowledge and multiple ways of knowing. To provide EBPC, nurses need a full understanding of the complexity and the uniqueness of each patient care encounter. Nurses can provide such care through inquiry and by using the principles, processes, and tools of DCI.

Phase 5: Evaluation

An iterative evaluation process is integral to the DCI model. Two strategies are used to evaluate the efficacy of the DCI model. The first approach is to elicit assessments from nursing staff regarding the extent to which DCI has empowered them in the following areas: competency, acculturation, productivity, and satisfaction. The second approach involves objective assessment of the EBP products developed by individual nurses using EBP skill sets and criterion-based reviews of EBP projects involving two or more clinicians.

Strategy 1: Empowerment Evaluation

Empowerment evaluation is used to determine nurses' satisfaction with the DCI journey. It has been argued that "to ensure that programs have a lasting effect, they need to be conceptualized, negotiated, run, and evaluated jointly by all stakeholders" (Van Vlaenderen & Nkwinti, as cited in Van Vlaenderen, 2001, p. 343). As such, empowerment evaluation is utilized alongside other objective measures. Nurses are periodically asked to conduct self-evaluations and reflect critically on both practice issues and the process of finding solutions and taking corrective actions. Empowerment evaluation is the use of evaluative concepts, techniques, and findings to foster improvement. It employs both qualitative and quantitative methodologies and is attentive to empowering processes and outcomes. A process is considered empowering if it helps individuals develop skills to become problem solvers and decision makers. Empowerment outcomes refer to consequences of participants' attempts to gain greater control of their practice or the effects of interventions designed to empower the participants.

Empowerment evaluation is designed to help people help themselves and improve their programs using a form of self-evaluation and reflection (Fetterman, Kaftarian, & Wandersman, 1996). Consistent with these principles, DCI offers self-evaluation tools that provide nurses with the ability to track their achievements and areas for improvement. The following tools may be used for evaluation purposes and are made available online as part of the DCI model.

Tool A: Evaluating the Culture. Nurses reflect on the factors that facilitate or hamper the evolution of an EBP culture based on their personal experience during the DCI journey using a five-point Likert-type scale. Objectively, the evolving culture is considered to be actualized in the practice arena when nurses start routinely reflecting on their day-to-day practice using systematic inquiry to identify problems, create solutions, and strategically initiate evidence-based action plans.

Tool B: Evaluating Competency. The second area of empowerment evaluation focuses on nurses' competencies in developing EBP abilities through

Web-based self-directed learning. The expected competencies correspond to the various sections of the learning journey: identifying clinical issues and determining priorities, asking a focused question, accessing the sources of evidence, appraising single studies, interpreting systematic reviews, interpreting clinical practice guidelines, mapping the best evidence, relating and interpreting the best evidence, alerting peers on the adaptation of new knowledge, action planning, and familiarity with EBP jargons. A Likert scale with four levels of competencies (awareness, beginning skills, independence, and mentorship) is used to quantify these competencies.

Tool C: Evaluating Productivity. Nurses' productivity is reported in terms of the nature and degree of their participation and capacity to develop strategies that facilitate the dissemination and application of best evidence. Nurses report in which capacity they participated: as a member, as a resource person, as a team leader, or as a mentor.

Tool D: Evaluating Satisfaction. This evaluation involves appraising the degree to which the learning journey met the nurse's personal needs and explores the satisfaction levels of patients affected by the initiative. Specific clinical impact is assessed using outcome evaluation or population-based research methods. Assessment of personal satisfaction includes reflection on competency within in a workplace that promotes a culture of excellence, becoming a collegial partner in caring, and other benefits gained as a result of an ongoing learning journey.

Strategy 2: Objective Evaluation

Self-evaluation and reflection are complemented by objective evaluation. Evaluation is conducted at various points of the DCI phases. At UTMB, objective evaluation is used in appraising nurses' achievement of the five EBP core competencies, EBP outcomes for each step of the learning process, and EBP products for clinical advancement. Criteria-based evaluation is used to assess evidence-based components of essential nursing functions (e.g., practice standards). One of the current challenges is developing reliable measures to objectively establish the correlation between EBNP and patient satisfaction and selected nurse-sensitive quality indicators.

CONCLUSION

This chapter reflects information gleaned from the authors' experiences in developing and implementing EBP for nurses in an academic medical center.

This process was initiated in 1999 as a unit-based project; in 2003, EBP was designated as a specific program within the department of Nursing Practice and Professional Advancement. Over the years, several pilot projects paved the way for the EBP program to expand as a well-defined component of individual nursing practice and essential functions of the nursing department. The parallel processes of individual and organizational development and the assessment of these processes were described in detail in this chapter.

The primary goal of the program was to embed EBP into the nursing culture. Although cultural change is an ongoing process that requires constant renewal, we have reason to believe that evidence-based nursing practice has become a normative factor in the UTMB culture. Specifically, feedback from nurses who have been involved in the program, the evidence-based products they have created, and the systems and functions developed as part of this process support the contention that EBP can prove effective in improving the care process. The most compelling evidence, however, has taken the form of the voices of the nurses who participated.

Change begins with the individual and their intent. We hope this chapter assists with your journey. "We must become the change we want to see" (Mahatma Gandhi, 1869–1948). People who change not merely the content of a particular discipline, but also its practice and focus, are not just innovators, but leaders (Bennis, 2000, p. 33).

REFERENCES

Allen, D., Benner, P., & Diekelmann, N. (1986). Three paradigms for nursing research: Methodological implications. In P. Chinn (Ed.), *Nursing Research Methodology: Issues and Implementations* (pp. 23–38). Rockville, MD: Aspen.

American Nurses Association (ANA). (2002). *Nursing's agenda for the future: A call to the nation.* Washington, DC: Author.

Bailey, S. (2004). Nursing knowledge in integrated care. *Nursing Standard, 18*(44), 38–41.

Benner, P. (Ed.). (1994). *Interpretive phenomenology: Embodiment, caring, and ethics in health care and illness.* Thousand Oaks, CA: Sage.

Bennis, W. (2000). *Managing the dream: Reflections on leadership and change.* Cambridge, MA: Perseus.

Bent, S., Shojania, K., & Saint, S. (2004). The use of systematic reviews and meta-analyses in infection control and hospital epidemiology. *American Journal of Infection Control, 32*(4), 246–254.

Berg, A. O. (2000). Dimension of evidence. In J. P. Geyman, R. A. Deyo, & S. D. Ramsey (Eds.), *Evidence-based clinical practice: Concepts and approaches* (pp. 21–28). Boston: Butterworth-Heinemann.

Bostrom, A-M., Kajermo, K., Nordstrom, G., & Wallin, L. (2008). Barriers to research utilization and research use among RNs working in the care of older people. *Implementation Science, 3*(24). Retrieved December 10, 2008, from http://www.implementationscience.com/content/3/1/24

Canadian Health Services Research Foundation (CHSRF). (2006). *Weighing up the evidence: Making evidence-informed guidance accurate, achievable, and acceptable.* A summary of the workshop held on September 29, 2005. Retrieved April 8, 2009, from http://www.chsrf.ca/other_documents/pdf/weighing_up_the_evidence_e.pdf

Carper, B. (1978). Fundamental patterns of knowing in nursing. *Advances in Nursing Science, 1*(1), 13–23.

Christman, L. (1987). The future of the nursing profession. *Nursing Administration Quarterly, 11*(2), 1–8.

Craig, J. V., & Smyth, R. (Eds.). (2002). *The evidence-based practice manual for nurses.* London: Churchill Livingstone.

Dicenso, A., Guyatt, G., & Ciliska, D. (2005). *Evidence-based nursing: A guide to clinical practice.* St. Louis, MO: Mosby.

Estabrooks, C. A. (1998). Will evidence-based nursing practice make practice perfect? *Canadian Journal of Nursing Research, 30*(1), 15–36.

Estabrooks, C. A., Scott, S., Squires, J. E., Stevens, B., O'Brien-Pallas, L., Watt-Watson, J., et al. (2008). Patterns of research utilization on patient care units. *Implementation Science, 3*(31). Retrieved December 10, 2008, from http://www.implementationscience.com/content/3/1/31

Fetterman, D. M., Kaftarian, S. J., & Wandersman, A. (1996). *Empowerment evaluation: Knowledge and tools for self-assessment and accountability.* London: Sage.

Feuerbach, R. D., & Panniers, T. (2003). Building an expert system: Systematic approach to developing an instrument for data extraction from the literature. *Journal of Nursing Care Quality, 18*(2), 129–138.

Finfgeld, D. L. (2003). Metasynthesis: The state of the art—so far. *Qualitative Health Research, 13*(7), 893–904.

Foxcroft, D. R., & Cole, N. (2004). Organisational infrastructures to promote evidence-based nursing practice. *Cochrane Database of Systematic Reviews, 3.* Retrieved November 2, 2004, from http://gateway.ut.ovid.com/gw1/ovidweb.cgi

Freire, P. (1970). *Pedagogy of the oppressed.* New York: Seabury.

Funk, S. G., Tornquist, E. M., & Champagne, M. T. (1995). Barriers and facilitators of research utilization: An integrative review. *Nursing Clinics of North America, 30*(3), 395–407.

Habermas, J. (1987). *The theory of communicative action* (Vol. 1). Boston: Beacon.

Hagel, J., III, Brown, J., & Davison, L. (2008, October). Shaping strategy in a world of constant disruption. *Harvard Business Review,* 81–89.

Institute of Medicine (IOM). (2003). *Health professionals' education: A bridge to quality.* Washington, DC: National Academies Press.

Institute of Medicine (IOM). (2008). *Evidence-based medicine and the changing nature of health care: Workshop summary roundtable on EBM.* Washington, DC: National Academies Press.

The Joint Commission. (2008). *Health acre at the crossroads: Guiding principles for the development of the hospital of the future.* Retrieved April 8, 2009, from http://www.jointcommission.org/NR/rdonlyres/1C9A7079–7A29–4658-B80D-A7DF8771309B/0/Hosptal_Future.pdf

Lewin, K. (1946). Action research and minority problems. *Journal of Social Issues, 2,* 34–46.

McCleary, L., & Brown, G. (2003). Barriers to pediatric nurses' research utilization. *Journal of Advanced Nursing, 42*(4), 364–372.

Newman, M., Papadopoulos, I., & Sigsworth, J. (1998). Barriers to evidence-based practice. *Intensive and Critical Care Nursing, 14*(5), 231–238.

Porta, M. (2006). Five warrants for medical decision making: Commentary on Tonelli's "Integrating evidence into clinical practice." *Journal of Evaluation in Clinical Practice, 12*(3), 265–268.

Retsas, A. (2000). Barriers to using research evidence in nursing practice. *Journal of Advanced Nursing, 31*(3), 559–606.

Rogers, E. M. (1995). *Diffusion of innovations* (4th ed.). New York: Free Press.

Sackett, D. L., Straus, S. E., Richardson, W. S., Rosenberg, W., & Haynes, R. B. (2000). *Evidence-based medicine: How to practice and teach EBM*. London: Churchill Livingstone.

Sanares, D., & Heliker, D. (2002). Implementation of an evidence-based nursing practice model: Disciplined clinical inquiry. *Journal for Nurses in Staff Development, 18*(5), 233–238.

Sanares, D., Waters, P., & Marshall, D. (2007). Mainstreaming EBP. *Nurse Leader, 5*(3), 44–49.

Silva, M. C., Sorrell, J. M., & Sorrell, C. D. (1995). From Carper's patterns of knowing to ways of being: An ontological philosophical shift in nursing. *Advances in Nursing Science, 18*(1), 1–13.

Strauss, S. E., Richardson, W. S., Glasziou, P., & Haynes, R. B. (2005). *Evidence-based medicine: How to practice and teach EBM* (3rd ed.). Edinburgh, UK: Elsevier Churchill Livingstone.

Swan, B. A., & Boruch, R. F. (2004). Quality of evidence: Usefulness in measuring the quality of health care. *Medical Care, 42*(2), II-12–II-20.

Thompson, C., Cullum, N., McCaughan, D., Sheldon, T., & Raynor, P. (2004). Nurses, information use, and clinical decision making: The real world potential for evidence-based decisions in nursing. *Evidence-Based Nursing, 7*(3), 68–72.

Thorne, S., Jensen, L., Kearney, M. H., Noblit, G., & Sandelowski, M. (2004). Qualitative metasynthesis: Reflections on methodological orientation and ideological agenda. *Qualitative Health Research, 14*(10), 1342–1365.

Van Vlaenderen, H. (2001). Evaluating development programs: Building joint activity. *Evaluation and Program Planning, 24*(4), 343–352.

Waters, P. (2003). *Nexus model for nursing practice and professional development*. Unpublished document.

White, J. (1995). Patterns of knowing: Review, critique, and update. *Advances in Nursing Science, 17*(4), 73–86.

Whittemore, R. & Knafl, K. (2005). The integrative review: Updated methodology. *Journal of Advanced Nursing, 52*(5), 546–553.

CHAPTER 3

From Nursing Process to Nursing Synthesis: Evidence-Based Nursing Education

Marcia K. Flesner, Louise Miller, Roxanne McDaniel, and Marilyn Rantz

Nursing education faces the daunting task of preparing registered nurses to participate in a healthcare environment where the pace of change is nothing less than breathtaking. The explosion of research-based information and easier accessibility of the information have led to the expectation that nursing staff will incorporate evidence-based knowledge into their practice settings—indeed, they are perceived to have a responsibility to do so.

Of course, the practice sites available to nurses today range from the traditional hospital setting to home health and hospice, a multitude of specialty areas, and long-term care settings. The nurse as teacher is a major function of the profession in those settings, and the skills required to teach effectively are technical and difficult (Van Hoozer et al., 1987). Today the practice environment for nurses is full of subordinate employees who perform delegated nursing functions that are the responsibilities of registered nurses, indicating that a level of supervisory knowledge is essential for a registered nurse to possess.

Delivering a graduate nurse who possesses advanced skills, as identified by Benner (1984), is an impossible task for nursing educators because expertise takes time to develop. Nevertheless, as Benner advised, "a strong educational preparation in the biological and psychosocial sciences and in nursing arts and science" (p. 184) provides the basis for safe care and the background knowledge needed to ask the right questions. In the scientific age in which we live today, new medical advances are reported weekly, bombarding nurses with new information that can quickly become overwhelming, regardless of the quality of the basic educational program. Graduation from nursing school is just the beginning of lifelong learning—a process that is essential to practice nursing competently and safely in the twenty-first century.

Since the 1970s, the nursing profession has been developing a scientific body of knowledge in the areas of nursing practice and nursing education (Polit & Beck, 2003). As this body of knowledge grew, the nursing community became aware of the importance of scientific evidence needed for practice decisions. The communication of research findings started to become more prevalent through the publication of journals devoted to nursing research. In the 1980s, the National Center for Nursing Research at the National Institutes of Health and the American Nurses Association Commission on Nursing Research were established to identify research priorities that focused on nursing practice.

In the 1990s, the development of clinical guidelines occurred as nursing specialty groups, the American Nurses Association, and the federal government responded to nurses' need for timely information for effective decision making. In 1997, the Agency for Healthcare Research and Quality (formerly the Agency for Health Care Policy and Research) established 12 Evidence-Based Practice Centers; a thirteenth evidence-based center was added in 2002 (AHRQ, 2008). These centers develop evidence reports and technology assessments on topics of clinical importance to healthcare organizations, including the following topics of interest to nursing: blood pressure monitoring, practice outside the clinic area, end-of-life care, best strategies for quality improvement, management of cancer-associated pain and related symptoms, and rehabilitation for traumatic brain injury.

Today, nurses can access research-based clinical information that provides guidance for clinical practice via a variety of media, including publications, journals, and Web sites. The educational preparation of registered nurses has responded to the proliferation of research findings since the 1970s by adding a research component of curricula in the undergraduate nursing curriculum, and by focusing on preparing master's-level nurses to conduct nursing research (Polit & Beck, 2003). Inclusion of informatics in nursing education programs has been yet another direct consequence of the rapidly changing healthcare environment.

The Institute of Medicine (IOM), Committee on Quality of Health Care in America, published the pivotal report *Crossing the Quality Chasm* (2001), which, in part, addresses the notion of evidence-based practice. This report uses the following definition of evidence-based practice, which was adapted from Sackett, Straus, Richardson, Rosenberg, and Haynes (2000):

> Evidence-based practice is the integration of best research evidence with clinical expertise and patient values. Best research evidence refers to clinically relevant research, often from the basic health and medical sciences, but especially from patient-centered clinical research into the accuracy and precision of diagnostic

tests (including the clinical examination); the power of prognostic markers; and the efficacy and safety of therapeutic, rehabilitative, and preventative regimens. Clinical expertise means the ability to use clinical skills and past experience to rapidly identify each patient's unique health state and diagnosis, individual risks and benefits of potential interventions, and personal values and expectations. Patient values refer to the unique preferences, concerns, and expectations that each patient brings to a clinical encounter and that must be integrated into clinical decisions if they are to serve the patient (Institute of Medicine, 2001, p. 147).

The rapid evolution of evidence-based practice, first in medicine and then other health fields, is influencing the design of nursing education programs of both today and the future. This chapter discusses educational changes that should be considered by nurse educators, so that nursing educational programs can respond to the changing fields where registered nurses will practice.

HISTORY OF EVIDENCE-BASED MEDICINE AND PRACTICE

Since the 1970s, U.S. nurses and physicians have developed and focused on evidence-based medicine (EBM) and evidence-based practices (Titler et al., 2001), especially as medical advances have proliferated at a pace that few professionals maintain. In addition, U.S. consumers have become better informed, with expectations subsequently growing that their healthcare providers would make recommendations on the best available scientific information. The opinions and intuition of nurses and physicians could no longer be as reliable as the latest systemic review of high-quality research.

Nursing practice and education have been influenced by the use of research in nursing practice. As more nurses with master's- and doctoral-level education entered the work force in the last 30 years, the research-based data produced by their scientific investigation acknowledged the integral role that nursing plays in health care (Polit & Beck, 2003). The National Center for Nursing Research at the National Institutes of Health and the American Nurses Association Cabinet on Nursing Research have promoted and provided guidance by focusing research on nursing practice and education issues.

Archie Cochrane, a British physician, has been closely associated with the movement of EBM (Reynolds, 2000). Cochrane suggested that because health resources are always limited, resources used to deliver services to patients need to be shown to be effective. From his personal physician–patient experiences, Cochrane described the problems associated with applying research principles to the field of health care as well as the difficulties of using research trials for individual patient care. To integrate research with medical practice, he advocated use of randomized clinical trials for evaluating treatment methods. In addition, Cochrane pioneered the use of systematic reviews and meta-analyses in medicine.

In 1989, a British medical group, headed by Murray Enkin, published a review of the "evidence" for effective care in pregnancy and childbirth (Enkin, Keirse, & Chalmers, 1989). This landmark work helped articulate the need for other healthcare professionals—and particularly physicians—to systematically collate best-practices information from research reports and make practice decisions based on the collective results.

Paralleling the developments in the United Kingdom, faculty at McMaster University in Canada, who had pioneered problem-based, self-directed learning, integrated the application of research findings into medical education (Reynolds, 2000). Central to this approach was the integration of clinical practice with research and use of research methods to make patient care decisions (diagnosis, treatment/therapy, and prognosis). This approach was named evidence-based medicine in 1992 by a group at McMaster University (Sackett et al., 2000).

The British and Canadian movements in EBM led to the development of databases for systematic reviews, meta-analyses, clinical guidelines, and best practices. Among these resources are the well-regarded Cochrane Library (*http://www.concrane.co.uk*), the Best Evidence Database (*http://www .evidence-basedmedicine.com*), and Bandolier (*http://www.jr2.ox.ac.uk/ Bandolier*).

Development of computer technology and the Internet has also influenced the evolution of evidence-based practice in healthcare settings. For example, the ability of computers to process large amounts of data (i.e., databases), retain historical records, and speedily access information led to the introduction of computerized clinical charting systems. The Internet has allowed healthcare professionals to access up-to-date research information and clinical guidelines based on systematic literature reviews, irrespective of their location. In the future, nurses will see nursing practice change on a regular basis as more evidence-based information is produced by nurse researchers.

In addition, the "gold standard" for evidence, which traditionally has been data gleaned from randomized clinical trials, has been broadened to include other types of systematically acquired information. These resources include other types of epidemiologic research as well as patient interviews, patient surveys, and data gathered using other qualitative methods.

Muir Gray (2001) identified four factors that typically influence healthcare delivery on a global scale:

- Increasing healthcare expenditures
- The inability of countries to pay for all the services demanded by professionals and patients

- Variation in the rates of delivery of health services within a country and among countries
- Delayed implementation of research findings into practice

One response to these challenges faced by healthcare organizations and healthcare providers has been the movement toward an evidence-based approach to the delivery of care. From the research studies conducted singly and the systematic reviews performed of multiple studies, the body of clinical knowledge has grown over the years, with best practices guidelines and treatment protocols emerging for use in the clinic (Roberts & Yeager, 2004). Evidence-based nursing practice results when nurses use the latest scientific evidence in their practice, targeting patient outcomes and best practice interventions.

STATUS OF NURSING EDUCATION

Formal nursing education in the United States began as hospital training programs that were under the direction and supervision of physicians. The main purpose of these schools was to prepare nurses by providing them with the skills necessary to care for hospitalized patients and to carry out physicians' orders (Kalisch & Kalisch, 1987). In hospital-based training schools, education took the form of an apprenticeship: Students were responsible for staffing the hospitals, with most of their time being devoted to working on the wards. Students learned by providing service to the patients in the hospital, but engaged in little or no formal classwork. Their "education" was based on ritual and tradition.

In 1893, the first organization for developing standards of nursing education was founded in the United States. This organization, which became the National League for Nursing, established the first standard nursing education curriculum in 1917. The curriculum provided the outline for the three-year diploma program, but was highly prescriptive and did not allow for diversity in education. In 1937, the guidelines were revised and named *A Curriculum Guide for Schools of Nursing*.

In the early 1900s, nursing education moved into a collegiate setting. Many of the early university programs were five-year programs. These programs initially prepared students to be nurse educators. In 1908, the American Hospital Association urged a return to the earlier educational practice of two-year courses to meet the increasing demand for nurses to staff the numerous hospitals that were opening throughout the country.

Nursing education was also influenced by major military conflicts. During World War I and immediately afterward, a marked increase in the demand for nurses occurred. To meet this demand, admission and training standards were lowered. In response to this trend, a committee, funded by the Rockefeller Foundation to study the education programs of nurses, published a report that recommended higher standards of education, special training for instructors, stronger associations with colleges and universities, and adequate financial support for nursing education programs.

World War II also brought about an increased demand for trained nurses. Once again, a committee was formed to study nursing education, but this time it was composed of representatives of the major nursing organizations. In 1948, the committee published the Brown Report, which contained major recommendations for nursing. Its recommendations included accreditation of schools, standards for faculty preparation, improved courses in hospital-based schools, and greater utilization of university teaching resources. The Brown Report also recommended using the term "professional" to designate those who studied in an accredited professional school and establishing two-year college-based programs to help relieve the shortage of qualified nurses. Following publication of this report, the number of baccalaureate programs in the United States steadily increased.

The associate degree education program was started in 1952, based on a research project by Mildred Montag. The associate degree nurse (ADN) was defined as a bedside nurse or "technical nurse." The ADN's education was originally based in community and junior colleges and could be completed in two years. Montag envisioned the ADN graduate to be a technician with a narrower scope of practice than the professional nurse. The education of the ADN included general education along with nursing content. These programs were not intended to include leadership and management or research, but rather focused on preparing the nurse to work under the guidance of a professional nurse. The original vision of the technical or associate nurse did not include integrating research into practice. According to the American Nurses Association (1965), the education of the ADN was to be scientifically based, but technically oriented, and was not concerned with developing theory.

Over the years, the idea of an associate degree in nursing as a terminal degree has evolved. Articulation agreements with baccalaureate nursing programs are now common throughout the country. Although ADNs account for 52% of nursing graduates, they represent only 40% of the RN work force (U.S. Department of Health and Human Services, 2000).

The first graduate program in nursing was established at Columbia University's Teachers College. This master's-level program was intended to prepare nurses for the role of educator or administrator. These roles dominated nursing master's education until the development of advanced practice roles, such as the clinical nurse specialist and the nurse practitioner. Currently, almost 85% of the students enrolled in master's programs are learning these advanced practice roles (American Association of Colleges of Nursing [AACN], 2003).

The curriculum of the master's program varies depending on the area of specialization, but should include core content for all advanced practice nurses. The content areas for core competencies include research, healthcare policy, ethics, role, theory, diversity and social issues, and health promotion and disease prevention (AACN, 1996). Because educational preparation and research experience include these core competencies, the master's-prepared nurse is able to provide leadership in evidence-based nursing practice. The coursework in research, theory, and specialty content areas allows advanced practice nurses to critically examine the research data and to use the latest scientific evidence in their practice.

Baccalaureate and master's nursing education programs continue to evolve in response to the demand for evidence-based practice. The need to instill the skills needed for registered nurses to practice in an evidence-based work environment will continue to place new demands on nursing educators. Indeed, the teaching methods and traditions of clinical nursing education are no longer sufficient to meet the needs of tomorrow's registered nurses. Instead, educational programs need to provide a new set of skills needed for evidence-based practice, as discussed next.

SKILLS NECESSARY FOR EVIDENCE-BASED PRACTICE
Critical Thinking Skills

"Critical thinking is defined... as the rational examination of ideas, inferences, assumptions, principles, arguments, conclusions, issues, statements, beliefs, and action" (Bandman & Bandman, 1995, p. 7). Alfaro-LeFevre (1999) advised that if we want to survive and thrive, we need to think critically. Critical thinking is an essential skill that student nurses must develop during their educational program. Purposeful and goal-directed thinking is needed to manage and direct the nursing care of people with chronic and complex diseases.

Pesut and Herman (1999) reviewed the evolution of nursing process that had provided the structure for thinking in nursing since the 1950s. The four-step model of nursing process (assessment, planning, intervention, and evaluation) represented an important development in clinical nursing, as it forced nurses to think before acting when providing care to patients. As use of the model allowed the profession to gather information on nursing care problems over the next 20 years, a need was identified to classify and standardize the nomenclature used to describe commonly occurring problems. To meet this need, work began in 1973 on the development of nursing diagnosis at the first Nursing Diagnosis Conference.

The second phase of the nursing process evolution identified by Pesut and Herman (1999) started in 1973 when the American Nurses Association expanded the model to five steps: assessment, diagnosis, planning, implementation, and evaluation. As researchers gathered information about processes and products of diagnostic reasoning in the 1980s, the complexity involved in information gathering and decision making by nurses became apparent. The advantages and disadvantages of the nursing process were debated by the profession, with problem identification and solving now being identified as hypothesis formulation and testing. Benner (1984) showed that thinking occurred differently among nurses, based on the experiences they had gained, and that intuition was another element of decision making.

Pesut and Herman (1999) developed what they called the third-generation nursing process. Known formally as the Outcome–Present State Test (OPT) Model of Reflective Clinical Reasoning, their new model of reasoning provides for a structure of iterative reasoning. Such new models of reasoning are clearly needed in the current outcomes-focused healthcare environment. The OPT model relies on the North America Nursing Diagnosis Association, Nursing Intervention Classification, and Nursing Outcome Classification taxonomies to provide a vocabulary for clinical reasoning. Three worksheets ("The OPT Model," "The Clinical Reasoning Web," and "The Thinking Strategies") are used to determine the focus of care for patients. Another key component of OPT is reflection, wherein nurses review their reasoning to discover flaws in their thinking. As the evolution of the nursing process continues, nursing faculty will need to continue their education so that they will be familiar with the developing models, thereby ensuring that future nurses will have exposure to the latest approach to clinical reasoning before they enter their own practice.

Nursing educators can no longer focus on the mastery of skills and content as the sole means to prepare nurses for jobs in the future. Completion of 10-page care plans will not prepare students to provide skilled care based on evidence-based knowledge. Research in the fields of critical thinking and nursing education has revealed a mixed bag of results, but overall has raised concerns about the ability of current curricula to foster development of critical thinking in students (Krichbaum, Lewis, & Duckett, 1997).

Figure 3-1 is an example of a critical thinking exercise used at the Sinclair School of Nursing at the University of Missouri–Columbia.

Exposure to Research Knowledge

Baccalaureate nursing programs require research as a component of the nursing curriculum. The goal of a research course is to introduce nursing students to the basics of the scientific approach of research, with the goal being that they develop the ability to use the information produced to guide their nursing practice upon graduation. It is certainly a challenging prospect to convince a

Figure 3-1   Sinclair School of Nursing critical thinking exercise.

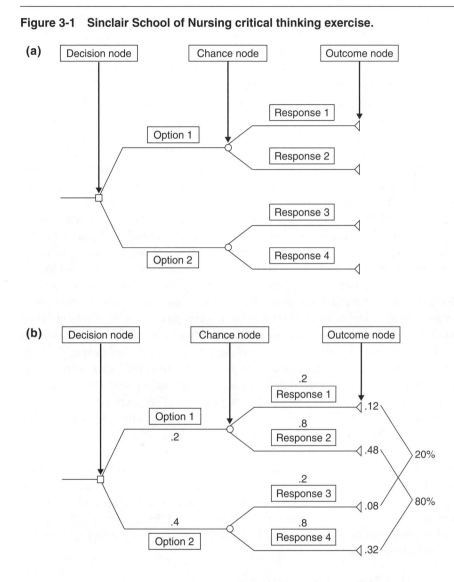

room full of busy students who are eager to learn clinical skills that nursing research can assist them in becoming proficient nurses in the future. The language, scientific concepts, constructs, and theories of research can be daunting to learn, and if a connection is not made between nursing students' clinical and classroom experiences, any knowledge from the course may soon be shelved in the part of the brain labeled "rarely used."

To improve the use of research knowledge by baccalaureate students, nursing research should be seamlessly integrated into the curriculum of nursing programs. When Wheeler, Fasano, and Burr (1995) surveyed National League for Nursing programs, they found that none of the 67 respondents reported integrating research into the curriculum. An example of integrating research into one course was provided by Kenty (2001). Named the Collaborative Learning Project (CLP), this adult health course was "designed to increase student's research knowledge and change attitudes, but more importantly to help students understand the importance of evidence-based practice" (p. 182).

Kenty designed CLP to follow the five research-related functions proposed by the American Nurses Association in 1989: "(1) identify a practice problem; (2) interpret and evaluate the applicability of specific practice problem; (3) implement the practice innovation; (4) evaluate the practice innovation using measurable outcomes; and (5) share research findings in an oral presentation" (p. 182). Evaluation of the project revealed significantly increased research knowledge in students who participated in CLP as compared to students who did not participate. Positive changes in the students' attitudes were also reported, with students demonstrating synthesis of research concepts.

Assisting students to critically examine research results is a basic skill needed for evidence-based practice. **Figure 3-2** is an example of a worksheet used in a master's course at the University of Missouri–Columbia, Sinclair School of Nursing. Students who use the worksheet are able to demonstrate their ability to understand research designs used to answer clinical questions.

Successfully integrating research into practice-based experiences requires the commitment of faculty and clinical sponsors, including development of collaborative relationships between the two groups. Practice setting issues will undoubtedly arise (as discussed by Kenty), but through planning and post-evaluation analysis with staff of the clinical site, these difficulties can be reduced or avoided. Integrating research into the coursework of a nursing program also requires a commitment by the nursing program leader and faculty members. The transition will necessitate additional work initially, but students who participate in such a nursing program will be well prepared for evidence-based practice.

Information Technology Knowledge and Skills

Students who enter college today are expected to have gained essential skills in the use of computers and software. Nursing students will use computerized information systems (IS) at their clinical sites throughout their nursing program. They must be prepared to handle different IS if they are to enter data correctly and efficiently. Patient and clinical encounters at all levels take place for the purpose of gathering and exchanging information that can be shared with other clinicians. Unfortunately, there is no uniform method of collecting data in the healthcare delivery system. Owing to the lack of a uniform data collection method, today's nursing educators are challenged to prepare students to work in healthcare systems where timely information sharing is needed, but a common nursing technology system does not exist as a base for nursing informatics programs.

Nursing educators must develop the skills necessary to include information technology (IT) content in their nursing curriculum and be able to teach the content, so that nursing students have adequate IT skills upon graduation. Research by McNeil and colleagues (2003) revealed that, of the faculty teaching IT courses in 166 baccalaureate and higher nursing degree programs, 39% of faculty were rated at the advanced beginner's level and 18% reported their faculty at the novice level. The information skills of nursing faculty need to advance beyond those levels if students are to be fully prepared upon graduation with a level of competence that is needed for evidence-based practice skills.

Clinical-decision support systems (CDSS) consist of software that integrates patient-specific information with a computer knowledge base (IOM, 2001). The goal of CDSS is to assist healthcare providers in making clinical decisions. Although development and evaluation of CDSS has had minimal impact on healthcare delivery systems to date, the 2001 IOM report advised that future systems might potentially enhance evidence-based practice. Nurses who are prepared to be computer proficient and capable of using new CDSS will be able to adapt to a rapidly evolving technology scene in the future, where handheld computers may become the norm in the work setting.

Information Literacy

Information literacy has been described as a prerequisite to evidence-based nursing practice (Shorten, Wallace, & Crookes, 2001). Information literacy means that a nurse is able to recognize when information is needed to plan and provide nursing care, and has the ability to find, evaluate, and effectively use the necessary information (American Library Association [ALA], 2001). For nursing students to become information literate, the skill of locating relevant clinical information should be incorporated into the nursing curriculum.

Educators in Australia have described such a curriculum-integrated model in several publications (Shorten et al., 2001; Wallace, Shorten, Crookes, McGurk, & Brewer, 1999; Wallace, Shorten, & Russell, 1997). In this model, an interdisciplinary partnership between a faculty librarian and nursing faculty led to the development of library-based learning activities and complementary assessment tasks that were integrated into a fundamental clinical nursing subject. The program was structured to ensure successful searching of the library's electronic databases, which improved students' self-confidence

Figure 3-2   Evidence-based practice worksheet used at the University of Missouri–Columbia.

To critique your article, answer the following questions. Be sure that you critique your article, rather than simply summarizing the information presented in the article. To critique a study, you make judgments of clarity, appropriateness, accuracy, and reliability of the components of the study. Begin the paper with a title page, listing the citation (i.e., title of the article, authors, and journal information). You need to include sections on the purpose/goal/hypothesis of the study, groups studied (sample), how the study was conducted (methods, tools used, how data were collected), results and conclusions, and, of course, the "so what" (i.e., the significance of the study: "What difference did this study make in the whole scheme of things?"). The information in italics under each point is discussion points to include in your critique.

PURPOSE

1. Choose some phrases from the abstract or first paragraphs that tell you what the study is about. Restate the question—don't copy it from the article.

2. Look at the information about the authors. Where are they from? What is their education and practice area (e.g., medicine, nursing, epidemiology, psychology)? How does their area of expertise affect the choice of the study question and how the question is asked?

3. Does it appear to be a relevant question? For example, is this question one that needs to be answered? Is there a need for more information about this topic in the practice world? Is this type of information already available? If so, is that information conflicting and does it need clarification, or does this study reinforce what is already known? Sort out the answers to these questions, and emphasize the strengths and/or weaknesses of the overall purpose.

4. Is there background information (other studies) included? Does it give you an idea of what is already known (or not known) about this particular issue? Does it lead you right into this current study—that is, does it "make the case" for doing this study? Is it clearly written? Are there some omissions about this issue that should have been included to better understand why these authors chose to do this study? Does the background information seem skewed (or twisted) based on what is known about this issue? In other words, have the authors been selective about which information they have included just to prove a point? Make a judgment about all of these issues and include a statement about the relevance of the background information and the relationship/importance to the current study question.

SAMPLE AND GROUPS STUDIED

5. Who is being studied? Describe the groups (e.g., by gender, by race/ethnic group) and the number of people included in the study. Now, forget about who the authors picked to study: Think instead about who *should* be included to

really understand the research question and make the results relevant. Compare the kinds of people you think should be included to the ones who were included. Which groups were omitted in the study that you included? Why are they important? How could the authors have included them—or could they? Which potential information would these "omitted" people add?

6. Is there a statement about protection of patient's rights? Things to consider include these issues:

   - Were participants informed of the study prior to participation?
   - Were participants informed that they could drop out at any time?
   - Were notes, interview transcripts, patient records, and the like protected from access to others and the chance of "falling into the wrong hands"?
   - Was patient information coded with numbers or other symbols that detached the patient's name from the information?
   - Was the coded number system with patient names kept separate from the actual patient information (patient data)?
   - Do the results have the potential of jeopardizing the health and well-being of the subjects?

All credible research must be approved by institutional review boards (known as IRBs). These boards protect the rights of human subjects. These boards came about as a result of the Nazi atrocities committed against the Jews, the Tuskegee experiments, and other horrible human experiments. On the one hand, it is important that patients who participate in research are fully informed of their rights. On the other hand, requirements for patient consent can pose some significant methodological issues for researchers, such those who seek out vulnerable groups who may be viewed as exploited subjects in research. Look for a statement in the article about the participants receiving informed consent and/or approval by the IRB.

STUDY DESIGN AND METHODS FOR COLLECTING PATIENT DATA

7. How was this study designed? Was there one group, or were the participants divided into two groups? Did the authors pick a readily accessible group to study (also known as convenience sample)? Or did the authors work hard to make it a random sample? A random sample means that everyone who has a possibility of participating has a chance to participate. For example, when studying people in the state of Missouri, everyone has equal chance to participate. How many groups were included in this study—one, two, or more? Should economic impact be considered as a component of the study? Were economic impact data included as a dimension of the study design? If not, should they have been, and how should the questions about costs have been asked?

8. Was there an intervention done in this study? This is common with more than one group—that is, one group receives a "treatment" and the other receives no treatment. Or was this study descriptive, meaning that the data describe

(continues)

Figure 3-2   Evidence-based practice worksheet used at the University of Missouri–Columbia. (Continued)

or "tell a story" about the people studied? Determine if the study is descriptive or includes an intervention/treatment. If you are familiar with types of epidemiological studies (e.g., prevalence or cross-sectional, case control, and clinical trials), specify the type.

9. Which methods did the authors use to collect information? Did they interview the participants? Did they survey the participants? Did they use patient records? Did they use other methods to collect information? Did they use a combination of methods (e.g., interviews plus patient records)? Did they give you a sample of the questions asked and/or the information (variables) collected? Did they use a standardized tool (e.g., blood pressure cuff, repeatedly used questionnaire)? Were these tools checked out to make sure they give the same answers over and over (also called "reliability")? Was the procedure (the step-by-step directions) for collecting the patient information explained in the article? Do you have a good idea of how this information was collected? Could you do the study again using the description given by the authors? Think about which information you think should be collected to answer the question (see Item 1). Did the authors collect the "right" information? What other questions should have been asked? How could you get that information? In your lesson instruction, this issue is explained as "outcomes" (see Item 5).

RESULTS, CONCLUSIONS, AND "SO WHAT"

10. Results and conclusions are different. Results are a listing of compiled data that has been analyzed. For example, data can be reported as statistics, as summary statements, or in tables. Conclusions are the next step beyond results. They represent judgments made by the authors about the significance of the results, applicability to the group(s) studied, and relevance to the research question. Refer to your lesson instruction (Item 6) for other ways to ask these questions. In your judgment, do the data reflect the conclusions the authors draw, or are they jumping to conclusions that should not be made? Are there alternative explanations for the data? What are those alternative explanations? Do the authors suggest alternative explanations?

11. So what? Does this study make a difference? Can you see its implications for a broader group of people? Does it make you think of more questions that should be asked about the problem/issue? What should the next steps be for this problem/issue? Is there an expression of economic impact, if appropriate, in the research study?

Source: From the online policy course of the Sinclair School of Nursing at the University of Missouri–Columbia. Reprinted with permission.

and contributed to student motivation and skill development. Evaluation of the model provided statistically significant evidence that students who participated in the program successfully developed information literacy skills and retained the skills at the end of the study. Nursing faculty members are encouraged to review the Australian group's experiences for guidance when working to design educational programs to develop information literacy skills in their own nursing students.

Role Modeling by Faculty

Nursing faculty are the first nurses who have an opportunity to influence nursing students. Initially, students learn through classroom experience, reading assignments, and interactions with faculty and other students. Faculty members serve as the key role models for student nurses throughout their educational program, and they influence how students learn and retain knowledge. It is no longer acceptable to ask students to memorize data about a clinical topic and then to test on the memorized data. Instead, application of the knowledge in a clinical setting should be the goal. Critical thinking can and must be taught, and nursing faculty need to be experts on the topic of critical thinking development.

At the undergraduate level, innovative approaches will be needed to develop learning experiences that promote outcome-oriented thinking. Alfaro-LeFevre (1999) offered critical thinking exercises and nursing research exercises at the end of each chapter in her book to assist nurses to improve thinking skills, with the goal of expanding the students' skill set beyond good problem solving to reflective thinking. Critical thinking is described succinctly as "a commitment to look for the best way, based on the most current research and practice findings" (p. 59). Faculty must assist novice learners to progress through the steps of learning how to think critically. As they mentor students, they need to interweave evidence-based data into the curriculum and learning experiences of the nursing program and the clinical setting.

Nursing faculty must also serve as role models in terms of promoting the value of nursing research in the clinical setting. In addition to learning the basic concepts of research, students need to learn how to apply those research findings into a practice setting. Several strategies can be used to actively engage students in research. One strategy to involve students in this process is to use a research proposal to demonstrate the principles of the research process and have students conduct the necessary data collection and analysis. Another strategy is to have students provide the data for a research study. Demographic data can be collected about the students and then compared with data gathered from previous classes and the literature.

One way to teach evidence-based practice in a research course is to put students in small groups and provide them with research articles to critique. The students share their critiques and then assess the studies in terms of the clinical settings in which the findings could be implemented. The next step is to discuss if the findings are ready for use or if additional research is needed. If the research could be implemented in clinical practice, the students discuss how to put the research findings into practice and how to evaluate their implementation. Actively engaging undergraduate students in the research process increases understanding and appreciation of the importance of research for evidence-based practice.

The importance of evidence-based practice in nursing is highlighted by the proposal for the master's-prepared clinical nurse leader that has been put forth by the American Association of Colleges of Nursing. In the education of this role, evidence-based practice is identified as an essential curriculum element, along with identified competencies and clinical experiences.

Selecting an evidence-based practice model for use in a nursing program will be a necessary challenge that must be met. Faculty members need to familiarize themselves with the various evolving models and integrate a model into their curriculum. Models help to clarify and visualize the process for students.

Mohide and King (2003) reported locating 23 distinct evidence-based practice models in a literature search of several databases. Pape (2003) reviewed the evolution of four evidence-based practice models: Iowa Model of Research-Based Practice to Promote Quality Care, Stetler Model, Rogers Model, and Academic Center for Evidence-Based Practice (ACE) Star Model. The Iowa Model was developed in 1994 to be used as a guide for nursing staff to use research findings to improve patient care (Titler et al., 2001). Revisions have been made to this model based on feedback from users and prompted by changes in the health care market. The Stetler Model, first reported on in 1976, and then refined and expanded in 1994, consists of six phases to use at the practitioner level to apply research finds to practice (Stetler, 1994).

The Rogers Model consists of five stages: knowledge, persuasion, decision, implementation, and confirmation (Burns & Grove, 1999). The ACE Star Model, developed by the University of Texas Health Science Center at San Antonio, consists of five knowledge transformation steps, which are represented by five points on the ACE Star Model. The ACE model framework organizes evidence-based practice processes and approaches, revealing the relationships between the five steps. The University of Texas Health Science Center at San Antonio is also a funded ACE, and information on its funded studies can be located at *http://www.acestar.uthscsa.edu*.

Finally, nursing faculty need to be cognizant of the differences between novice thinking and expert thinking. Faculty have experiences and expanded knowledge that allows them to generate better hypotheses when problem solving with a patient situation. Novice students are eager to act before assessing and have limited knowledge. Learning about evidence-based practice can occur when faculty are supportive and knowledgeable about how critical thinking is taught.

Communication Skills

The availability of evidence-based practice guidelines does not guarantee that practicing nurses will use them. When nursing graduates enter the work world, they will be confronted with a work force encrusted in the practice models of the institution. Unfortunately, many nursing practices are not based on facts, but rather reflect routines and traditions of the institution. Graduates should be prepared to be greeted with resistance from co-workers who may have had minimal exposure to research principles or minimal opportunities to develop critical thinking skills. Obviously, it is easier to do a job when you just follow the rules instead of analyzing each situation and do what is appropriate for each individual patient.

Graduate nurses will need to be effective and skilled communicators when introducing evidence-based practice information in their work setting. They will need skills for working with groups, managing change, and disseminating information. The first year of nursing practice is a difficult time for recent graduates, and the challenge of introducing a new approach of problem solving while developing their clinical skills merely adds to the stress and anxiety levels of the individual.

Understanding why nurses resist technology is also important for graduate nurses. Introduction of evidence-based practice information can be unsettling for nursing staff. A common fear among practicing nurses is that obtaining the needed information will be time-consuming, and there is little time available in a work setting where nurses are already overloaded. Being an advocate for evidence-based practice is a challenging endeavor if the nurse is not prepared to communicate and advocate on behalf of evidence-based practices within the work setting and among team members.

Educational Preparation

Nurses who graduate from baccalaureate nursing programs are knowledgeable about basic research methods and principles. Put simply, the nursing graduates who participate in educational programs at the collegiate level are the nurses who will be prepared to practice in an evidence-based practice environment.

Pape (2003) advocates for the introduction of the role of knowledge broker when implementing evidence-based nursing practice. The knowledge broker is viewed as the change agent who can facilitate a team in collaborating to meet a common goal. Master's-prepared nurses are ideal candidates for the role of knowledge broker. Their advanced education, specialization in a clinical area, and research participation at the collegiate level should have thoroughly prepared them for the demands of evidence-based practice.

FUTURE CHALLENGES

Nursing educators face numerous challenges as they seek to adapt nursing programs to match the same pace of change that occurs in the real world. Learning transmission increasingly occurs by electronic communication methods, and this transition is changing the way nursing education is delivered. A time of rapid change can be scary, but it can also be a time of wonderful growth, if individuals are willing to be risk takers. Their ability and willingness to work with the new technology of today and the future will allow those risk takers to help design the new structure of nursing education. The teaching of evidence-based practice in nursing programs is but one of many innovations that faculty will use to prepare future nurses to close the gap between research and practice.

Practicing health care from an evidence base has become essential as more information is generated and becomes available via rapid access technology. To adequately prepare future nurses to perform their jobs, educators must offer educational opportunities to explore and use various data sources and technologies that will become routine and mandatory in the worksite. Nurses will need critical thinking and decision-making skills as they implement "evidence" in practice—considering whether, for example, a guideline is appropriate or a prescribed treatment is supported by the most current research practice. These skills are best taught while nurses are in school—for example, in simulated situations, where discussion can occur, options can be considered, and outcomes evaluated. This goal can be accomplished by assignments such as structured critiques of research articles, with follow-up application of findings and implications to clinical practice situations.

REFERENCES

Agency for Healthcare Research and Quality (AHRQ). (2008). *Evidence-based practice centers.* Retrieved May 26, 2009, from http://www.ahrq.gov/clinic/epc

Alfaro-LeFevre, R. (1999). *Critical thinking in nursing: A practical approach* (2nd ed.). Philadelphia: W.B. Saunders.

American Association of Colleges of Nursing (AACN). (1996). *The essentials of master's education for advanced practice nursing.* Washington, DC: Author.

American Association of Colleges of Nursing (AACN). (2003). *Enrollment and graduations in baccalaureate and graduate programs in nursing, 2003–2004.* Washington, DC: Author.

American Library Association (ALA). (2001). *Objectives for information literacy instruction: A model statement for academic librarians.* Retrieved September 1, 2004, from http://www.ala .org/ala/acrl/acrlstandards/objectivesinformation.htm

American Nurses Association (ANA). (1965). *Position paper on education.* Kansas City, MO: Author.

American Nurses Association (ANA). (1989). *Education for participating in research.* Kansas City, MO: Author.

Bandman, E. L., & Bandman, B. (1995). *Critical thinking in nursing* (2nd ed.). Norwalk, CT: Appleton & Lange.

Benner, P. (1984). *From novice to expert: Excellence and power in clinical practice.* Menlo Park, CA: Addison-Wesley.

Burns, N., & Grove, S. K. (1999). *Understanding nursing research* (2nd ed.). Philadelphia: W. B. Saunders.

Enkin, M., Keirse, M. J. N. C., & Chalmers, I. (1989). *A guide to effective care in pregnancy and childbirth.* Oxford, UK: Oxford University Press.

Institute of Medicine (IOM). (2001). *Crossing the quality chasm: A new health system for the 21st century.* Washington, DC: National Academies Press.

Kalisch, P., & Kalisch, B. (1987). *The challenging image of the nurse.* Lebanon, IN: Addison-Wesley.

Kenty, J. R. (2001). Weaving undergraduate research into practice-based experiences. *Nursing Educator, 26*(4), 182–186.

Krichbaum, K., Lewis, M., & Duckett, L. (1997). Critical thinking: What is it and how do we teach it? In J. C. McClosky & H. K. Grace (Eds.), *Current issues in nursing* (5th ed., pp. 169–179). St. Louis, MO: C. V. Mosby.

McNeil, B. J., Elfrink, V. L., Bickford, C. J., Pierce, S. T., Beyea, S. C., Averill, C., et al. (2003). Nursing information technology knowledge, skills and preparation of student nurses, faculty, and clinicians: A U.S. survey. *Journal of Nursing Education, 42*(8), 341–348.

Mohide, E. A., & King, B. (2003). Building a foundation for evidence-based practice: Experiences in a tertiary hospital. *Evidence-Based Nursing, 6*(4), 100–103.

Muir Gray, J. A. (2001). *Evidence-based healthcare* (2nd ed.). Edinburgh, UK: Churchill Livingstone.

Pape, T. M. (2003). Evidence-based nursing practice: To infinity and beyond. *Journal of Continuing Education in Nursing, 34*(4), 154–161.

Pesut, D. J., & Herman, J. (1999). *Clinical reasoning: The art and science of critical and creative thinking.* Albany, NY: Delmar.

Polit, D. F., & Beck, C. T. (2003). *Nursing research: Principles and methods.* Philadelphia: Lippincott.

Reynolds, S. (2000). The anatomy of evidence-based practice: Principles and methods. In L. Trinder & S. Reynolds (Eds.), *Evidence-based practice: A critical appraisal* (pp. 2–18). Malden, MA: Blackwell Science.

Roberts, A. R., & Yeager, K. (2004). Systematic reviews of evidence-based studies and practice-based research: How to search for, develop and use them. In A. R. Roberts & K. R. Yeager (Eds.), *Evidence-based practice manual: Research and outcome measures in health and human services* (pp. 3–14). Oxford, UK: Oxford University Press.

Sackett, D. L., Straus, S. E., Richardson, W. S., Rosenberg, W., & Haynes, R. B. (2000). *Evidence-based medicine: How to practice and teach EBM* (2nd ed.). London: Churchill Livingstone.

Shorten, A., Wallace, M. C., & Crookes, P. A. (2001). Develop information literacy: A key to evidence-based nursing. *International Nursing Review, 48*(2), 86–92.

Stetler, C. B. (1994). Refinement of the Stetler/Marram model for application of research findings to practice. *Nursing Outlook, 42*(1), 15–25.

Titler, M. G., Kleiber, C., Steelman, V. J., Rakel, B. A., Budreau, G., Everett, L. Q., et al. (2001). The Iowa Model of evidence-based practice to promote quality care. *Critical Care Nursing Clinics of North America, 13*(4), 497–509.

U.S. Department of Health and Human Services (DHHS). (2000). *The registered nurse popula-tion, March 2000: Findings from the National Sample Survey of Registered Nurses.* Retrieved September 22, 2004, from http://bhpr.hrsa.gov/healthworkforce/reports/rnsurvey/rnss1.htm

Van Hoozer, H. L., Bratton, B. D., Ostmoe, P. M., Wienholtz, D., Craft, M. J., Albanese, M. A., et al. (1987). *The teaching process: Theory and practice in nursing.* Norwalk, CT: Appleton-Century-Crofts.

Wallace, M. C., Shorten, A., Crookes, P. A., McGurk, C., & Brewer, C. (1999). Integrating infor-mation literacies into an undergraduate nursing programme. *Nurse Education Today, 19*(2), 136–141.

Wallace, M. C., Shorten, A., & Russell, K. G. (1997). Paving the way: Stepping stones to evidence-based nursing. *International Journal of Nursing Practice, 3*(3), 147–152.

Wheeler, K., Fasano, N., & Burr, L. (1995). Strategies for teaching research: A survey of baccalau-reate programs. *Journal of Professional Nursing, 11*(4), 233–238.

CHAPTER 4

Linking Structure and Healing: Building Architecture for Evidence-Based Practice

Rosalyn Cama

The concept of designing buildings that engage our senses, envelope our psyche, and affect our well-being is nothing new. A well-designed building that influences human behavior is often noted, but rarely measured. This chapter addresses the link between structure and healing. It demonstrates how a process known as evidence-based design (EBD) builds the strongest argument to design healing facilities in an informed way. We consider the historical links between structure and healing.

HISTORICAL PERSPECTIVE

In a dark place the sick indulge themselves too much in various fancies, and are harassed by imaginings devised in an alienated mind, since no external phenomena can fall on the senses; but in a bright place they are prevented from being wholly in their own fancies, which are rather weakened by external phenomena.

Asclepiades of Bithynia, circa 50 b.c. (Green, 1955)

Second only to fresh air... I should be inclined to rank light in importance for the sick. Direct sunlight, not only daylight, is necessary for speedy recovery. I mention from experience, as quite perceptible in promoting recovery, the being able to see out of a window, instead of looking against a dead wall; the bright colours of flowers; the being able to read in bed by the light of the window close to the bed-head. It is generally said the effect is upon the mind. Perhaps so, but it is not less so upon the body on that account.

Florence Nightingale, 1820–1910

77

The concept that our surroundings affect our well-being is not new. The recovery environment for patients described by Asclepiades and Nightingale amply demonstrates the importance of environmental attributes on patients' healing process. With such notable historical references to the healing environment, why has relatively little attention been given to this subject in contemporary design practices?

From a more modern perspective, the economy has played a significant role in the approach a professional designer takes to a healthcare project. Hearken back to the recent past of the 1970s—during that period, the healthcare design specialty was known as "institutional design." The interior products available were nothing more than that, "institutional." In fact, many were standard products from medical supply houses. During this same decade, much innovation was taking place in the corporate segment in terms of the development of new building materials, interior finishes, textiles, and furnishings. The downturn in the economy in the early 1980s slowed production of those high-end products and sent a starving corporate sales force calling on the institutional design community. The beautiful finishes and expensive "bells and whistles" of products for the corporate sector, however, were not acceptable to the emerging managed healthcare market. Healthcare designers instead turned to European suppliers, who were ahead of the U.S. manufacturers in terms of design issues, and ordered Scandinavian and German products from those vendors that understood the ergonomic and maintenance issues of the healthcare environment. Unsurprisingly, it was not long before U.S. office furniture makers retooled their product lines and stimulated competitiveness in the healthcare product industry.

Simultaneously, the entire economic structure of the healthcare industry changed. The cry from the newly formed Facilities Department was to deliver a much more hospitable environment for patients, who were turning into "customers." It is said that it was the baby boomers, just starting their families, who demanded a new experience in birthing babies—and labor and delivery units across the country have not been the same ever since. Market pressures forced many hospitals to renovate and create a more home-like environment for their obstetrical units that encouraged participation from the father and extended family. As hospitals began to compete for this customer base, more market research was conducted. When support was found for this trend, hospitable amenities became standard hospital fare. The emergence at this very time of hospice care was also no coincidence, as it, too, was driven by the same demographic needs of baby boomers preparing their parents for death and dying.

In 1988, a group of savvy professionals engaged in hospital consulting and design realized that the building and renovating of hospitals, primarily driven by the needs of medical practitioners and their new technologies, was missing an important participant in the final design solution. Put simply, patients and the host of caregivers, either clinical or family, were not being thoughtfully factored into the final design solutions. This band of innovators decided that those trying to take a broader approach to healthcare design should be highlighted in an annual conference. Thus the Symposium on Healthcare Interior Design (Ripple, Inc., 2000) was born. This design conference focused on the areas of related research and aimed to educate a growing number of professionals already practicing in or entering this specialty. The originators of the Symposium have since created a more comprehensive learning experience. In 2003, they premiered Healthcare Design—an annual conference that draws in administrators, clinicians, practitioners and their project teams, and advocates who are making a difference in the way patients and caregivers are accommodated in their hospital experience, with the goal of positively impacting health, organizational, and economic outcomes.

The Center for Health Design, whose founders started the Symposium on Healthcare Design and produced it until 1998, was formed in 1993 as a research and advocacy organization. Through its research-based approach, the Center sought to find and sponsor some of the best research in the area of healthcare design. Today this effort continues to bring to light a host of emerging topics, as the healthcare industry continues to grow and become much more complex. The mission of The Center for Health Design is to "transform healthcare settings into healing environments that improve outcomes through the creative use of evidence-based design" (2004, p. 1). To that end, the Center's vision is to "[d]evelop a future where healing environments are recognized as a vital part of therapeutic treatment, and where the design contributes to health and does not add to the burden of stress."

This nonprofit agency operates through the diligent efforts of a volunteer multidisciplinary board of directors and a committed host of dedicated committee members, who work toward a common goal of improving the settings in which health care is delivered. This group consists of researchers, architects, interior designers, healthcare chief executive officers (CEOs), physicians, nurse executives, quality improvement professionals, futurists, marketing, and fund-raising professionals. This is precisely the interdisciplinary team make-up one would expect to find on a healthcare project's building team.

The list of new hospital building projects in the United States is remarkable. In 2004, approximately $17 billion of healthcare-related construction took place in the United States. In 2008, that amount rose to $50.5 billion, and the anticipated growth is to $71.5 billion by 2011 (Jones, 2008). "This is the strongest construction market in health care," said Robert Levine, Vice President of Turner Construction: Healthcare (Brandrud Company, 2003).

This increase in new building projects is attributed to a variety of factors: the lack of capital investment in the most recent years; a shortage of hospital beds in most markets; bottlenecks in emergency departments, surgical suites, and intensive care units; and an increase in acuity levels as technology moves less complicated case procedures into the outpatient arena. In addition, an aging population will tax this system as baby boomers, who have already proven their power to instigate change in this and many other industries, enter an age of increased medical need. Taken together, these forces are driving a stronger desire to have this discussion now and to build a body of knowledge that will help shape future projects. As Leland R. Kaiser, PhD, healthcare futurist, noted, "the hospital is a human invention and can be reinvented at any time" (Personal communication).

LOOKING TO THE PAST TO DETERMINE THE FUTURE

Three years after it began, The Center for Health Design engaged Haya Rubin, MD, PhD, to lead a team at Johns Hopkins University. The team's task was to conduct a literature search and analyze 30 years of research that had measured how the built environment and other environmental factors affected patient health outcomes. Accepting only those studies that had followed rigorous scientific methodologies, the Johns Hopkins team performed a meta-analysis of 78,761 publications, of which only 84 studies met their criteria.

Armed with this knowledge, the Center identified five areas that needed field study work (The Center for Health Design, 1998):

- Access to nature
- Control of one's personal space
- Positive distractions
- Social support
- Elimination of environmental stressors

The Center, along with Rubin's team, published these findings in an article entitled "Status Report: An Investigation to Determine Whether the Built Environment Affects Patients' Health Outcomes," which is available on the Center's Web site (*http://www.healthdesign.org*).

The Center for Health Design next decided to explore consumer opinion to determine the best place to begin its research. In partnership with the Picker Institute (Cambridge, Massachusetts), patients and their families were asked two questions: Which design strategies should be used to improve the quality of the physical environment? and What matters in the environment?

This topic was not new to the Picker Institute. In their book *Through the Patient's Eyes*, Gerteis, Edgeman-Levitan, Daley, and Delbanco (1993) had previously described the way in which the design of a facility affects the perception of the quality of care. "Patient experiences and their perceptions of that experience, according to Picker and The Center for Health Design, should matter to not only patients and their families, but also to healthcare planners, policymakers, and managers" (The Center for Health Design, 1997).

Nine two-hour focus groups were conducted that included three specific user groups: acute care, ambulatory care, and long-term care. The objective was to collect insights, attitudes, opinions, and perceptions from consumers about the physical environment of their hospital. The Center for Health Design and the Picker Institute recognized the need to capture the patient and family perspective, as defined by them, as a means to facilitate, integrate and accelerate the creation of life-enhancing environments. Patients and family members are increasingly being viewed as the experts in telling us what quality means to them—what matters, what makes them feel better and what things they need to support their recovery, healing and adaptation to significant life changes (The Center for Health Design & Picker Institute, 1998).

Seven common themes emerged from this research. Consumers asked for a physical environment that met the following criteria:

- Facilitates connection to staff
- Is conducive to well-being
- Is convenient and accessible
- Is confidential and private
- Is caring for the family
- Is considerate of people's impairments
- Is close to nature

Eight years later, the Robert Wood Johnson Foundation funded a project for The Center for Health Design to engage Roger Ulrich at Texas A&M University and Craig Zimring at Georgia Tech to update the meta-analysis survey that had been done by Rubin and her team. The intent of this project was to raise awareness in an industry that was investing a significant amount of money into capital improvements. This time, approximately 600 studies were discovered that met the standards for research rigor (Ulrich & Zimring, 2004). The updated survey found that the documented areas of evidence-based research primarily fell into three categories:

- Environmental psychology, or how a building environment affects stress levels
- Clinical research, or where the built environment impacts the medical and scientific approach to care
- Administrative studies, or how the built environment affects the management of their institution

A small body of research in the areas of evolutionary biology and neuroscience was also discovered.

In the environmental psychology studies, the researchers found outcomes related to areas where social support was needed to promote health and healing. The degree of control persons had over their environment influenced not only their own health outcomes, but also performance issues related to their caregivers. Positive distractions were found to be a factor that eliminated stress. Indeed, countless studies showed a direct correlation between access to nature and health outcomes, particularly when considering the length of stay. Ulrich's landmark 1984 study set the standard for what a patient views from his or her bed: Those patients who had a view of nature versus a brick wall had a shorter length of hospital stay (Ulrich & Zimring, 2004).

In a paper published in 2008, Ulrich and Zimring conducted a follow-up review of the research literature on evidence-based healthcare design. This review found 1250 studies and organized the results into three general types of outcomes:

- Patient safety problems, such as infections, medical errors, and falls
- Other patient outcomes, such as pain, sleep, stress, depression, length of stay, spatial orientation, privacy, communication, social support, and overall patient satisfaction
- Staff outcomes, such as injuries, stress, work effectiveness, and satisfaction

Ulrich and Zimring found that especially strong evidence (converging findings from multiple rigorous studies) supports the view that single-bed rooms, access to daylight, appropriate lighting, views of nature, noise-reducing ceilings, and ceiling lifts improve a health outcome. The presence of a family zone in patient rooms, carpeting, nursing floor layout, decentralized supplies, and acuity-adaptable rooms also affected healthcare outcomes, either directly or indirectly, in the empirical studies reviewed in this report (Ulrich & Zimring, 2008).

WHAT IS EVIDENCE-BASED DESIGN?

EBD is the process of basing decisions about the built environment on credible research to achieve the best possible outcomes (The Center for Health Design, 2008). In a survey of The Center for Health Design's board, members identified six factors as being most likely to influence building design:

1. Patient outcomes
2. Staff recruitment and retention
3. Quality of service

4. Improved medical safety procedures
5. Operational efficiency
6. Financial performance

Rationale for Evidence-Based Design

A visit to a healthcare facility is often one of the most stressful events in a person's life. People entering a facility are typically anxious about their illness and often in pain. In spite of these known stresses, finding their way through the facility for patients and their families is often confusing, with navigation through one of the most complex structures in the community being considered at best a self-service process. Further, once the patient is admitted, information about planned activities and services is limited, further increasing patient and family stress. Add clinicians who are overworked and may need an attitude adjustment because of a recently missed replenishment break, and you have a perfect recipe for overwhelming frustration and stress. These and a myriad of other factors add to the recipe for stressful environments.

For both patient and relatives, these factors have notable psychological effects, often engendering a sense of helplessness, anxiety, and/or depression. Physiologically, blood pressure increases, and increased muscle tension and higher levels of circulating stress hormones are noted. Behaviorally, a patient may respond with a verbal outburst, social withdrawal, passivity, sleeplessness, and/or noncompliance with medication orders.

Few studies have examined healthcare workplace performance, but much can be learned through the research done in other design industries. In 1998, the American Society of Interior Designers (ASID) conducted a study entitled "Workplace Performance" to explore how design can influence performance and change corporate culture. Its results led to a deeper understanding of how interior surroundings can contribute to an improved work life. Although it was conducted in corporate environments, this study identified five key components to creating a productive workplace:

1. People performance
2. Designed environment
3. Workflow
4. Technology
5. Human resources

When the designed environment was explored further, four design factors were noted to improve productivity (ASID, 1998):

1. Access to people and resources
2. Comfort in one's surroundings

3. Privacy
4. Flexibility of the environment

Inclusion of these four design factors not only contributes to improvements in staff productivity, but also enhances recruitment and retention efforts. In a subsequent ASID study entitled "Retaining and Recruiting Employees through Design," researchers found that after compensation, design of the work environment was tied for second with benefits as a factor determining an employee's decision to accept or stay with a job. In both of these studies, the built environment is known to influence productivity and reduce work force turnover (ASID, 1998).

These early qualitative studies conducted by The Center for Health Design and ASID in the late 1990s served as a flashpoint for thinking about how design is perceived to influence human behavior and determining how best to educate the design profession about the way in which current research can inform design solutions. One important outcome was a joint venture between ASID and the University of Minnesota, which created a Web-based clearinghouse for all research being conducted in all design specialties. The resulting Web site is known as "Informedesign" (*http://www.informedesign.com*). Intended to be a communications tool, it is updated on a weekly basis. The goal of the Web site's founders is to make the process of finding research to support design issues as easy as the process of searching for a product. In this sense, the clearinghouse represents a starting point for making a behavioral change in the design process.

At the same time the Informedesign effort was under way, the American Institute of Architects, working with the American Academy of Neuroscience for Architecture, undertook a study of how the brain responds to the built environment (Noble, 2008). The partners' goal was to determine how the application of neuroscience research might facilitate understanding the impact of architectural settings on human emotions, moods, and behaviors. This effort marked an important collaborative step, in which multiple specialties were brought to bear on the impact the built environment has on human behavior. (More information can be found at *http://www.aia.org*.)

In a follow-up to the Robert Wood Johnson Foundation research, a conference was convened in June 2004 that spoke directly to the transformation needed in the hospital work environment. Using a holistic approach that addresses the "mind, body, and spirit" of hospitals, Project Leader Victoria Weisfeld made the connection clearly. The "mind" part of the equation refers to work design and process in hospitals; the "body" focuses on the physical design of the hospital workplace; and the "spirit" refers to the soul of an organization, which encompasses its vitality, values, and attitudes, or, simply put, its culture ("Designing the 21st Century Hospital," 2004).

In 2008, The Center for Health Design and the Global Health and Safety Initiative funded by Kaiser Permanente and the Robert Wood Johnson Foundation launched Ripple. Ripple is an open-source, searchable database containing usable and relevant information from multiple health systems. It allows for interaction with colleagues to discuss best ways to use this base of knowledge and leverage current and anticipated exemplary practices so as to design an informed hospital of the future (Ripple, Inc., 2008).

THE REVOLUTIONARY PEBBLE PROJECT

The Center for Health Design found that in approaching this important design issue, a multiyear field research project was needed to fill the gap in knowledge needed to build the healthcare facility of the future. Field research in this area has traditionally been difficult because of the numerous variables that can influence outcomes. Working with a group of academic researchers, however, the Center devised a way to overcome most of these variables.

"The Pebble Project," as this amazing research project is known, aims to work with progressive healthcare organizations throughout the world that are engaged in significant building projects, and that believe in the potentially beneficial relationship between the facility design process, the ultimate facility design, and organizational behavior. The Center for Health Design believes that, just as a pebble tossed into a pond creates a ripple effect, so the lessons learned from well-researched and documented examples of projects demonstrating the benefit of these relationships will ripple throughout the healthcare and design communities.

There are two unique components to this Pebble Project. The first is its emphasis on understanding how organizational behavior changes because of the planning and design process. The second is its development of a standardized evaluation methodology, which in turn leads to the following possibilities:

- Comparison of outcomes
- Identification of best practices
- Continuous improvements in healthcare design

Timing Is Everything

When a number of people begin to feel the same pain about a topic at the same time, a movement often begins. In healthcare design, such a convergence of thinking began in the late 1990s. In 2000, the Institute of Medicine (IOM) issued a "Statement on Quality of Care" for the U.S. healthcare system. In this statement, IOM described quality care as care that is patient centered, efficient, effective, safe, equitable, and timely. Although the focus of this thinking was about how a system of health delivery could improve its culture and, therefore, its behavior, The Center for Health Design (1998) examined this mantra in an effort to understand how the built environment can support such behavioral changes. The questions raised helped to form the research matrix of the Pebble Project (**Table 4-1**). The results currently being gathered in the Pebble Project support the Center's initial hypotheses.

Table 4-1   Pebble Project Research Matrix

Comparative Group → Outcome Research ↓	Patients (S, G or A)	Employees/ Physicians (S, G or A)	Family/Visitors (S, G, A)	Community	Organization/ Institution
Clinical/Technical Outcomes		N/A	N/A	N/A	N/A
Economic/Financial Resource Utilization					
Operational Improvements				N/A	
Satisfaction, Quality of Life, Cultural Assessment					
Safety/Error Reduction Outcomes			N/A		N/A
Environmental/ Sustainability					
Other Measurable Outcomes					

Project Name: _____

Explanation of S, G or A:
Research studies can be designed to look at the effects as follows:

1. **S = Same** (identical) group of patients, families or employees pre and post intervention.
   a. Sickle cell patients admitted to an old unit vs. the same patients admitted to a new unit
   b. Patients undergoing knee replacement of one knee in old unit vs. other knee in new unit
   c. Same mothers giving birth in old unit vs. new unit

2. **G = Group** (type/group) of patient, families or employees pre and post intervention.
   a. Patients of a particular diagnostic type
   b. Patients treated in a particular unit or in a particular office
   c. Employees in a particular work group
   d. Families of hospitalized children

3. **A = All** (the entire population) of patient, families or employees pre and post intervention.

The research matrix depicted in Table 4-1 is now being used to advise hospitals on research possibilities. It is also used by The Center for Health Design to determine when multiple hospitals are reporting on the same hypotheses. The correlation between the IOM's "Statement on Quality of Care" and the Pebble Project's initial results is described in the following sections.

Patient-Centered Care

In 2004, we asked, "In a customer-driven society, why would we even consider less than a private room?" At first glance, the answer given might be "the costs to deliver care." But do we really know the effect that the sharing of a space has on a health outcome, on the effectiveness of family-provided care, or on the flexibility a room designed for variable acuity can have on operational costs? If the facility provides positive distractions, will the experience be less stressful? If access to information using resource libraries or computer terminals answers more questions, will the patient feel a partnership in his or her care?

By 2004, the Pebble Project research had yielded great support for a patient-centered approach. When the first four Pebble Projects reported their collected data, the following findings were noted:

Saint Alphonsus Regional Medical Center, Boise, Idaho

"Noise levels have been reduced by designing larger private rooms, adding carpet to the hallways, putting acoustical tiles on the walls and ceilings, and relocating machinery and nurse charting away from patients."

"Average decibel rate per patient room was less than 51.7."

"Quality of sleep improved from 4.9 to 7.3 (on a scale of 0–10)."

"Patient satisfaction scores improved during a three-month comparison period."

Bronson Methodist Hospital, Kalamazoo, Michigan

"Private patient rooms have resulted in decreased patient transfers because of the elimination of conflicts among patients that necessitated moves and an increase in patient sleep quality."

"Built environment survey found that private rooms made for a better patient experience and that it enables higher quality of patient care."

The single-patient room has since been accepted into the AIA Guidelines for Design and Construction of Healthcare Facilities. Subsequent Pebble projects have focused on proving the effectiveness of additional amenities for care delivery, family involvement, and patient communication.

Timely Care

In any service-based business, timing is everything. In health care, the key questions is this: How can we deliver quality care in an environment that supports redundancy of motion, yet which does not support increased access to patients or seek to improve communications between staff and patients and their family members? By understanding the tasks at hand to deliver care, studying the time and motion required to deliver that care, challenging conventional delivery models, and improving visual and physical access, the quality of care improves. The amount of bedside care delivered increases, thereby improving staff satisfaction among nurses—after all, bedside care is why they went into nursing in the first place. The net result is a reduction in turnover rates.

Technology has increased the patient's access to medical knowledge at home, so why restrict that flow of information in a health setting? Communications can be timely and can be delivered not only at the bedside, but also in community conference centers, patient- and family-accessible resource libraries, and Internet-accessible dataports to a hospital Web-based information center located in waiting rooms. As more hospitals offer private rooms, waiting rooms will become obsolete; these sites are perfect locations to create patient floor resource centers.

Evidence from Pebble research includes the following findings:

Bronson Methodist Hospital, Kalamazoo, Michigan
"Overall satisfaction increased to 95.4%."
"Nursing turnover rates are less than 12%."
"Market share has increased 6%."
"Employee satisfaction has improved."

Methodist Hospital/Clarian Health Partners, Indianapolis, Indiana
"Overall patient dissatisfaction dropped from 6% in 1998 to 3% in 2001."

Barbara Ann Karmanos Cancer Institute, Detroit, Michigan
"Patient satisfaction rose 18%."
"Nurse attrition fell from 23% to 3.8%."

Efficiency

When dealing with the health of humankind, why would we, as a society, expect less than efficient work processes in the setting that delivers our care? Yet most facilities are antiquated and ridden with processes that were the best in their day, but need serious redefinition given today's technology. Do patients need to be transferred to services that are now mobile?

Pebble research includes the following findings on efficiency:

Methodist Hospital/Clarian Health Partners, Indianapolis, Indiana
"Patient room layout, equipment integration, and other design features have helped push patient transfers down 90%."

Methodist Hospital/Clarian Health Partners, Indianapolis, Indiana
"Caregiver workload index has been reduced, resulting in improvements in nursing efficiency."

Barbara Ann Karmanos Cancer Institute, Detroit, Michigan
"Lower daily variable costs per case."

Equitable Care

Is health care different for the "haves" and the "have-nots"? We all know that should not be true, but a recent Yale University study found that African Americans and Hispanics suffering severe heart attacks must wait significantly longer than whites for emergency treatment at hospitals. The delays are largely due to the poor quality of the hospitals that minorities typically use. These hospitals (i.e., those that serve largely minority populations) may lack up-to-date communications and diagnostic equipment and could be poorly organized (Bradley et al., 2004).

Efficacy

If the goal of medicine is "to do no harm," then in addition to filling the role of caregiver, which responsibilities do healthcare facility managers have? It has been proven that the amount of disruption in an environment directly affects a patient's quality of sleep and has a direct effect on healing. Likewise, the design of private rooms, the location of sinks, and the rate of air exchange are all factors in decreasing infection rates. The elimination of environmental stressors such as noise, glare, odor, and poor air quality, as well as the inclusion of adequate way-finding measures, also lower stress.

Pebble research shows that the following result is possible with improved design:

Barbara Ann Karmanos Cancer Institute, Detroit, Michigan
"Reduced pain medication requirements and decreased medication variances."

Safety

A facility that is designed to deliver care for a person's health should also be a safe environment—but that is not always the case. Obstacles contribute to patient falls; medical orders are misunderstood because of acoustical distractions; there is a lack of physical organization; storage for just-in-time material delivery reduces efficiency in the delivery of care; and lack of proper hand-washing or air exchange rates increases the risk of hospital-borne (nosocomial) infections.

Pebble research evidence found the following results:

Bronson Methodist Hospital, Kalamazoo, Michigan
"Private rooms, location of sinks, and air flow design have resulted in an 11% overall decrease in nosocomial infections."

Methodist Hospital/Clarian Health Partners, Indianapolis, Indiana
"Patient falls are down 75% due to the unit's decentralized design, which allows for better observation."
"A decrease in patient transfers and nurses' more consistent knowledge of each patient's condition have contributed to an improved medication error index."

Barbara Ann Karmanos Cancer Institute, Detroit, Michigan
"A 30% reduction in medical errors [was the] result of increased space in the medication room, location of the medication room, organization of medical supplies, standardized visual cues, and acoustical panels to decrease noise levels."
"A 6% reduction in patient falls [resulted from] better visualization of patients due to the angle of doorway, improved lighting, and room layout."

A GROWING BODY OF EVIDENCE

Timing is everything. When a group of innovators presents a strong enough case to push a new concept forward, others will follow suit as soon as the risk level is diminished. The previously mentioned research results support the notion that the built environment does, in fact, affect behavior. Indeed, enough evidence is available that this concept is no longer a hypothesis. In the healthcare segment of design, more than 50 organizations are now participating in the Pebble Project's ongoing work to build the case for irrefutable proof. As more healthcare facilities add to this body of knowledge, we will see what futurist Daniel Burrus (1993) refers to as a "flashpoint"; ultimately, what is now seen as a solution to spend discretionary dollars may, in fact, become code. This transformation in thinking offers hope for those who have learned to rely on an evidence-based approach to hypothesize, measure, and then design outcome-driven solutions.

In their literature search, Ulrich and Zimring (2004) found four basic assumptions where there is a compelling amount of research to drive design decisions:

- By reducing staff stress/fatigue, the effectiveness in delivering care increases.
- By changing design, patient safety and quality of care improve.
- By reducing patient stress, the quality of life and healing for patients and families improves.
- By improving overall health quality, costs are reduced.

In support of their first assumption ("By reducing staff stress/fatigue the effectiveness in delivering care increases"), Ulrich and Zimring found overwhelming evidence that reducing noise levels in the work environment and improving job satisfaction create positive outcomes. To a lesser degree, improving medication processing and delivery times, improving work effectiveness, and increasing patient care time per shift achieve the same outcome. Other studies show a correlation between improvements in the workplace and higher job satisfaction, reduced fatigue, and lower turnover rates.

Ulrich and Zimring's second assumption ("By changing design, patient safety and quality of care improve") is most assuredly achieved by reducing the rates of airborne and contact nosocomial infections. Improving communication between all parties involved in care, reducing the number of patient falls and medication errors, improving confidentiality of patient information, and increasing hand-washing compliance by staff are all measures that have proven positive outcomes.

In support of Ulrich and Zimring's third assumption ("By reducing patient stress, the quality of life and healing for patients and families improves)" a tremendous amount of work demonstrates a direct correlation with improved outcomes when noise is reduced, spatial disorientation is minimized, sleep quality improves, and social support increases—all measures that reduce patient stress (emotional, duress, anxiety, and depression). Fewer studies are offered in support of the idea that reducing depression, improving circadian rhythms, reducing feelings of helplessness, and empowering patients and families, providing positive distractions, and reducing pain (intake of pain drugs and reported pain) affect outcomes.

In regard to Ulrich and Zimring's final assumption ("By improving overall health quality, costs are reduced"), reducing the number of patient transfers and improving quality of care clearly lead to the best results. To a lesser degree, patient outcomes are affected by staff work effectiveness or increased patient care time per shift, reduction in the length of stay, reduction in the administration of drugs, patient satisfaction as it relates to staff quality, and finally, rehospitalization or readmission rates (The Center for Health Design, 2004).

Ulrich and Zimring's 2008 review of the literature helps quantify where much work has already been completed. These studies offer clues about sources for informing design hypotheses and, subsequently, design solutions. Although a prescriptive solution is not so easy to devise, the Pebble Project nevertheless provides a framework through which to begin to understand how best to create structured, individual research projects that can achieve the right solutions in each of these areas for a given design problem. The Center for Health Design also offers guidance in this process.

A TRADITION BASED ON TRUST

Even with better ideas and products, if they come to market before their time, their impact will be lost on a society that is just not ready to accept them. Likewise, results gained from these early healthcare-based research projects face a challenge: They must now be introduced into practice to inform upcoming design decisions. This process—an evidence-based approach—is not new to the design field; it is just uncommon outside of the ivy halls of academia.

Much research has already proven that the built environment does have an impact on human behavior. The problem, however, is that design profession-als (including architects, interior designers, landscape architects, and graphic designers) have tended to rely mostly on an interview process, time-honored design principles, and experience to justify solutions. Over time, building codes and regulatory guidelines have ensured that the most obvious and sometimes proven solutions that pertain to health, safety, and welfare have been applied. Within the confines of a building project, it is rare that the processes of hypoth-esis, measurement, and outcome determination are integrated and supportive of an evidence-based approach. It is ironic that in the healthcare field, where medical practice is built on measurement and improving outcomes, the same does not hold true for its design consultants.

But things may be changing. In an August 2000 *Lancet* article, Colin Martin wrote, "Although the premise that the physical environment affects well-being reflects common sense, evidence-based design is poised to emulate evidence-based medicine as a central tenet for health care in the twenty-first century."

Selection Process of Qualified Design Consultants

Most design consultants come to a new client's table by presenting the best examples of their previous projects. A portfolio of similar projects, an under-standing of the client's goals, the design process, decision-making skills, an ability to build consensus, an ability to manage both budgets and schedule, and team compatibility are often the qualifiers for project awards. This practice is a blatant example of a "trust me" model. Although this approach does not fail outright, it is devoid of measurement and lacks quantifiable results that might prove the building's impact on health outcomes and workplace performance.

A good design practitioner is trained in interviewing skills and will take a soft approach toward introducing a more rigorous scientific model to mea-sure, draw conclusions, and develop intuitive hypotheses that will prove that a proposed solution is sound. Is this wrong? Many great buildings and memo-rable interiors have been built in this less than scientific way, but many great opportunities in design also have been missed because of a misunderstanding of a design feature's effects on the behavior of the building's occupants. The real sacrifice is made when a project's budget needs to be shaved—a process we irreverently call "value engineering," wherein decisions are made to arbi-trarily remove a value-added feature with no justification other than to cut the project's capital expenditure. Because very little evidence exists to support the design's operational impact, the feature is deleted.

If the "trust me" model were, in fact, replaced with a "show me" model for the design process, then decision making would refer to past evidence in similar scenarios to help predict the results of a new scenario. This new scenario would have to be tested again to reveal whether it proved worthy in the new situation. When enough data are gathered to support a supposition, the design feature should inform a new code or design guideline. With the number of building projects that occur on an annual basis, it would not be long before a substantial body of knowledge would engender a more evidence-based approach to project decisions.

A note of caution is in order, however: These individual research projects do not lead to "cookie cutter" solutions. Instead, the intent—and this is an important point—is that the process should lead to an evolutionary way to improve the design of healthcare facilities. Just as myriad advances in medical care, technology, and societal needs lead to an ever-changing healthcare environment, so shall our design solutions evolve and not remain stagnant.

In a November 2003 *Healthcare Design* article, Hamilton best described the roles of design consultants. He defined the practitioner's tasks as follows (p. 18):

- Study the available research and interpretation of the implications for design.
- Hypothesize the intended results of a design intervention and measure the outcomes.
- Share the results publicly to advance the field.
- Subject the results to peer review and the validity of academic rigor.

Table 4-2 expands on these "four levels" by outlining a few practical ways that designers can achieve a better practice.

A PROCESS DEFINED

The process of planning, programming, designing, and building a new facility is well established and proven to deliver award-winning results. The idea of using an evidence-based approach is not intended to challenge that methodology, but rather to enhance it. In *Evidence-Based Healthcare Design* (Cama, 2009), a book I wrote to teach design teams how best to adopt this method of practice and facility managers how best to request this method of practice, I define evidence-based design as an iterative decision-making process that begins with the analysis of current best evidence from an organization as well as from the field. The intersection of this knowledge, behavioral, organizational, or economic clues, when they are aligned with a stated design objective, can be hypothesized as a beneficial outcome.

This approach does not provide prescriptive solutions to design, but rather a platform from which to add to an existing base of knowledge or to launch

Table 4-2   Four Stages of Evidence-Based Practice

Activity	Level 1	Level 2	Level 3	Level 4
Read material to stay current on emerging research	H	H	H	H
Use critical thinking to interpret implications of research on current projects	H	H	H	H
Collect success stories and historical data on completed projects	H	H	H	H
Perform applied research as a practitioner on real projects		H	H	H
Hypothesize intended results of design interventions	H	H	H	
Measure the results associated with design interventions		H	H	H
Report unbiased project results in the public arena, by both writing and speaking			H	H
Perform independent third-party post-occupancy evaluations			H	H
Obtain advanced educations to improve understanding of research methods			H	H
Collaborate with credible academic researchers and social scientists				H
Publish research results in peer-reviewed journals			H	
Complete an academic thesis or dissertation on an evidence-based design topic			H	

innovation. It espouses an ethical obligation to measure outcomes and share knowledge gained for a particular design's successes and failures, ideally in a peer-reviewed fashion, as is common in academia (Cama, 2009). The process is divided into four components:

1. Gather qualitative and quantitative intelligence.
2. Map strategic, cultural, and research goals.
3. Hypothesize outcomes, innovate, and implement translational design.
4. Measure and share outcomes.

The best way to begin a project is with a clear expectation of what is to be accomplished in the effort of building a new facility or renovating the existing facility. It is here that the partnership between consultant and client needs to be strong. Time and time again, it has been shown that what makes a project great is that it is client driven by a strong vision. This vision must be more than just an inspiring phrase crafted during an administrative retreat—it must be an image emotionally owned by all who are involved in a building project for what is being created for an institution's future. It is this insight that will make a consultant's role in hypothesizing design and, therefore, behavioral outcomes more realistic. The financial investment, when measured and evaluated, will be justifiably clear.

In his book *Discovering the Soul of Service* (1999), Berry identifies nine drivers of successful leadership:

1. Value-driven leadership
2. Strategic focus
3. Executional excellence
4. Control of destiny
5. Trust-based relationships
6. Investment in employee success
7. Acting small
8. Brand cultivation
9. Company's generosity

Berry's ingredients for such leadership will empower an interdisciplinary design team (outside consultants as well as internal committees) to produce their best work. Add to this mix a willingness and ability to conduct literature searches to identify a proven outcome, develop a hypothesis for the project's outcome, and then measure unique differences in the subject's environment. It is then that the conventional design process can be transformed so that a noteworthy project can be built in which behaviors will be changed with clear and full understanding of the intended outcomes.

FUTURE EXPECTATIONS ARE FOREVER CHANGED

In 2004, Leonard L. Berry, Derek Parker, Russell C. Coile, Jr., D. Kirk Hamilton, David D. O'Neill, and Blair L. Sadler (all current or past board members of

The Center for Health Design) developed a futurist's perspective of a hospital, suggesting how it could function after applying the known principles learned from the Pebble Project. This compilation of known outcomes was written as a fictitious parable entitled "Fable Hospital," where a fable is defined as a form of imaginative literature constructed in such a way that readers are encouraged to look for meanings hidden beneath the literal surface of the fiction (Berry et al., 2004).

These authors described Fable Hospital as a 300-bed regional medical center built to replace a 50-year-old facility that had 250 beds. Located on an urban site, the new facility provides a comprehensive range of inpatient and ambulatory services with a cost for replacement of $240 million. The assumption was made that leadership and operational core values were outstanding and clearly administered, that the design protocol was truly evidence based, and that research was ongoing throughout the design process.

Added features include those assets now proven to improve outcomes— oversized rooms maximizing outdoor views and daylight exposure; acuity-adaptable rooms with state-of-the-art monitoring and communications technology; double-door bathroom access; decentralized barrier-free nursing; alcohol-rub hand hygiene dispensers as needed; HEPA filtration; built-in flexibility for future technology growth; peaceful settings creating necessary distractions; noise-reducing measures; private consultation areas; patient education centers on each floor; and staff support facilities that reduce stress. These design upgrades cost the project an additional $12 million. In a CEO report to the hospital board, after the first year of operation where outcomes were carefully measured, the incremental costs were virtually recovered after one year and significant financial benefit began to accrue year after year.

This initial work is now supported by ongoing research in an ever-growing number of Pebble Projects, such as OhioHealth's Dublin Methodist Hospital, that are currently developing their own business cases. The report fully describes the cost expenditures and savings, and it is certainly worth studying if your organization plans to engage in a building project. This database of knowledge will only grow as this movement continues.

JOIN A PROVEN MOVEMENT

This chapter has only begun to hint at the possibilities inherent in linking structure and healing. Evidence-based design is an exciting new field that is now drawing the attention it so richly deserves. If you are engaged in designing or building a healthcare facility, then it is important to fully understand the evidence-based approach to design, embrace it, and invest in the methodology before your next building project is launched. This body of knowledge is evolving daily and can change—for the better—a life-altering, health-related event, of the type that we will all experience personally or through a loved one at some time during our lives.

Close your eyes and imagine the place where you like to escape to after a stressful period. Focus on those elements of that environment that support your sense of well-being. Design your hospital of the future with those qualities in mind, using the known evidence to justify their expenditures and without value-engineering out those factors that make us heal.

REFERENCES

American Society of Interior Designers (ASID). (1998). *Productive workplaces: How design increases productivity: Expert insights*. Washington, DC: Author.

Berry, L. (1999). *Discovering the soul of service: Nine drivers of sustainable business success*. New York: Free Press.

Berry, L., Parker, D., Coile, R., Hamilton, D. K., O'Neill, D., & Sadler, B. (2004). *Can better buildings improve care and increase your financial returns?* Chicago: ACHE/HAP.

Bradley, E. H., Herrin, J., Wang, Y., McNamara, R. I., Webster, T. R., Magid, D. J., et al. (2004). Racial and ethnic differences in time to acute reperfusion therapy for patients hospitalized with myocardial infarction. *Journal of the American Medical Association, 292*(13), 1563–1572.

Brandrud Company. (2003). *Transforming medical institutions into cultures of caring* [brochure].

Burrus, D. (1993). *Technotrends: How to use technology to go beyond your competition*. New York: Harper Business.

Cama, R. (2009). *Evidence-based healthcare design*. Hoboken, NJ: John Wiley & Sons, Inc.

The Center for Health Design. (1998). *Status report: An investigation to determine whether the built environment affects patients' medical outcomes*. Martinez, CA: Author.

The Center for Health Design. (2004). *Preliminary report for Designing the 21st Century Hospital Symposium*. Washington, DC: Author.

The Center for Health Design. (2008). *Definition of evidence-based design*. Retrieved April 14, 2009, from http://www.healthdesign.org/aboutus/mission/EBD_definition.php

The Center for Health Design & the Picker Institute. (1997). *Consumer perceptions of the healthcare environment: An investigation to determine what matters*. Martinez, CA: Author.

Designing the 21st Century Hospital [conference sponsored by Robert Wood Johnson Foundation and Center for Health Design], Washington, DC, June 2004.

Gerteis, M., Edgeman-Levitan, S., Daley, J., & Delbanco, T. L. (1993). *Through the patient's eyes: Understanding and promoting patient centered care*. San Francisco: Jossey-Bass.

Green, R. M. (1955). *Asclepiades: His life and writings*. New Haven, CT: Licht.

Hamilton, D. K. (2003, November). The four levels of evidence-based practice. *Healthcare Design, 3*(9), 18–26.

Jones, H. (2008, February). FMI's construction outlook: First quarter 2008. *FMI*. Retrieved April 14, 2009, from http://www.fminet.com

Martin, C. (2000). Transported by the architecture of London's new Underground. *Lancet*, *356*(9233), 947–948.

Noble, C. (2008). *Neuroscience and courthouse design workshop: Understanding cognitive processes in the courthouse.* Retrieved May 29, 2009, from http://www.aia.org/professionals/groups/nac/AIAS074909?dvid=&recspec=AIAS074909

Nightingale, F. (1860/1969). *Notes on nursing: What it is and what it is not.* Mineola, NY: Dover.

Ripple, Inc. (2008). Symposium on Healthcare Design [sponsored by Imark Communications and Center for Health Design], Anaheim, CA, 2000. Retrieved January 31, 2009, from http://ripple.healthdesign.org

Ulrich, R., & Zimring, C. (2004). *The role of the physical environment in the hospital of the 21st century: A once in a lifetime opportunity.* Concord, CA: The Center for Health Design.

Ulrich, R., & Zimring, C. (2008). A review of the research literature on evidence-based healthcare design. *Health Environments Research and Design Journal, 1*(3), 61–125.

CHAPTER 5

Living Evidence: Translating Research into Practice

Marie P. Farrell

The Calf-Path

One day, through the primeval wood,
A calf walked home, as good calves should;
But made a trail all bent askew,
A crooked trail, as all calves do.

Since then three hundred years have fled,
And, I infer, the calf is dead.
But still he left behind his trail,
And thereby hangs my moral tale.

* * *

The years passed on in swiftness fleet.
The road became a village street,
And this, before men were aware,
A city's crowded thoroughfare,
And soon the central street was this
Of a renowned metropolis;
And men two centuries and a half
Trod in the footsteps of that calf.

Each day a hundred thousand rout
Followed that zigzag calf about,
And o'er his crooked journey went
The traffic of a continent.
A hundred thousand men were led

By one calf near three centuries dead.
They follow still his crooked way,
And lose one hundred years a day,
For thus such reverence is lent
To well-established precedent.

A moral lesson this might teach,
Were I ordained and called to preach;
For men are prone to go it blind
Along the calf-paths of the mind,
And work away from sun to sun
To do what other men have done.
They follow in the beaten track,
And out and in, and forth and back,
And still their devious course pursue,
To keep the path that others do.

They keep the path a sacred groove,
Along which all their lives they move,
But how the wise old wood-gods laugh,
Who saw the first primeval calf!
Ah! Many things this tale might teach—
But I am not ordained to preach.

—*Sam Walter Foss (1858–1911)*

Ancient chronicles tell how, for a thousand years, the Kazakhstan city of Alma-Ata gave a friendly welcome to the trade caravans that journeyed along the Great Silk Road between Europe and the Far East. For centuries, traders followed the old familiar path to Alma Ata until the discovery of new sea routes. Then the old path was gradually abandoned. It was in this city of this most ancient of trade routes that in 1978, the World Health Organization (WHO) held its summit on the future of global health care. Financial experts, governmental officials, attorneys, health officials, nurses, physicians, and other health providers from more than 168 countries gathered to map out new paths for health care into the next century.

The result of their efforts was a call for perhaps the most revolutionary healthcare reforms ever made: the Alma Ata Declaration and *Health for All by the Year 2000* (HFA 2000; Primary health care, 1978). Health care, the delegates declared, had to be universally accessible to individuals and families in the community by means acceptable to them, through their full participation, and at a cost the individual, community, and country could afford ("Primary Health Care," 1978, p. 34). This declaration became the cornerstone of the WHO regional and worldwide efforts to think globally and act locally.

The local version of the declaration in the United States was *Healthy People 2000* and, more recently, *Healthy People 2010*. The European regional version was *Thirty-Eight Regional Targets for Health*. Regardless of region, however, the approach to health was envisioned as occurring through primary health care (PHC). Nursing was to play a major role in PHC, mapping this discipline's path from the time of Florence Nightingale, through the years of the Alma Ata Declaration, through a century of practice and research to the present—a time some characterize as a chaotic period in health care.

This chapter examines how nursing has evolved within the context of a tumultuous period of events, both within and outside the healthcare industry, and how it has distinguished itself from "doing what other men have done" by carving out its unique contribution through a series of developmental steps. One of these steps—and the subject of this chapter—is the linkage between research and evidence-based practice. This relationship has brought both opportunities and challenges to the nursing discipline as well as to the patients and communities served by nursing.

IMPLICATIONS OF THE ALMA ATA DECLARATION

The Alma Ata Declaration has considerable implications for the delivery of nursing and the movement toward evidence-based practice. Major shifts in thinking had to occur, because millions of people throughout the world had little or no access to care despite the burgeoning health-related industries in many countries (Parker, 2002). The intent was to ensure quality care and to place the individual at the center at that care, to have access to knowledge, information, and resources for treating diseases and maintaining high levels of wellness, for a life span that might extend into one's nineties. This goal was to be accomplished in ways that would be appropriate, culturally acceptable, and affordable.

This affordable health care was to shift from the top down, from large bureaucratic institutions to locally managed health services, or through PHC. At the time when the Alma Ata Declaration was published, governments were struggling with the burgeoning costs of their health services, in part owing to the advances under way in computer technology, genetic engineering, organizational development, communication technology, and thinking about ways to work smarter at a lower cost. As the health community worked to integrate the explosion of knowledge and technology, a similar pattern of change was apparent in Japan, in a field unrelated to health care.

THE 1980s

A worldwide transformation occurred after World War II, when Deming (2000) traveled to Japan to help rebuild the country after its war-time devastation. This initiative launched the total quality movement, which eventually evolved into the drive for continuous quality improvement (CQI). (The name most associated with quality, however, was Donabedian [1980, 1988], who emphasized the key elements of structure, process, and outcome—the traces of which can be found in today's literature on evidence-based practice.)

Throughout the 1980s, various organizations adopted new goals for health care: WHO promoted HFA 2000; Europe, its *Thirty-Eight Regional Targets for Health* (Targets for HFA, 1991); and the United States, its *Healthy People 2000*. These initiatives, in part, helped to focus attention on a concrete, albeit medically oriented, set of healthcare outcomes. The inspired initiatives of WHO also emphasized an inductive process from the primary level of individual clients and their healthcare providers, to the secondary level of the community hospital, to the tertiary levels of specialized hospitals—a trajectory that moved through local, regional, national, and international levels of health care. PHC providers developed the PHC system to support their services. Now they would use the same system to process their surrogate measure of success: data.

Data as Evidence

Data would be central to this process, along with the measurement, transferability, and generalizability of those data. As Pirsig observed in his cavalier analysis of the metaphysics of quality, "Data without generalization is just gossip" (1991, p. 5). Clearly, the importance of data as evidence, its measurement, and its application would be critical, as would its generalized use beyond the immediate research setting. Nevertheless, effective measurement would, in turn, depend on the knowledge of exactly what should be measured, and this knowledge would be generated from the bottom up. Data would be used to compare best practices and to support innovation across hospital units, cities, regions, countries, and continents. With increasing sophistication, countries could compare the relative number, type, and intensity or "dose" of interventions carried out as well as their costs; ultimately, funding of practices could be awarded based not on intuition, but on evidence. In this regard, the very essence of practice became an issue of concern at the governmental level, and the business of funding evidence-based practices would emerge as a transformative force to promote best practices as financial transactions, with the goal being to benefit from them or, as some fear, to control them (Winch, Creedy, & Chaboyer, 2002).

Research, Evidence, and Costs

A precursor of evidence-based practice was the quality movement. After Japan, quality initiatives appeared in the United States at Florida Power and Light and then found leadership in Dr. Brent James at Intermountain Health Care in Utah. Gradually, total quality management (TQM) was replaced by total quality improvement or CQI. Dr. Don Berwick in Massachusetts, among others, demonstrated unique approaches in regard to healthcare data, their quality, and their measurement. Deming, Juran, and others who wrote during this period insisted that management was responsible for outcomes and had to assume a leadership role to ensure these outcomes throughout the healthcare system (Juran, 1989, 1992).

The effects of this movement were widespread. The insurance industry saw reduced premium payouts and advocated approaches to lowering the enormous healthcare costs that had put some employers out of business. Administrators in the healthcare industry found a reduction in lawsuits, as timely response rates satisfied clients and attended immediately to the presented health issue. The European Union established funding sources for projects in this area and worked to "normalize" practices across the European region. Canada and Australia made similar changes. In addition, government agencies came to recognize the role played by nursing as a major force in the quality initiative. In nursing, the major countries in the forefront of these initiatives were Australia, Belgium, Canada, Great Britain, and the United States.

During the 1980s, European researchers undertook the most extensive study of nursing care ever funded at national levels in Europe (Farrell, 1987a, 1987b), and European nursing programs developed projects on quality improvement. In the United States, the National Institute of Nursing Research was launched in 1983 under Dr. Ada Sue Hinshaw's leadership. Funded studies focused on the practice of nursing that met the criteria of PHC, and advocates encouraged nursing practices that would yield the greatest results at costs that were affordable.

Organizations throughout the United States, including healthcare organizations, created quality teams. As part of these efforts, hospitals held numerous meetings during which healthcare providers were trained as leaders and facilitators. Tired pediatricians, unit secretaries, nursing's clinical specialists, group leaders, and facilitators sat through hours of discussions regarding the flow-through of a piece of equipment from the loading dock to the patient's bedside, all in the name of reducing the territorial mentality of vertical "product lines" and strengthening horizontal processing. The goal: to ensure the right equipment, at the right bedside, for the right patient, under the right conditions. Quality teams described these efforts in words not unlike the PHC philosophy—that is, care provided in a manner that was appropriate, and delivered in a manner that was culturally appropriate, acceptable, and cost-effective.

Soon, however, hospitals found that the discipline-packed teams grew weary of endless meetings that spanned extended periods. Teamwork activities took precious time from other duties. Most importantly, many participants in these efforts recognized that the crucial element in practice was not time on task, but rather the best practice that resulted and was amenable to other practices determined through a comparative analysis called benchmarking.

Comparing Evidence

While hospitals and health services were comparing best practices, patients were comparing worst practices. Over time, these patients and their advocates became vocal and persistent critics of certain healthcare practice. As the acquired immune deficiency syndrome (AIDS) epidemic galloped through the 1980s and into the 1990s, bright, articulate, young people who had been infected with human immunodeficiency virus (HIV) insisted on being involved in their care and, in part, contributed to the sweeping changes among consumers (Shilts, 1987). The Internet emerged with a consumer movement that was to change the way all parties were to view health and its ownership. Government, insurers, hospitals, healthcare providers, and consumers were all simultaneously moving toward ways of knowing that were unprecedented in health care's history.

In industry, just-in-time philosophies invaded manufacturing and other organizations that sold products (Goldratt & Fox, 1986). Just how many greeting cards did Hallmark have to keep ready in its storehouse, anyway? And who were the people who really made a difference to a company? Did a bank really need all those tellers? Why not improve the way banking services were delivered and at the same time (or so went the argument) reduce costs by placing workers in part-time positions, thereby reducing, or eliminating altogether, their healthcare coverage? Why does a surgical intervention require a hospital stay? Why not provide these services on an outpatient basis? And how many beds does a city need to support this burgeoning outpatient trend? The number of beds in Worcester, Massachusetts, which had been spread over three hospitals, was reduced to one fourth of the original number during this period. Along with this reduction in beds came a concomitant reduction of nursing staff in all three institutions.

Health care was now at a premium, and only those practices that were classified within the diagnostic-related group (DRG) were reimbursed. Further, this evidence was to be located at the site of the interface between the customer (read: patient) and the organization (read: nurse).

During this time, the locus of control was shifting. In banking, the traditional model of teller and customer evolved into a wall of a bank building with an ATM attached, which was accessed through an ATM card used by a banking customer who plugged it in from a drive-through window. In health care, the locus of control shifted such that a patient at an emergency department came directly face-to-face with the point-of-contact provider: the nurse. For better or worse, decisions that mimicked the just-in-time philosophy in the manufacturing and selling of a product were now being applied to the decision-making processes of the professional services delivered by a nurse as front-line worker.

Research versus Evidence-Based Practice

In summary, the quality movement of the 1980s brought a new sensibility to what had been exclusively nursing research into the early part of the 1990s, instilling an awareness of the brevity of time considered acceptable in the quality movement and the need for "good enough data." The intersection of these three dimensions suggested the need for a distinction between research and evidence-based practice, with the latter seen as the new, everyday fare of teams in healthcare organizations.

Armed with their control charts and fishtail exercises, nurses marched to the rhythm of their flip charts. Teams could be observed staring at the graphs of dubious, yet concrete numbers that indicated an increase or decrease in some purported set of variables of interest. The debates about what a quality initiative was, what did not meet the criteria of research, and what evidence-based practice actually meant were core issues that distinguished research and evidence-based practice from each other. For the research-minded practitioner, the traditional route of generating findings for the sake of generating knowledge was one thing; to articulate, deliver, and evaluate concrete practices that would lead to concrete evidence was another (McSherry, Simmons, & Abbott, 2002). If these results could be combined with other studies' results, in systematic reviews called meta-analysis, all the better. And if these studies and their clear evidence could be documented and placed in easy-to-read formats (preferably pictures), then the chances would be enhanced of using the results in places far removed from the location of the original study, and at a reasonable cost and in a manner acceptable to the user.

THE 1990s AND BEYOND

By the mid-1990s, the term "evidence-based practice" had begun to appear in the healthcare literature (Stetler, Brunell, Giuliano, Morsi, Prince, & Newell-Stokes,

1998). The Agency for Health Care Policy and Research (AHCPR) coined the term and created steps that would help researchers identify healthcare initiatives for specific clinical conditions.

Subsequently, an epistemological debate took place about evidence-based practice as a viable construct. Its origins and precursors, as described earlier in this chapter, were derived from a variety of sources, including professional practice, research findings, information technology, and managed care (French, 2002). This consideration of evidence-based practice as a viable construct or as a process, French observed, was questionable; indeed, he suggested that no evidence exists to support the notion of "evidence" as a stable construct. Further, he questioned whether evidence-based practice is a distinct process, a political construction, or simply another iteration of quality. Several meanings had been associated with the term "evidence-based practice," and the challenge was to distinguish the practice from personal, subjective informed perception or opinion (French, 2002, p. 255).

Opportunities and Challenges

Throughout the 1990s, nursing continued to evolve as a major force (Prescott, 1993), as a major cost center, and as a national resource that demanded funding. Nurses understood well and promoted graduate programs that examined the role of the front-line bedside nurse as decision maker who had become all the more powerful given the ever-expanding integrated healthcare systems spread over multi-mile campuses. Decision making, George (1999) argued, belonged at the local level, with the bedside nurse. With this perspective, interventions now had to lead to evidence that met the 24-hour turnaround for an overnight hospital stay. Babies and mothers bonded in one day through some miraculous process that Reva Rubin and others asserted constituted not an event, but an evolution that they presumed occurred over several days, weeks, or months. Intensive psychotherapy that once took a lifetime was now reduced to 12 sessions of cognitive therapy and perhaps a book that presumably alleviated depression through a 10-step process of recovery. Some confrontation, a book on the topic of angst, and some generic antidepressant medication became the silver bullet for providing "mental health services."

In nursing during these years, the discipline's literature databases had extensively documented the empirical, positivist approach to research and simultaneously embraced the post-modern, post-empirical studies that acknowledged the interaction of the researcher with the researched. These qualitative studies questioned underlying assumptions about the processes that occurred when people, despite all odds, did *not* die—when they survived and *flourished*. The studies examined the place of action research, the imperative of which was to alter the research processes to accommodate changes that occurred during the life of the research study, and put reputations at risk as researchers examined the relationship between getting well and experiencing music and art as part of the caring process. These qualitative studies appeared in peer-reviewed journals in nursing as well as in what some would character-ize as enlightened journals in medicine.

Outside of nursing, other disciplines were telling another story. Social sci-entists were forging other ways of viewing people's lives and experiences. The social constructionists and anthropologists insisted that contrary to general-izing results, meaning and experience were local, and not applicable beyond the immediate area of study. In research, cultures of inquiry now included positivism, participatory action research (PAR), interpretive social science (ISS), and critical social science (CSS) (encompassing feminism, critical race theory [CRT], and queer theory). Local knowledge emerged because people from local areas developed a language to communicate with others about their own text; they could tell their own stories. Some asserted that the findings from one institution could not be generalized to another institution because the culture of each institution was unique. In fact, some suggested, one clinical unit's culture might be strikingly different from another clinical unit's culture within the same hospital.

As time progressed, evidence-based practice, like its predecessors TQM and CQI, attracted some notable critics. Some, including Mitchell (1997), sug-gested that after 50 years of nursing research, little direction was forthcoming in helping nurses enhance patients' quality of life and assisting them to deal with the human responses of loss, despair, and suffering. Not only were the studies conducted at that time perceived as unhelpful, but the move toward evidence-based practice, Mitchell asserted, removed the individual approach to participation between the patient and the nurse (p. 154). Evidence-based prac-tice, she said, may call for "decontextualized, menu-driven directives, based on diagnoses or generalized situations" (p. 155). However, the characteristic of generalizability is acknowledged as the very goal of evidence-based practice, so that research results can be used in other places without the arduous task of conducting the research again.

Perhaps somewhat predictably, these debates and the data generated by research into evidence-based practice continued to produce mixed sentiments. Some asserted that evidence-based practice was not new—that nurses had, in fact, been engaged in it for years. DiCenso, Cullum, and Ciliska (1998) exam-ined the major constraints applied to this concept within nursing. As with other innovations, the definition of evidence-based practice was questioned (so vague as to be meaningless), its theoretical source was questioned (the frame-work lacked scientific verification), its methods (randomized control trials) were criticized (too narrow in focus), and its sampling frames (with narrow inclusion criteria) were questioned (so restrictive as to prevent generalization to large mixed groups of patients) (Deaton, 2001). Some critics even suggested that researchers, as data collectors, were promoting "cookbook nursing."

These perceived drawbacks were compounded by the nursing research environment, which presented its own constraints on implementation of evidence-based practice. Specifically, the environments in which nurses worked were such that the staff could not access research data. Nurses found nursing research theories to be presented at an unhelpful level of abstraction, and they experienced a gap between the ways in which results were presented and the ways in which the lives of their patients and their illnesses remained unexamined (DiCenso et al., 1998; McCaughan, Thompson, Cullum, Sheldon, & Thompson, 2002).

Thus, despite the advances in nursing research over the previous 20 years, some asserted that much of the research went unused for a variety of reasons, which were collectively classified as "barriers to research utilization" (Funk, Champagne, Tornquist, & Wiese, 1995). These obstacles to evidence-based practice included heavy workloads, aspects of the setting, nurses' lack of time (Ervin, 2002; Funk et al., 1995; Wallin, Bostrom, Wikblad, & Ewald, 2003), awareness of and access to research that might alter practice (Ervin, 2002), nurses' isolation from knowledgeable colleagues (Funk et al., 1995), inability to translate research into practice (Ervin, 2002), and feeling incapable of understanding the implications for practice (Funk et al., 1995).

Nurses, however, were not the only disenfranchised group. Patients and their families also struggled to make sense of a healthcare system they felt did not listen to them, did not understand them, did not teach them about their health conditions, and had no time for them. In the United States, then-First Lady Hillary Clinton heard these concerns and emerged as the champion of healthcare reform. While Clinton stomped through the country listening to the horror stories of healthcare needs gone unattended, ministries of health in the rest of the world watched the healthcare budget in the United States soar and its major health indicators receive mediocre ratings among the world's countries.

Europe continued to push for PHC and the avoidance, at all costs, of becoming like the U.S. healthcare system. The World Bank funded privatization and the U.S. Agency for International Development (USAID) sponsored projects in Eastern Europe and elsewhere that sought to spur private practice among physicians and nurses. (Never mind that most Eastern European citizens did not have the wherewithal to pay for private services, and that entire healthcare systems in Eastern Europe, Africa, and Asia were based on a totally different set of assumptions about health and healthcare delivery.) If these conditions were not enough, the resurgence of other factors would exacerbate the situation.

The world was under siege during this time, as many populations dealt with a resurgence of the infectious disease era, less developed countries joined developed countries in the quest to address the chronic disease era, and vast numbers of nations pondered the effects of the social health era. Large populations experienced a resurgence of tuberculosis and bacterial infections; the costly, long-term chronic illnesses of heart disease, cancer, and HIV; and the emerging social conditions of drug abuse, adolescent unwed pregnancy, and gang behavior. By this time, the populations of both India and China passed the 1 billion mark in population. For good reason, the search to determine which healthcare practices were and were not effective became an imperative on the minds of most concerned governments—yet progress was slow.

The Language and Alignment of Nursing

Evers (2001) suggests that the purported slow rate of progress toward evidence-based practice reflected incongruence between nursing terminology and the terminology of the health community. He argued for a better fit, for example, between WHO's (1980) *International Classification of Impairments, Disabilities and Handicaps* (ICIDH), which asserts the classification not of disease, but rather of the consequences of disease (Evers, 2001, p. 138), and other nomenclatures. Evers noted the similarity of the ICIDH nomenclature with Orem's inability for self-care and Henderson's focus on health deviations and self-care requisites. These observations underscored his plea for collaboration among researchers and the developers of taxonomies, and for classifications that document nursing practices, interventions, and outcomes. They also underscored the need for centers of excellence to develop guidelines for these conditions, described as occurring through a process of research utilization (Stetler et al., 1998).

Theories in Use

Other arguments challenged the uptake of evidence-based practice. A major reason for the slow adoption of this approach, some asserted, was that nursing theories provide an abstract view of nursing (Evers, 2001). The resulting generic statements are at odds with the highly specific results produced through evidence-based practice guidelines and experimental studies that explicate targeted evidence for narrowly defined conditions. This discrepancy may have been due, in part, to the restricted inclusion and exclusion criteria that studies adopted so that the results did actually emerge as clear evidence. However, the specificity of the targeted study subjects often precluded the application of the results to large, homogeneous groups of patients and demanded a sophisticated reader of research results.

Researchers conducted studies to examine nurses' clinical decision-making processes and to identify the sources of information and other measures they found useful in reducing the uncertainty associated with their clinical decisions (Nagy, Lumby, McKinley, & Macfarlane, 2001). In one study, researchers examined the commentaries of 108 nurses in three large acute hospitals in England (Thompson, McCaughan, Thompson, Cullum, Sheldon, & Thompson, 2002). They found that for information to be useful, it had to provide direction, experiential knowledge, organization support for practice, and a combination of research technology and experience. Further, these researchers identified overwhelming support for human information sources—namely, for the role of the clinical nurse specialist (CNS), whom they characterized as having extensive networks and clinical and research expertise. Importantly, nursing textbooks and information files were not found to be particularly useful. Based on these findings, the researchers concluded that research knowledge was neither the issue nor the problem; rather, the core element was the *medium* through which research knowledge was delivered (Thompson et al., 2002).

These findings may be generalizable only to the United Kingdom, but hospitals in the United States had already begun hiring nurses with titles addressing evidence-based practice. In addition, nursing administrators were extending their support and expectations for research-based nursing delivery to evidence-based practices. Like other innovations, evidence-based practice had to meet certain criteria for adoption. These criteria constituted what USAID suggests are requisite qualities of an innovation: It is sustainable, has absorptive capacity, and can be transferable. That is, the efforts can be maintained after the initial seed money has been spent; the organization can integrate the materials, concepts, and actions into its existing systems; and the ideas, framework, and practices can be applied in settings other than the test sites. To ensure that evidence-based practice met these criteria, healthcare organizations oriented nurse leaders; hired, retrained, and renamed CNSs as "specialists for evidence-based practice" (Stetler et al., 1998); and developed processes, workgroups, and data collection instruments to implement the innovations.

A NEW MILLENNIUM

The end of the twentieth century came and went. By any measure, the world did not achieve Health for All by the turn of the century. In fact, some would assert, the world's scorecard for health was worse than it had been a decade earlier. One factor that underscored this lagging status was the move of the public debate on health care to center stage, where critics highlighted the high costs of health care and the disappointing health indicators in the United States, despite the vast sums of money invested in U.S. healthcare programs

(15% of the gross national product). Some countries with far less resources managed to achieve far better scores than the United States on the major indicators of a community's and nation's health status—specifically, mortality rates for neonates, infants, and children younger than age 5 years.

In the meantime, insurers, drug companies, health maintenance organizations, physician groups, and individual practices had undergone major changes. Physician groups specialized in "product lines" that brought them superior incomes, insurance companies insured the healthy, and abandoned consumers fled to the Internet for information, consolation, and support groups of like-minded folks who shared their illnesses and discussed topics that patients would otherwise be discussing with their healthcare providers.

Consumers were becoming sophisticated in the ways of their bodies and minds. They debated the opportunities and risks of over-the-counter medications, Canadian drug prices, and the interaction effects of herbs and food supplements on longevity. Huge patient samples in longitudinal investigations yielded data in mega-research studies where data were crunched by laptop computers the size of telephones. The Human Genome Project erupted onto interconnected computer systems, and Dolly, the world's first cloned sheep, died.

Thus, while remarkable advances occurred, political and other forces continued to blind the world to obvious issues that had profound effects on populations. The AIDS epidemic had eliminated entire populations in Africa, while thousands of people with AIDS in the United States did not succumb to the disease after all. A quarter of a century after Case #1 was identified, AIDS emerged as a chronic illness, and persons with the disease with it lived to fight another day—just as had the survivors of cancer, the trisomies, and many other illnesses that a century ago would have spelled almost immediate death. Paradoxically, the illnesses that were once thought to be conquered made their way back into public consciousness. As noted earlier, tuberculosis and other bacterial, viral, and infectious diseases returned with a vengeance, along with the emotional conditions exacerbated by family and community violence and the ever-impending threat of terrorism.

These remarkable events had affected every part of people's lives. They focused attention on the brevity of life, the vulnerability of entire nations, and the staggering, domino effects of catastrophic events on a region's physical, social, financial, and community structures. While the creativity, energy, and intelligence of so many had clearly brought about mind-boggling changes to everyday lives, the seductive notion persisted that researchers might eventually find silver bullets for what were, in earlier times, formidable challenges for even the bravest of hearts.

While conceptual models, theories, methods, data collection instruments, Web sites, and Call-a-Nurse services were more readily available than ever, more nurses were asked to find answers to their practice questions in highly specialized databases that extend to near infinity through the World Wide Web. These same nurses (mostly women) were working 12-hour shifts, supported by an army of traveling nurses, and absorbing the ever-present threats of litigation as clinical areas became increasingly unsafe and dangerous.

Nurses in this new century were tempted with generous sign-on bonuses. On the education front, baccalaureate graduates were asked to teach undergraduate students who, only a year before, had been their college chums. What ordinarily was perceived as a fairly long career path was now considered a novice-to-expert trajectory that could be taught in a fraction of the time required for most mortal nurses.

Almost a decade into the new millennium, the way nurses seek evidence continues to work at cross-purposes with the ways in which care is conceptualized and practiced. For example, Eisenberg asserts that "the brain is no longer conceptualized as a hardwired telephone switchboard (with a ghost in the machine for its operator)" (2005, p. 46). A practitioner at Harvard Medical School, he notes that while genomic specifications shape the central nervous system, "experience molds the brain in a process that continues throughout life and is reflected in measurable changes in brain function" (p. 46). Eisenberg also suggests that talking with a person can change brain metabolism. That is, when a client undergoes psychotherapy, not only are the symptoms of his or her condition (for example, obsessive-compulsive disorder) reduced, but changes also occur in the individual's glucose metabolic rate.

These relationships are not conjectural. Indeed, brain imaging has revealed linkages between mind and brain not imagined a decade ago (Eisenberg, 2005, p. 46). These findings once again underscore the linkages between the individual, his or her context, the kinds of interpersonal interactions that person experiences, and the changes that occur in other parts of the body and personality. These experiences can result in distortion from the self-constructed personal narratives people tell themselves. As a consequence, a major focus of therapy is defined as "helping patients to reconstruct their autobiographies in such a way as to foster growth rather than to impair it" (Eisenberg, 2005, p. 51). As Eisenberg notes, today people receive interventions through brief visits, during which they focus no longer on irrelevant topics such as syndromes and disease, but rather on individual and family dynamics (p. 49). So much for a neat, precise DRG designation.

This reframing of care and the sophistication of computers and the dazzling array of techniques available to researchers require quite the opposite sort of context, thinking frame, and clinical focus. The decision-making exercise involved in developing an internally coherent piece of research is, indeed, painstakingly slow and simply does not lend itself to a linear process, to generalizations, and to the opportunity for benchmarking. Most importantly, individual and family dynamics tend to constitute local phenomena and cannot be extrapolated to other families and populations. In addition, the cultures of inquiry used to investigate these kinds of phenomena are descriptive in nature and are challenging to document in a form suitable for evidence-based approaches. In short, the very evidence needed to inform practice in this fast-paced, high-risk environment of nursing is found in the data derived from this emerging use of a variety of cultures of inquiry.

All of these contemporary issues in this new millennium serve to focus our attention on the nursing practices that can be delivered in the most parsimonious way, yet yield the greatest benefit—not unlike the very characteristics promoted in the Alma Ata Declaration.

Ongoing Tensions

Clearly, the oft-voiced impediments to evidence-based practice are powerful forces. Nevertheless, they pale in comparison to the critical need for practices that are based on sound evidence and can be carried out with fewer and fewer resources. Not surprisingly, the tensions persist between this imperative and the worry that the adoption of evidence-based practice will lead to regimentation (Winch et al., 2002) and government control.

Australian nurse researchers contextualize the concern over evidence-based practice within the framework of Foucault's concept of governmentality (Winch et al., 2002). That is, Foucault views science as a form of social control through discipline and normalization. For nursing, practitioners can now conduct systematic reviews, cull and rank evidence, create practice guidelines, determine which interventions work and which don't, and identify the research that is needed. The government can then determine the programs, types of thought, and actions that seek to guide nurses' conduct (Cochrane, 1989; cited in Winch et al., 2002). Likewise, the interventions that do not lend themselves to scientific evidence are discounted, producing a form of rationing. Proponents of this view suggest that this kind of development might also coincide with a loss of nursing's rich intuitive base. Further, the narrow range of research methods deemed acceptable—including randomized control trials and other empirical methods—would preclude the methodological pluralistic approach seen as prohibitively costly. Most importantly, in the Foucaultian framework, a potential exists to influence nurses politically and personally. To counter this possibility, the Australians invite nurses to reframe and reshape the "truth taxonomies" (Winch et al., p. 160) they cherish, and to sustain their ability to preserve the intuitive experiences that are a central part of nursing practice.

THE WAY FORWARD

The new millennium and the creativity inherent in the nursing field have led to proposals aimed at distinguishing research from evidence-based practice (Reigle et al., 2008). The same forces have also begun to provide the structure, processes, mechanisms, and documentation to promote both streams of development. This creative process is being spurred on by three major imperatives: the genuine concern for the patient, the pressure to ensure competent care, and the need to attract and retain well-prepared nurses. As part of these efforts, each of the challenges raised in the mid- and late-1990s continues to be addressed.

The new era has engendered an emphasis on innovation and an insistence on not doing "what other men [and women] have done" (Foss, 1911). Just a few years from the inception of evidence-based practice, three models of research utilization are now used in nursing: the Conduct and Utilization of Research in Nursing (CURN) Project, the Stetler Model of Research Utilization, and the Iowa Model for Research in Practice (*http://www.enursescribe.com/ebnart .htm*) (Sisk, 2002). Other advances have occurred as well.

Ervin (2002) has established an Organizational Model of Evidence-Based Practice; the physicians who coined the term "evidence-based medicine" have developed a journal with the same moniker. The United Kingdom has seen the birth of a journal with this name (*Evidence-Based Nursing: Linking Research to Practice*), and Sigma Theta Tau has created the *Online Journal of Knowledge Synthesis for Nursing International.*

Centers have been established to promote evidence-based practices; library and information literacy skills have been developed to strengthen the abilities of those interested in following evidence-based approaches to nursing practice (Shorten, Wallace, & Crookes, 2001); and librarians have harnessed their skills to develop a curriculum-integrated model to produce "research connoisseurs" (p. 87). Excellence in evidence-based practice is now a hallmark of nursing practice in the United States, Canada, the United Kingdom, Germany, New Zealand, Germany, and Australia (Sisk, 2002).

The Cochrane Collaboration (Fullerton-Smith, 1995) in England has developed *The Online Journal of Knowledge Synthesis.* Likewise, the Cochrane Library has developed holdings of randomized controlled and clinical trials (French, 2002).

Researchers have developed data collection instruments and protocols to examine the differences between evidence-based nursing and evidence-based medicine. Specifically, two scales are available: the Evidence-Based Nursing Scale (Lavin et al., 2002) and the Contribution to Nursing Scale. Protocol development is ongoing through the Conduct and Utilization of Research in Nursing

(CURN) Project, which is being funded by the Division of Nursing, U.S. Department of Health Education and Welfare, under the auspices of the Michigan Nurses Association.

Grossman and Bautista (2002) delineate approaches to developing evidence-based nursing protocols. Some universities are now offering courses and workshops on both a face-to-face and online basis to train educators in teaching evidence-based clinical practice ("How to Teach Evidence-Based Clinical Practice," 2004). Health Links, an Internet resource the University of Washington (2005), provides an impressive list of resources on the topic, including the following tools and documents: meta-search engines, evidence guidelines, clinical research critiques, case report/series/practice guidelines, evidence-based statistics, research centers' calculators, and literature (*http://healthlinks.washington.edu/ebp*).

EPISTEMOLOGY OF EVIDENCE-BASED PRACTICE

To date, evidence-based practice has followed its own epistemological path. As noted earlier, it has already undergone a process of definition (AHCPR), the aim of which is to distinguish it from other kinds of activities, including research; to harness the methods that best address it; and to facilitate pilot testing. Evidence-based practice is now being applied in a variety of settings. To ensure that this upward trajectory continues, researchers, healthcare providers, librarians, and information technology specialists have established these journals, programs, data collection instruments, protocols, and centers of excellence for evidence-based practice in various parts of the world.

North American researchers have taken the lead in the documentation of research on evidence-based practice, followed by their European counterparts. More than 1000 journal entries have been published on evidence-based practice in Southern Europe, hundreds of articles in Northern and Western Europe, and considerably fewer publications in Eastern Europe. Canada follows Europe in terms of the number of cited publications, with relatively few entries appearing for authors from the Middle East and Africa. A search for "evidence-based medicine," depending on the databases accessed, might list 35,000 studies worldwide. Nursing studies and projects in this area number in the thousands.

Throughout the United Sates, faculties of nursing have embraced projects, research studies, and grants geared toward evidence-based practice, with some schools of nursing emerging as centers of excellence. Here are a few of these sites:

- Northeast: Boston College, Yale University, Seton Hall University, University of Pennsylvania
- West: Arizona State University
- Midwest: University of Wisconsin and Case Western Reserve
- South: University of North Carolina at Chapel Hill and University of Kentucky

An emerging theme among these sources is the notion that evidence-based practice is not only needed for patients and families, but is also essential if healthcare institutions are to attract and retain qualified nurses. This idea has emerged, in part, as a result of the link nurses and their employers see between an institution's embrace of evidence-based practice, nurses' perception of what qualifies as a safe work environment, and the visible evidence of these qualities—namely, achievement of Magnet status (Goode, Krugman, Smith, Diaz, Edmonds, & Mulder, 2005; Turkel, Reidinger, Ferket, & Reno, 2005).

The pathway from Donabedian, to Juran, to the centers of excellence in U.S. universities, to the plethora of research in Europe, represents a trajectory spanning almost a century. During the next decade, men and women will *not* hew to the beaten track and keep the path that others followed. Sam Walter Foss, one would imagine, might be utterly amazed as creative researchers, legislators, policy makers, and practitioners manage the information infrastructure, educational processes, legislation, systems development, leadership, and healing—the very elements that formed the structure of this text and the living evidence that supports research into practice—by turning evidence-based practice into reality.

REFERENCES

Centre for Health Evidence. (2004). *How to teach evidence-based clinical practice.* Retrieved February 17, 2005, from http://www.cche.net/ebcp/info.asp

Cochrane, A. L. (1989). Effectiveness and efficiency: Random reflections on the health service. *Controlled Clinical Trials, 10*(4), 428–433.

Deaton, C. (2001). Outcomes measurement and evidence-based nursing practice. *Journal of Cardiovascular Nursing, 15*(2), 83–86.

Deming, W. E. (2000). *Out of the crisis.* Cambridge, MA: MIT Press.

DiCenso, A., Cullum, N., & Ciliska, D. (1998). Implementing evidence-based nursing: Some misconceptions. *Evidence-Based Nursing, 1,* 38–40. Retrieved February 17, 2005, from http://ebn.bmjjournals.com

Donabedian, A. (1980). *Explorations in quality assessment and monitoring.* Ann Arbor, MI: Health Administration Press.

Donabedian, A. (1988). The quality of care: How can it be defined? *Journal of the American Medical Association, 260*(12), 1743–1748.

Eisenberg, L. (2005). The "ecology" of psychiatry and neurology. In *The convergence of neuroscience, behavioral science, neurology, and psychiatry* (pp. 45–78). New York: The Josiah Macy Junior Foundation.

Ervin, N. E. (2002). Evidence-based nursing practice: Are we there yet? *Journal of the New York State Nurses Association, 33*(2), 11–16.

Evers, G. C. M. (2001). Naming nursing: Evidence-based nursing. *Nursing Diagnosis, 12*(4), 137–142.

Farrell, M. (Ed.). (1987a). *People's needs for nursing care: A European study.* Copenhagen, Denmark: WHO.

Farrell, M. (Ed.). (1987b). *Nursing care: Summary of a European study.* Copenhagen, Denmark: WHO.

Foss, S. W. (1911). *The calf-path.* Retrieved May 21, 2005, from http://www.giga-usa.com/gigaweb1/quotes2/qutopprecedentx%20001.htm

French, P. (2002). What is the evidence on evidence-based nursing? An epistemological concern. *Journal of Advanced Nursing, 37*(3), 250–257.

Fullerton-Smith, I. (1995). How members of the Cochrane Collaboration prepare and maintain systematic reviews of the effects of health care. *Evidence-Based Medicine, 1*, 7–8.

Funk, S. G., Champagne, M. T., Tornquist, E. M., & Wiese, R. A. (1995). Administrators' views on barriers to research utilization. *Applied Nursing Research, 8*(1), 44–49.

George, V. (1999). *An organizational case study of shared leadership development in nursing.* Unpublished doctoral dissertation, Marquette University, Milwaukee, WI.

Goldratt, E. M., & Fox, R. E. (1986). *The race.* Croton-on-Hudson, NY: North Rivers Press.

Goode, C. J., Krugman, M. E., Smith, K., Diaz, J., Edmonds, S., & Mulder, J. (2005). The pull of magnetism: A look at the standards and the experience of a western academic medical center hospital in achieving and sustaining Magnet status. *Journal of Nursing Administration, 29*(3), 202–213.

Grossman, S., & Bautista, C. (2002). Collaboration yields cost-effective, evidence-based nursing protocols. *Orthopaedic Nursing, 21*(3), 30–36.

Juran, J. M. (1989). *Juran on leadership for quality: An executive handbook.* New York: Free Press.

Juran, J. M. (1992). *Juran on quality by design.* New York: Free Press.

Lavin, M. A., Meyer, G., Krieger, M., McNary, P., Mals, R. N., Carlson, J., et al. (2002). Essential differences between evidence-based nursing and evidence-based medicine. *International Journal of Nursing Terminologies and Classifications, 12*(3), 101–106.

McCaughan, D., Thompson, C., Cullum, N., Sheldon, T. A., & Thompson, D. R. (2002). Acute care nurses' perceptions of barriers to using research information in clinical decision-making. *Journal of Advanced Nursing, 39*(1), 46–60.

McSherry, R., Simmons, M., & Abbott, P. (2002). *Evidence-informed nursing: A guide for clinical nurses.* London: Routledge.

Mitchell, G. J. (1997). Questioning evidence-based practice for nursing. *Nursing Science Quarterly, 10*(4), 154–155.

Nagy, S., Lumby, J., McKinley, S., & Macfarlane, C. (2001). Nurses' beliefs about the conditions that hinder or support evidence-based nursing. *International Journal of Nursing Practice, 7*(5), 314–321.

Parker, J. (2002). Evidence based nursing: A defence. *Nursing Inquiry, 9*(3), 139–140.

Pirsig, R. M. (1991). *Lila: An inquiry into morals.* New York: Bantam Books.

Prescott, P. (1993). Nursing: An important component of hospital survival under a reformed health care system. *Nursing Economic$, 11*(4), 192–199.

Primary health care. (1978). (Alma Ata, 1978). *Health for All Series No. 1.* Geneva, Switzerland: WHO.

Reigle, B. S., Stevens, K. R., Belcher, J. V., Huth, M. M., McGuire, E., Mals, D., et al. (2008). Evidence-based practice and the road to Magnet status. *Journal of Nursing Administration, 38*(2), 97–102.

Shilts, R. (1987). *And the band played on.* New York: Bedford/St. Martin's Press.

Shorten, A., Wallace, M. S., & Crookes, P. A. (2001). Developing information literacy: A key to evidence-based nursing. *International Nursing Review, 48*(2), 86–92.

Sisk, B. (2002). *Evidence-based nursing.* Retrieved February 17, 2005, from http://www.enursescribe.com/ebnart.htm

Stetler, C. B., Brunell, M., Giuliano, K. K., Morsi, D., Prince, L., & Newell-Stokes, V. (1998). Evidence-based practice and the role of nursing leadership. *Journal of Nursing Administration, 28*(7/8), 45–53.

Targets for HFA. (1991). Copenhagen, Denmark: WHO.

Thompson, C., McCaughan, D., Thompson, C., Cullum, N., Sheldon, T. A., & Thompson, D. R. (2002). Research information in nurses' clinical decision-making: What is useful? *Journal of Advanced Nursing, 36*(3), 376–388.

Turkel, M. C., Reidinger, G., Ferket, K., & Reno, K. (2005). An essential component of the magnet journey: Fostering an environment for evidence-based practice and nursing research. *Nursing Administration Quarterly, 29*(3), 254–262.

University of Washington. (n.d.). Evidence-based practice: Health links. Retrieved February 17, 2005, from http://healthlinks.washington.edu/ebp

Wallin, L., Bostrom, A. M., Wikblad, K., & Ewald, U. (2003). Sustainability in changing clinical practice promotes evidence-based nursing care. *Journal of Advanced Nursing, 41*(5), 509–518.

Winch, S., Creedy, D., & Chaboyer, W. (2002). Governing nursing conduct: The rise of evidence-based practice. *Nursing Inquiry, 9*(3), 156–161.

World Health Organization (WHO). (1980). *International classification of impairments, disabilities, and handicaps.* Geneva, Switzerland: Author.

CHAPTER 6

The Journey to Evidence: Using Technology to Support Evidence-Based Practice

Robert C. Geibert

The diffusion of technology into every aspect of the healthcare system and the realization of the powers of the Internet are perhaps the most significant factors that have supported the integration of evidence-based practice (EBP) into the provision of patient care. With 24/7 access to clinical data, clinicians can search for information from a growing number of online resources sponsored by organizations worldwide and incorporate findings into their clinical decision-making process. The availability of electronic networks provides access to data at the point of care, whether that location is the clinic exam room, the hospital bedside, or a patient's home. It is no longer necessary to visit a medical library during its limited hours of operation to find answers to clinical questions. This chapter discusses how the integration of technology and enhanced access to data can support EBP and improve patient care.

THE EXPANDING ROLE OF TECHNOLOGY

Healthcare practitioners are not the only beneficiaries of this wealth of information. Healthcare consumers—our patients and their families—can also access a significant amount of factual health-related data via the Internet at sites such as those operated by WebMD (*http://www.webmd.com*), the Mayo Clinic (*http://www.mayoclinic.com*), and PubMed (*http://www.ncbi.nlm.nih. gov/pubmed*). PubMed is a service sponsored by the U.S. National Library of Medicine that includes nearly 18 million journal article references from Medline, some of which are available in full-text versions. More than 900 million searches of Medline are performed each year by health professionals, scientists, librarians, and the public (National Library of Medicine, 2008). With this enormous availability of online health-related resources, consumers have an opportunity to be better-informed participants regarding their care.

According to Internet World Stats (2008), in June 2008 an estimated 72.5% of the U.S. population were Internet users, a percentage that equates to more than 220 million users. The Pew Internet Project (Fox, 2008) estimates that 75–80% of Internet users have looked online for health information. A Harris Interactive study (2007) unearthed similar findings, suggesting that 71% of Internet users have searched for health-related information. Harris Interactive refers to these 160 million users as "cyberchondriacs." Its researchers report that, on average, a cyberchondriac searches the Internet nearly six times per month. (See **Table 6-1**.)

Although Harris Interactive uses the label "cyberchondriac" to describe a person who uses the Internet to obtain health or healthcare information, this terminology has a negative connotation and implies that the information seekers are hypochondriacs—that is, persons who imagine that they have a particular disease based on information found on the Internet. Although that definition may apply to some people, the majority of users who seek health-related

**Table 6-1   Trends Related to Cyberchondriacs, 1998–2007[a]
(percentage based on all U.S. adults)**

	1998	1999	2001	2002	2003	2004	2005	2006	2007
All adults who are online[b]	38	46	63	66	67	69	74	77	79
All online adults who have ever looked online for health information	71	74	75	80	78	74	72	80	84
All adults who have ever looked online for health information	27	34	47	53	52	51	53	61	71
All adults who have looked online for health information in the last month	NA	NA	27	32	NA	31	45	51	53
All adults who have ever looked online for health information[c] (millions)	54	69	97	110	109	111	117	136	160

[a] No data available for the year 2000.
[b] Includes those who looked online from home, an office, a school, a library, or another location.
[c] Based on the July 2006 U.S. Census estimate, released January 2007 (225,700,000 total U.S. adults aged 18 or older).
NA = not asked.
Source: Used with permission. The Harris Poll®, #76, July 31, 2007, "Harris Poll shows number of cyberchondriacs—adults who have ever gone online for health information—increases to an estimated 160 million nationwide." Harris Interactive, Inc. All rights reserved.

information on the Internet are likely able to use the information in a positive way. Perhaps another, more positive term would be appropriate.

In the Harris Interactive poll, 86% of the cyberchondriacs found the online information to be reliable, 26% very reliable, and 60% somewhat reliable. Approximately 58% of the adult users who were surveyed had discussed their findings with their physician at least once in the last year. In addition, 55% of cyberchondriacs had searched the Internet for health information based on discussions with their physicians (Harris Interactive, 2007).

It is unfortunate that the Harris Interactive study did not identify users by age, race, gender, or socioeconomic level. However, a Pew Internet Project survey (Fox, 2008) found that Internet users who were living with a disability or chronic disease were more likely than other Internet users to search widely and report significant impacts. The researchers discovered that 75% of e-patients (their term) with a chronic condition reported that their last health search affected their decisions about treatment. This percentage far outstrips the 55% of other e-patients who reported treatment decisions based on Internet-discovered information. The Internet Project also found that newly diagnosed e-patients and those who had experienced a health crisis in the past year accounted for 59% of users who asked their doctor new questions or got a second opinion. By comparison, 48% who did not have a recent diagnosis or health crisis reported this behavior.

In summary, the number of Internet users who seek health-related information online is growing rapidly. The results of these searches have encouraged many users to enter into dialogue with their physicians in decision making related to their care. The use of technology is clearly providing useful tools that enable patients to become more fully involved in their health care. Nurses are in a unique position to assist patients and their families in accessing both useful and reliable online health information as a part of the patients' and families' self-care strategies.

THE DECADE OF HEALTH INFORMATION TECHNOLOGY

As our healthcare system continues to advance, technology will play an ever-increasing role in its expansion; however, as many have noted, funding remains a major hindrance to providing care for all. Tommy Thompson, former U.S. Health and Human Services Secretary, speaking at the July 2004 Secretarial Summit on Health Information Technology, stated, "[O]ur healthcare system needs all the help it can get, and health information technology is the best medicine we can get" (Beck, 2004). A report entitled *The Decade of Health Information Technology: Delivering Consumer-centric and Information-Rich Health Care* was released at the summit. This report was prepared by David J. Brailer (2004), who was the first National Coordinator for Health Information Technology; it laid out the broad steps needed to achieve always-current, always-available, electronic health records for Americans. The report provides a vision for consumer-centric and information-rich care, which includes the following features:

- Medical information will follow the consumer.
- Information tools will guide medical decisions.
- Clinicians will have appropriate access to a patient's complete treatment history, medical records, medication history, and laboratory and radiographic results.
- Computerized medication orders will eliminate handwriting errors, automatically check for doses that are too high or too low, check for harmful drug–drug interactions, and check for allergies.
- Prescriptions will be checked against a health plan's formulary, and out-of-pocket costs will be compared with alternative treatments.
- Electronic alerts will remind clinicians about treatment procedures and medical guidelines (Brailer, 2004).

Taking an even broader perspective is the American Health Information Community (AHIC Successor, Inc.), which is an independent, nonprofit, public–private enterprise whose role is to bring together the best public, nonprofit, and private sectors for the creation and use of a secure interoperable nationwide health information system. This group posits that the broad use of health-oriented IT will improve healthcare quality, safety, and efficiency by enabling the secure exchange of information. It will also enable improvements at the point of care and in public health, and provide an opportunity for researchers to more efficiently collect and analyze data to improve quality and affordability of care (AHIC Successor, 2008).

Electronic systems that incorporate these features are available now and are already being implemented in organizations around the world. It is clear that technology is an important tool that supports clinicians and consumers in making sound, evidence-based healthcare decisions.

THE ELECTRONIC HEALTH RECORD

The electronic health record (EHR) is known by many names: computer-based patient record, electronic medical record, and automated medical record. EHR is used here because it is consistent with the U.S. Department of Health and Human Services' terminology in reference to its Framework for Strategic Action. In addition, "EHR is believed to represent the most comprehensive vision of an information system that would support all types of caregivers, in all settings, including the individual who may be using it to record personal health status information" (Amatayakul, 2007, p. 9).

Amatayakul (2007) identifies three key criteria for an EHR as presented by the Computer-based Patient Record Institute (CPRI), an early advocacy group. An EHR should (1) integrate data from multiple sources, (2) capture data at the point of care, and (3) support caregiver decision making.

EHR Advantages

Many factors affect the integration of technology into healthcare environments. According to Brailer and Terasawa (2003, p. 18), factors that increase adoption fall into two categories: administrative and clinical. Major *administrative* drivers (and the percentage of respondents in Brailer and Terasawa's study who identified them as such) include the following issues:

- Need to share comparable patient data among different sites within a multi-entity healthcare delivery system (75.7%)
- Need to improve clinical documentation to support appropriate billing service levels (75.3%)
- Requirement to contain or reduce healthcare delivery costs (66.3%)
- Need to establish a more efficient and effective information infrastructure as a competitive advantage (64.3%)
- Need to meet the requirements of legal, regulatory, or accreditation standards (60.4%)
- Need to manage capitation contracts (21.8%)

Major *clinical* factors that drive EHR adoptions include the following issues:

- Need to improve the ability to share patient record information among healthcare practitioners and professionals within the enterprise (90%)
- Need to improve the quality of care (85.3%)
- Need to improve clinical processes or workflow efficiency (83.8%)
- Need to improve clinical data capture (82.6%)
- Need to reduce medical errors—that is, increase patient safety (81.9%)
- Provision of access to patient records at remote locations (70.9%)
- Facilitation of clinical decision support (70.4%)
- Need to improve employee/physician satisfaction (62.8%)
- Need to improve patient satisfaction (60.2%)
- Need to improve efficiency via pre-visit health assessments and post-visit patient education (39.9%)
- Support for and integration of patient healthcare information from Web-based personal health records (30.3%)
- Retention of health plan membership (8.5%)

A Medical Records Institute survey conducted in 2007 identified the top priorities in three settings: information technology (IT), hospitals, and medical practices. The top priorities for strategic *decisions in IT* were

- The need to improve clinical processes or workflow efficiency by making them more reliable, up-to-date, and efficient
- The need to improve quality of care

Major factors driving EMR adoption in the *hospital setting* were

- Patient safety considerations
- Efficiency and convenience
- Satisfaction of physicians and clinician employees

Major factors driving EMR adoption in the *medical practice* were

- Improved patient documentation
- Efficiency/convenience
- Remote access to patient information (Brailer & Terasawa, 2003)

Consumers are playing an important role in moving the EHR initiative forward by devoting their healthcare spending dollars to organizations that provide 24/7, technology-supported care. Just as they are accustomed to receiving customer-focused recommendations based on their past purchases or profiles from online retailers such as Amazon.com (*http://www.amazon.com*), so consumers are beginning to expect this same type of personalized service from their healthcare providers.

Kaiser Permanente (KP), a leading integrated healthcare system in the United States, reported that as of October 2008 its EHR project (KP Health-Connect) was providing all of its 14,000-plus physicians with electronic access to their patients' medical records in all of KP's 430 medical offices and clinics (Kaiser Permanente, 2008). The number of users is actually considerably higher when other clinicians (e.g., nurse practitioners and registered nurses) are included. The report also noted that Kaiser's 8.7 million members have access to "My Health Manager," whereby they can manage their health online. In 2007, KP members viewed more than 10 million test results and sent more than 3.6 million emails to their physicians. KP is currently implementing KP HealthConnect in its hospitals.

This approach stands in stark contrast to the more familiar visit to the paper-based medical office where, even with an appointment, the chart was not available when the patient arrived. The clinician had to take valuable time to elicit the patient's history, allergies, medications, and other pertinent information, and then needed to make decisions with limited, or perhaps even incorrect, patient- or caregiver-provided information.

Barriers to EHR Adoption

EHRs are technologically complex and very expensive systems to implement. They also require significant changes throughout an organization. Thus many barriers must be overcome during the planning and implementation processes. Lack of funding and resources have frequently been reported as the largest barriers to adoption of EHRs (Brailer & Terasawa, 2003; DesRoches et al., 2008). Other barriers include (1) anticipated difficulties in changing to an electronic system, (2) the inability to find an electronic solution at an affordable cost (Medical Records Institute, 2007), and (3) lack of support by medical staff, as reported by 35.4% of those responding to a Medical Records Institute study (2004).

EHR implementations require an enormous amount of time that far exceeds many—if not most—organizations' expectations. Bria (2006) tells us that the time needed to implement an electronic medical record (EMR) is roughly proportional to the size of the organization. He suggests that implementing an EMR system in a facility with 200 or more beds may take the same order of magnitude of time as it takes to construct a new hospital of that size (p. 779). Even at the end-user level, the amount of time to implement an EHR is challenging. A participant in a study by Terry et al. that examined implementations in primary care practices reported, "The time [for family doctors] has been amazing... Astounding, astonishing, overwhelming" (Terry, et al., 2008, p. 733). This author has personally experienced and observed the severe underestimation of time projections in multiple implementations in which he has participated as well as in many organizations he has observed.

When a 2002 Dorenfest study reported by Brailer and Terasawa (2003) reviewed spending on IT as a percentage of hospitals' budgets, the researchers found that 44% of hospitals spent less than 2% of their budgets on IT, and 93% spent less than 4%. Only 7% of hospitals spent 4% or more of their budgets on IT. Some respondents suggested that a 7% expenditure is the threshold that must be met to accommodate rapid IT adoption in hospitals.

Physician resistance has also been identified as a significant barrier to adoption of EHRs. This resistance is frequently expressed as refusal to use the EHR system after its implementation, and is a common finding in organizations that do not require use of the technology. A study by Ash et al., for example, found that, in more than half of the hospitals that had installed computer-based provider/prescriber order entry (CPOE) systems, only 10% (or less) of their medical staffs used the system (Brailer & Terasawa, 2003, p. 22). Of those hospitals, only 13.7% required use of the system, while 23.7% encouraged it. Use was optional in the remaining facilities.

These figures correlate with this author's experiences in observing organizations that have implemented EHRs. If use of the technology is not made mandatory, and the prior systems (often paper-based) remain available, clinicians will often resort to the familiar. Although it is difficult to deal upfront with physician resistance, administrators must notify end users early on in the process that technology use will be required. This approach provides clinicians with an opportunity to retire early, change organizations, or, most often, acquiesce to the changes. Because EHRs can improve patient care and offer the potential for reducing medication errors, an organization should consider adding language to its medical privilege bylaws that requires providers to use such a system when it is adopted.

Unfortunately, the integration of technology into healthcare systems lags behind the practice in most other industries. According to a HHS Fact Sheet (2004), hospitals' use of EHRs in 2002 was estimated to approach 13%; for physicians' practices, this percentage ranged from 14% to a possible high of 28%. A 2006 report by Jha et al. (2006, p. w496) found that in 2005, approximately 23.9% of physicians used EHRs in the ambulatory setting and only 5% of hospitals used CPOE. According to a report released in June 2008 by the Office of the National Coordinator for Health Information Technology, physician adoption of health IT has risen slowly from 10% in 2004 to 14% in 2007 (ONC-Coordinated Federal Health, 2008). The variance in statistics is likely due to the lack of a standard regarding the meaning of "EHR adoption." In addition, many studies on EHRs have included only a small number of respondents.

To provide a more precise estimate of adoption rates, the Office of the National Coordinator for Health Information Technology of the Department of Health and Human Services supported a survey by DesRoches et al. (2008) that was based on a clearly identified definition of an EHR. The group defined a "fully functional" EHR as one that would contain four domains: (1) recording the patient's clinical and demographic data, (2) viewing and managing results of laboratory tests and imaging, (3) managing order entry (including electronic prescriptions), and (4) supporting clinical decisions (including warnings about drug interactions or contraindications) (p. 51). These authors further described a "basic" EHR system as one that does not include certain order entry capabilities and clinical decision support—a constraint intended to clarify the extent of EHR adoption within an organization.

DesRoches et al.'s survey, which was conducted in 2007 and early 2008, found that 4% of physicians had adopted a fully functional electronic records system. The availability of basic systems was reported by 13% of respondents. In addition, the researchers found that primary care physicians, and those who practiced in large groups and in hospitals or medical centers, particularly in the western region of the United States, were more likely to use EHRs. Of the 83% of respondents who did not have EHRs at the time of the survey, 16% indicated that their organization had purchased but not yet implemented an EHR system. An additional 26% responded that their practice intended to purchase an EHR within two years.

In his 2004 State of the Union Address, President George W. Bush outlined a plan for (and subsequently issued Executive Order 13335 to enforce) widespread adoption of interoperable EHRs to ensure that most Americans would have electronic health records available at the time and place of care within the next 10 years (Brailer, 2004). To meet this goal, standardization of data structure and data architecture is imperative. Ensuring consistency across systems will enable consumers to have their medical information move seamlessly with them when they change clinicians or geographic locations. Without this interoperable infrastructure, the vision cannot be achieved.

The executive order resulted in a big boost for healthcare IT; however, questions arose concerning the ability of healthcare organizations to meet this goal. Ford, Menachemi, and Phillkips (2006) applied a statistical "Technology Diffusion Model" to project the potential for achieving a universally paperless health system by 2014; their findings suggest that the goal will not be met. Based on their empirical projections, 86.6% of physicians in small practices will be using EHRs in 2024! The period required to achieve this level is twice as long as the initial projection. Keep in mind, however, that a definition of EHR was not described in the Ford et al. study. In addition, at the time of the study, the authors used data that suggested fewer than 18% of physicians used EHRs in their offices (Ford et al., 2006, p. 106).

President Barack Obama is infusing new life into the area of healthcare reform and supports the use of health IT. In January 2009, he called for spending "to ensure that within five years, all of America's medical records are computerized." Obama wants to immediately start spending on health IT as part of his economic recovery plan. He said that health IT "will cut waste, eliminate red tape, and reduce the need to repeat expensive medical tests." He also indicated that "it will save lives by reducing the deadly but preventable medical errors that pervade our healthcare system" (Ferris, 2009). Senator Edward Kennedy, chairman of the Health, Education, Labor and Pensions Committee also supports the advancement of health IT, noting that "Modernizing our healthcare system through better use of information technology is the key to easing the heavy burden of healthcare costs" (Connolly, 2009).

CLINICAL INFORMATION-SEEKING NEEDS

When considering the adoption of an EHR system to improve patient care and clinical decision making, it is prudent to examine the information-seeking needs of clinicians. The literature in this area is limited, albeit informative. Research indicates that internal medicine clinicians need clinical information approximately twice for every three patients seen (Covell, Uman, & Manning, 1985). A 1995 study by Gorman (reported by D'Alessandro, Kreiter, and Peterson, 2004) found that rates of information needs varied from 0.013 to 5.044 questions per patient encounter.

Information resources at the point of care have a positive impact on clinical decision making. For example, drug–allergy or drug–drug interactions can be avoided when prescribing medications. Unfortunately, numerous obstacles to accessing information exist, and the lack of time is one of the most commonly encountered (D'Alessandro et al., 2004; Ely, Osheroff, Ebell, Chambliss, Vinson, & Stevermer, 2002; Jerome, Giuse, Rosenbloom, & Arbogast, 2008). Other obstacles include a lack of knowledge about appropriate answer sources and a reliance on convenient information sources, even when more appropriate resources were available (Osheroff, Forsythe, Buchanan, Bankowitz, Blumenfeld, & Miller, 1991). It is not surprising that answers are difficult to find, because the amount of clinical information that is available has exploded in recent years. For example, the National Library of Medicine added more than 670,000 completed references to its Medline database in 2007, or 2000–4000 new references each working day (National Library of Medicine, 2008).

In a 2003 systematic review of information-seeking behavior, researchers discovered that the most frequent resource consulted for information by physicians was text sources such as PDRs or journals that were readily available in clinicians' offices. The second most commonly consulted resource was a colleague. Only one study found electronic databases to be the primary resource for healthcare providers (Dawes & Sampson, 2003). In this study, the researchers reported that convenience of access, habit, reliability, high quality, speed of use, and applicability contributed to the likelihood of a successful search. They also discovered that a lack of time to search, the huge amount of material, forgetfulness, the belief that there is likely to be no answer, and the lack of urgency hindered the information-seeking process. Searching for information is clearly time-consuming. A 2007 study by González-González et al. (2007), who observed primary care physicians in Spain, found that the physicians had time to answer only one in five of their questions.

Because of the enormous amount of new information that is generated and made available each day, it is increasingly difficult for healthcare providers to remain current. Today's experienced clinician needs nearly 2 million pieces of information to practice medicine (Mark, 2008, p. 16). When identifying a gap in knowledge, clinicians must decide whether to do the best they can with their current knowledge or whether to expand their knowledge base by formulating and answering a question. The applicability of this finding is not limited to healthcare environments, of course. Any worker in an occupation that depends on on-demand information to perform his or her work duties experiences similar challenges. Rae and O'Driscoll (2004) refer to information availability as "proximity," and to the likelihood that what is provided will meet the needs of the information seeker as "relevancy." Providing clinical decision support systems (CDSSs) that are easily accessible and reliable is a strong contributing factor that may encourage clinicians to seek information to unanswered questions, rather than relying on their current knowledge.

As clinicians become accustomed to searching for and displaying data with the press of a few keys, it is unlikely that they will want to return to the often-tedious task of shuffling papers or searching through charts to find individual pieces of data.

CLINICAL DECISION SUPPORT SYSTEMS

Research has shown that physicians incorporate the latest medical evidence into their treatment decisions approximately 50% of the time (McGlynn et al., 2003). In a busy work environment, doing the best one can is often the only practical approach, even though this strategy can have enormous ethical, practice, and economic consequences. The following scenario described by Walker and Tingley (2004, p. 68) may explain why the incorporation of evidence into practice is so difficult.

> A 52 year-old woman with diabetes and a history of heart attack two years ago comes to her doctor's office. The patient reports that she would like a routine check-up, but also notes a week of ankle pain. In the 15 to 20 minutes the physician has to spend with this patient, the physician must consider many questions: Has the patient had a recent Pap test, mammogram, and colorectal cancer screening? When was her latest hemoglobin A1c test, and what was the result? Is it flu season and, if so, does the patient need vaccination? Does the practice have any more doses of vaccine available? What is the patient's pneumococcal vaccine status? Has she had eye and foot exams within the last year? What is the patient's cholesterol status and blood pressure control? What are appropriate targets for this patient and her actual risk if she doesn't meet them? Is the patient taking appropriate medicines to protect her heart and kidneys? Has she had her urine checked for protein in the last year? Has she had any symptoms of low blood sugar? What is her risk of having osteoporosis? Is she taking calcium and vitamin D in appropriate doses to prevent it? Has she been tested? Has she had any recent symptoms that might indicate worsening heart disease? Oh, and by the way, what's causing that ankle pain?

Fortunately, when the systems are programmed properly, and when clinicians have adequate training in their use, CDSSs can provide valuable assistance and guidance for the clinician. When the systems are programmed properly, and when clinicians have adequate training in their use, CDSSs can provide valuable assistance and guidance for the clinician. Clinical decision support systems provide clinicians with health knowledge at the point of care, which may be used to enhance patient care and safety. Wyatt and Spiegelhalter further define medical decision-aids as "active knowledge systems which use two or more items of patient data to generate case-specific advice" (p. 3). With this definition in mind, the viewing of laboratory results or a patient's current medication history is not considered decision support.

Although EHRs can capture, transform, display, and analyze some data, they may not filter and abstract information to the extent needed for complex decision making. By comparison, CDSSs take this process one step further. As detailed individual patient data are entered into a computer program, they are sorted and matched to programs or algorithms in a computerized knowledge base, resulting in the generation of patient-specific assessments or recommendations for clinicians (Randolph, Haynes, Wyatt, Cook, & Guyan, 2001). Denekamp (2007) offers a schematic representation of the components of a typical CDSS. (See **Figure 6-1**.)

In their literature review, Bryan and Boren (2008) noted that the most commonly identified components of a CDSS are (1) an automated process for delivery of alerts or reminders, (2) patient-specific content resulting from the comparison of patient information against a set of knowledge "rules" or guidelines, and (3) delivery of alerts or reminders at the point of care. Pryor (1990) defined six major generic uses of clinical decision support: (1) alerting, (2) interpretation, (3) assisting, (4) critiquing, (5) diagnosing, and (6) managing. **Table 6-2** provides examples of each of these applications.

Figure 6-1   Schematic representation of the components of a typical CDSS.

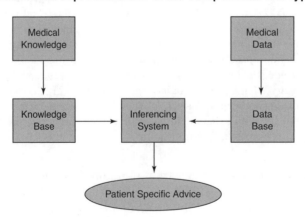

Source: Used with permission. Denekamp, 2007, p. 772.

Table 6-2   Clinical Decision Support Systems (CDSS) Components

Alerting	Notification of a critical laboratory value
Interpretation	A computerized EKG interpretation
Assisting	System calculation of a pediatric weight-based medication order
Critiquing	System reviews a clinician's orders for an asthma patient, compares it to guidelines, and provides recommendations
Diagnosing	System provides a list of potential diagnoses based on clinical symptoms, laboratory values, and other patient data as compared to medical literature
Managing	Automatic creation of nursing care plans

VALUE OF CLINICAL DECISION SUPPORT SYSTEMS

In 2004, after reviewing 37 million patient records, HealthGrades (an independent healthcare rating company) reported that an average of 195,000 people in the United States died as a result of potentially preventable, in-hospital medical errors in each of the years 2000, 2001, and 2002 (HealthGrades, 2004). The study found nearly double the number of deaths from medical errors as documented by the Institute of Medicine in its 1999 well-known and much publicized *To Err Is Human: Building a Safer Health System* report. According to Dr. Samatha Collier, HealthGrades' Vice President of Medical Affairs, "[T]he equivalent of 390 jumbo jets full of people are dying each year due to likely preventable, in-hospital medical errors, making this one of the leading killers in the United States" (HealthGrades, 2004). Both the HealthGrades and Institute of Medicine reports resulted in significant press coverage and public alarm. Unfortunately, the public's interest and level of distress soon subsided.

Another Institute of Medicine report, *Crossing the Quality Chasm: A New Health System for the 21st Century* (Institute of Medicine, 2001, p. 1), tells us that with the growing complexity of health care today, there is "more to know, more to do, more to manage, more to watch, and more people involved than ever before." A growing field of evidence supports the use of health information technology to enhance patient safety, quality, and continuity of care. The contribution that CDSSs make to better outcomes is being studied. Because so much variation exists in terms of which CDSS capabilities are available and how the systems are used (primarily in ambulatory settings), studying this topic is difficult and drawing statistically significant conclusions is challenging.

Bryan and Boren (2008) reviewed the literature regarding the use and effectiveness of electronic clinical decision support tools in the ambulatory/primary care setting. They examined data published from 2000 to 2006 and gathered via either nonrandomized observational or randomized controlled trials that used CDSSs in a single intervention, took place in a primary care ambulatory setting, and included quantifiable outcome measures. These authors validated the idea that CDSSs have the potential to produce statistically significant improvements in outcomes; at the same time, they noted the extensive variability among the types and methods of CDSS implementations and their effectiveness. The reviewers discovered that CDSSs are used for a variety of purposes: (1) prevention/screening, (2) drug dosing, (3) medical management of acute diagnoses, and (4) chronic disease management. The most common use of a CDSS was for chronic disease management. Bryan and Boren noted that these findings stand in contrast to the results of studies published prior to 2000, which found that CDSSs were most often used for prevention/screening and drug dosing.

Garg et al. (2005), in their review of 100 studies, found that CDSSs improved practitioner performance in 62 out of 97 studies, and that 7 out of 52 trials reported improved patient outcomes with use of such systems. They noted that improved practitioner performance was enhanced when prompts were automatic, as compared to when prompts required users to activate the system. Kawamoto, Houlihan, Balas, and Lobach (2005) found that CDSSs significantly improved clinical practice in 68% of trials. Their analysis identified four features that were independent predictors of improved clinical practice: (1) automatic provision of decision support as part of clinician workflow, (2) provision of recommendations rather than just assessments, (3) provision of decision support at the time and location of decision making, and (4) computer-based decision support.

Balas and colleagues (2000) reviewed and performed statistical analyses of 33 studies that took place between 1966 and 1996. They examined the result of performance prompts for physicians at the time of care and found that they were an effective method in improving preventive care. These authors suggest that healthcare organizations could use prompts, alerts, or reminders to provide information to clinicians when patient care decisions are made.

A common finding in all documented reviews is that more research is necessary and an important topic for study is the impact that CDSS usage has on patient outcomes. Nevertheless, a CDSS is clearly an important tool for supporting clinician decision making. It is not designed to replace the clinician, however. As David Eddy has stated, "The complexity of modern medicine exceeds the inherent limitations of an unaided human mind" (Scherger, 2006). As the availability of clinical information continues to grow exponentially, clinicians will most likely come to appreciate the power of a CDSS and fully integrate it into their everyday practice. In fact, they will soon become lost without it.

TECHNOLOGY SUPPORTS EVIDENCE-BASED PRACTICE

Evidence-based medicine (EBM) entails the conscientious use of current best evidence in making decisions about patient care. David Sackett, an early pioneer of EBM, states, "[T]he practice of evidence-based medicine means integrating individual clinical expertise with the best available external clinical evidence from systematic research (Sackett, Rosenberg, Gray, Haynes, & Richardson, 1996, p. 312). Barnsteiner and Prevost (2002), as reported by Melnyk and Fineout-Overholt (2005), suggest that EBP takes into consideration the expertise of the practitioner as well as patient preferences and values.

Interest in EBM is growing. Wells (2007) reported that a PubMed search in October 2006 using the keywords "evidence-based medicine" yielded 22,965 citations. This author performed the same PubMed search in January 2009 and turned up 51,879 citations; a search for "evidence-based practice" yielded 43,318 citations; and a search for "evidence-based nursing yielded 8,247 results. A January 2009 Google search for "evidence-based medicine" yielded 3,990,000 hits and a Google search for "evidence-based nursing" resulted in 2,060,000 items.

It takes a significant amount of time for proven medical advances to be incorporated into common practice. Liang (2007) posits that adoption of EHRs should drastically reduce the length of time it takes a new evidence-based practice to become daily practice. She further suggests that new practices and evidence might be in the hands of clinicians within hours, instead of taking years to make their way into practice. Liang also notes that decision support tools such as patient safety alerts or practice guidelines that are automatically triggered at the point of care could reduce clinicians' burden to learn and apply all the latest evidence, enabling them to focus on critical human factors related to changing behaviors and, ultimately, outcomes of care.

Hurwitz and colleagues, in describing orthopedic surgeons' evidence-seeking behaviors, indicate that it is far easier for a busy surgeon to call a colleague and ask for an expert opinion, or to read a textbook or journal article, than to formulate answerable questions and search the body of orthopedic literature (Hurwitz, Tornetta, & Wright, 2006). Unfortunately, opinion-based practice may not always provide best practice advice. Hurwitz et al. confirm that the amount of surgical literature can be overwhelming and propose that the literature should be systematically reviewed to identify the best evidence. In this regard, they identify practice guidelines as particularly useful tools.

Hurwitz, Tornetta, and Wright make an interesting observation about the final step in evidence-based practice, suggesting it "requires surgeons to adopt better evidence by changing their opinions and, more importantly, their practice, when confronted with good evidence" (Hurwitz et al., 2006, p. 187). How true! However, change for most clinicians is not easy.

Robert Hayward, director of the Centre for Health Evidence, has developed a framework for understanding the process of practicing evidence-based care, which he calls the "Evidence-based Information Cycle." He informs us that the first step is to *assess* clinical or policy problems and to identify key issues. Then, the clinician should *ask* well-built questions that can be answered using evidence-based resources. The next steps are to *acquire* the evidence and *appraise* its validity, importance, and applicability. The final step is to *apply* the evidence. (See **Figure 6-2**.)

Technology is the bridge that will facilitate integrating EBP into patient care. It is the electronic highway that enables information dissemination and access that is neither time nor place dependent. It is a lifeline to the external clinical evidence that Sackett describes.

DEVELOPING THE INFRASTRUCTURE

Infrastructure is defined by the *American Heritage Dictionary* (2001) as "an underlying base, especially for an organization or system." Creating a technologic infrastructure that will support EBP is a challenging undertaking. Infrastructure has three basic components: (1) strategy, (2) people, and (3) architecture. Without considering and planning for each of these components, organizations run the risk of not achieving their desired outcomes.

Figure 6-2   Evidence-based information cycle.

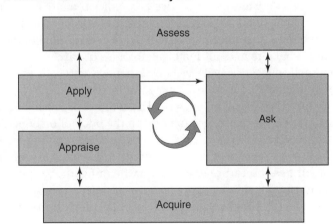

Source: Used with permission. Hayward, n. d.

The healthcare literature offers limited guidance on developing an infrastructure. Although an abundance of resources describe why an integrated, technology-rich healthcare system is needed and identify the challenges that an organization may face when implementing technology-based solutions, few sources provide insight into the systems that must be in place to achieve these goals. Amatayakul, a leading authority on EHR strategies, offers the most comprehensive guidance in her 2007 book, *Electronic Health Records: A Practical Guide for Professionals and Organizations.* She discusses strategic planning, assessments of healthcare process, functional needs, data infrastructure, and IT and systems infrastructure. In addition, she provides guidance in EHR selection, project management, implementation, and maintenance.

Describing each of these activities, including development of the appropriate architecture, is beyond the scope of this chapter; instead, the focus here is on strategy and people components. Based on this author's experience in implementing Web-based instruction and EHRs into organizations, the e-learning literature is a valuable parallel resource. The goals and challenges for both ventures are similar—for example, moving from a paper-based classroom to a technology-based online model.

Strategic Planning

A strategy is a plan of action. Rosenberg (2001) offers a strategic foundation for e-learning that can be applied to creating a strategy that is applicable to EBP. This author indicates how Rosenberg's concepts relate to the EHR.

- **A new approach to e-learning:** in the healthcare environment, online training (the instructional strategy) and knowledge management (the informational strategy), which provides informational databases and performance support tools to support EBP.
- **Learning architecture:** the coordination of e-learning with the rest of the organization's learning efforts. EBP must not be a stand-alone project, but rather must be integrated and coordinated with other initiatives.
- **Infrastructure:** using the organization's technological capabilities to deliver and manage computerized decision support. Rosenberg suggests that the lack of a good infrastructure can stop e-learning in its tracks. Inadequate or ineffective technology capabilities coupled with a weak infrastructure will, without doubt, negatively affect the implementation of EBP.
- **Learning cultures, management ownership, and change management:** the creation of an environment that encourages learning as a valuable business activity. The integration of technology and clinical decision support must be perceived as providing value to the organization, as evidenced by management support.

- **Sound business case:** a case that supports technology-based EBP.
- **Reinventing the training organization:** the adoption of an organizational and business training model that supports EBP.

Hunter-Harvey and Geibert (2003) inform us that it is important to examine the integration of the Web into organizations from a systemic perspective. The same is also true when implementing technologic solutions that support EBP. Notice the focus on people who will be involved in an implementation in the following components:

- **Rationale:** What is the rationale for incorporating technology to support EBP?
- **Skill preparedness:** Does the organization have human resources who are ready to support the transition from a paper-based model to the electronic world?
- **Technology issues:** Is a suitable technology infrastructure present to achieve the organizational goals?
- **Resistance to change:** Are front-line users prepared to make the necessary changes and to accommodate the paradigm shift?
- **User preparedness and user support:** Is appropriate support available for users?
- **Professional development opportunities:** Will users receive adequate training to enable them to effectively achieve desired outcomes?
- **Technology support:** Is 24/7 technology support available? Are the support system personnel conversant with the issues involved with electronic delivery? Do support staff understand the clinical workflow of the users they support?

It is important for organizations to carefully assess each of these components as they relate to developing an infrastructure to support technology-assisted patient care. Lack of attention to, and significant planning for any one of these items will have a negative impact on a successful implementation.

Integrating an EHR system into an organization is frequently identified as a new technology project on which the organization will embark. Although this is a true statement, the more closely the EHR can be linked to the organization's mission, goals, objectives, and other strategic initiatives, the more likely it will be viewed as an integral part of them (Amatayakul, 2004). George (2002) has suggested that one of the biggest risks new initiatives face is the prospect of becoming "collateralized." In other words, the initiative doesn't become "doing business as usual," but rather is seen as a program, or something that is being done with spare time or resources. According to George, failures of previous programs to reach sustainability create a strong paradigm that must be broken.

After observing several failed initiatives, individuals who are scheduled to use the new systems often respond with a weary "Here we go again" or "I wonder what the next one will be?" Changing these attitudes is extremely difficult and adds to the challenge of ensuring a successful implementation.

Planning strategically, and with infinite detail, is critical to achieving success. Amatayakul (2004, p. 93) has discussed a study of chief technology officers that found that 10% did not do strategic planning for technology. Their rationale: Strategic planning was frustrating and time-consuming, and it interfered with their real work of building and maintaining a technology infrastructure. However, the same respondents indicated that good planning did help achieve impressive outcomes and did so with a minimum of frustration.

These respondents are correct: Strategic planning for technology implementations is, indeed, frustrating and time-consuming. This is especially true for EHR implementations, for five reasons:

- They are generally among the largest technology integrations that an organization will ever experience.
- They are implemented in phases over an extended period of time.
- They involve and affect multiple departments and people.
- They require substantial financial investments.
- They require changes in the way business will be done.
- Implementing an EHR system is no simple task. Nevertheless, having a clearly defined strategy and implementation plan that has input from end users will contribute significantly to the chance of achieving a successful outcome.

Knowledge Management

CDSSs incorporate *knowledge management* (KM), which Rosenberg defines as strategies for delivering knowledge in the digital age. KM supports the "creation, archiving, and sharing of valued information, expertise, and insight within and across communities of people and organizations with similar interests and needs" (Rosenberg, 2001, p. 70). Rosenberg suggests that KM can be divided into three levels (depicted as a pyramid in **Figure 6-3**): (1) document management; (2) information creation, sharing, and management; and (3) enterprise intelligence. He also indicates that the KM system becomes more tightly integrated with actual work the higher that one climbs on the pyramid.

The concept of KM can be easily applied to EHR functionality. Basic EHRs are built on three capabilities: access, retrieval, and online storage of documentation. This feature set evolves to a higher level, where information is managed in real time, in more complex systems. Finally, the top of the pyramid is represented by EHRs that provide performance support and are built

Figure 6-3   Knowledge management pyramid.

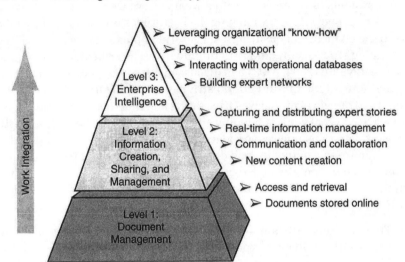

Source: Used with permission. Rosenberg, 2001.

upon expert networks. The next section in this chapter explores levels of EHR functionality.

In level 1, document management involves digitized copies of paper documents, such as signed consent forms. Data available for access and retrieval equate to online laboratory or radiology results.

The second level in the pyramid (information creation, sharing, and management) involves clinicians contributing information to the system, creating new content, and adding to the data contained in the knowledge database. Examples include efforts to document patient encounters, allergies, medications, family and social history, and demographics. Data are easily updated and communicated at level 2.

In level 3, the actual operation of the business depends on the expertise that is embedded in the system. People rely on it in the performance of their jobs, and the resulting experiences are captured and added to the system in a way that increases the collective intelligence of the business. An example might be the collection and mining of data to determine "best practice" interventions in treating certain medical conditions, or providing nursing care.

People

When developing an infrastructure, significant attention must be focused on the people who will be involved. Doncaster and Hunter-Harvey (2003) refer to this task as "peopling" the effort. Implementing EHRs requires a significant investment of human resources that begins many months—if not years—prior to the actual implementation of the system. The need for enhanced levels of human resource will continue throughout—and beyond—the initial implementation as upgrades or additional functionalities are later applied. Leaders must be instrumental in shaping organizational culture and obtaining alignment within the organization to ensure that support is available to sustain technology-based initiatives.

Unfortunately, when implementing technologic solutions, it is the technology—rather than the people—that frequently receives the most attention. Admittedly, the "gee whiz" factor of the systems is difficult to ignore, as vendors and others demonstrate the many features of the products that are to be implemented. In reality, however, it is the people who make or break a successful implementation.

Everett Rogers, an expert in the diffusion of innovations (DOI), tells us that when done properly, the implementation process must allow sufficient time for the organization and its end users to adapt to the innovation, while simultaneously allowing the innovation to adapt to the organization. He identifies five main characteristics of the DOI process: (1) relative advantage, (2) compatibility, (3) complexity, (4) trialability, and (5) observability of the innovation (Rogers, 2003). Each characteristic is described here briefly:

Relative advantage: The end user will inevitably perceive the new innovation in comparison to prior practice. For example, does the innovation provide more speed, efficiency, effectiveness, safety, and defragmentation of care? Even though the innovation may objectively have an advantage, the end user must perceive that the innovation is better.

Compatibility: The end users must determine how the innovation is compatible with their needs, professional norms, and values (e.g., to do no harm). This process will take time.

Complexity: A goal of innovation is to provide a solution that is easy to use and does what an end user thinks it should do. If end users perceive the innovation to be too complex and difficult to learn, an implementation will be adversely affected.

Trialability: End users must have an opportunity to experience what the innovation means to them. If their perceptions are negative, the innovation's relative advantage and compatibility will be affected.

Observability: End users need to see how an innovation will improve patient care, enhance safety and patient satisfaction, and control costs. Peer leaders such as "black belts" may be utilized to demonstrate these advantages and provide a powerful support to end users who are making the transition.

As application end users, clinicians will need a new knowledge base and skill sets to enable them to use EHRs effectively. In many cases, however, advances in technology have rapidly outpaced the capabilities of end users to use them effectively. It is a common perception that, in this technological age, everyone knows how to use computers. Unfortunately, this is not true. Although many clinicians are computer savvy, and newly graduated clinicians enter the work force with technology skills, large numbers of practicing clinicians and other staff members are, at best, technology novices. Some will be familiar only with mainframe systems that use keyboards for data entry and will need to learn how to navigate with a mouse. Others have poor typing skills and cannot enter information at rates either equal to or faster than writing by hand. Still others are "computer phobic," and may even consider retiring early or changing to a work environment where the use of technology to complete everyday tasks may not be as integrated into the workflow. Each of these groups deserves attention to achieve a successful implementation.

A recommended activity prior to an EHR implementation is to survey end users regarding their personal computer (PC) skills. The findings can then be used to determine how many individuals will need PC training prior to the implementation. Although the results may provide valuable information, they may not be adequate to meet the desired objectives. For example, Rick Raker, an EHR trainer at Kaiser Permanente in Honolulu, Hawaii, reported to this author that when surveyed participants entered their EHR training, the trainers noted a discrepancy between actual PC skills and survey results. Some respondents overestimated their PC skills, perhaps because they were embarrassed and didn't want others to know that their computer skills were limited. Other respondents underestimated their skills, because they thought there would be some aspect of PC knowledge they did not possess and, therefore, perceived that they would not be able to perform effectively during the EHR implementation.

Because accurate data were needed to ensure that end users had the requisite PC skills to be successful in the EHR implementation, the Honolulu trainers contacted department managers for input. In most cases, managers were aware of those individuals who were "PC challenged." In addition, the managers could identify those experienced staff members to whom colleagues frequently turned for help when computer-related issues arose during the workday. As this example demonstrates, a combination of a self-reporting survey coupled with department manager validation is highly recommended and may provide more reliable data than simply using a survey alone.

Roles and Responsibilities

Establishing clearly defined roles and responsibilities for everyone involved in a project is critical to any project's success. Although there is great variety among organizations in labeling various roles, the five roles as described by George (2002) in Lean Six Sigma are a good fit with an EHR implementation. George suggests the following structure: (1) chief executive officer (CEO)/ president, (2) business unit managers, (3) line managers, (4) champions, and (5) belts. The same roles may be applied to the EHR implementation, as described next.

CEO/President: This person must decide that adopting the EHR system is of strategic importance to the company. He or she must consistently communicate the strategic priorities to the top-level management staff as well as to the organization as a whole. Monitoring the project's results against the plan and taking corrective action are other duties within this person's realm of responsibility.

Business Unit Managers: These individuals work with the champions to articulate the implementation strategy. They provide input and guidance regarding the EHR functionality that will best support business needs. They also recommend when functionality should be added to the implementation timeline. The business unit managers work with the champions to (1) identify, develop, and support "Black Belts" (George's term for experts) and other resources; (2) create a deployment plan for their unit; (3) solve business problems; and (4) inspire and drive the initiative during the rollout.

Line Managers: Line managers report to the business unit managers and own the processes that will be affected by the implementation of the EHR. They are sometimes referred to as "process owners." Their specific responsibilities include (1) aiding in project selection by contributing their intimate knowledge of the processes; (2) contributing to the selection of Black Belts; (3) creating an environment that will contribute to project success; (4) working with the unit champion and Black Belts to provide data and insight; (5) monitoring project progress; and (6) sustaining the improvements after Black Belts move on to another project.

Champions: Two types of champions are distinguished: company or group champions, and business unit champions. George recommends that company champions should report to the CEO, the chief operating officer (COO), or president. Their roles include (1) leading the design team; (2) helping to develop the strategy; and (3) monitoring the execution of the project. Their primary responsibility is to ensure that the organization executes a consistent and rapid deployment. Business unit champions are responsible for (1) developing the schedule and deployment plans for a unit in conjunction with the unit manager and the implementation team; (2) overseeing the deployment in their business unit; (3) providing communication and ensuring that best practices are shared; (4) ensuring business unit engagement, not compliance; (5) tracking and reporting business unit results to the corporate champion; and (6) providing integration for cross-business unit processes.

The value that champions can bring to an EHR implementation is often overlooked. However, the role is of such importance that Miller and colleagues, in their report entitled "Electronic Medical Records: Lessons from Small Physician Practices," stated, "Identify an EMR champion—or don't implement" (Miller, Sim, & Newman, 2003, p. 7). These authors' advice is equally appropriate to any size implementation. A champion's efforts greatly influence the implementation process, not only in leading the project forward, but also in providing support to those colleagues who may not be so enthusiastic about the implementation. Effective champions—generally physicians—who are valued and respected as leaders, and who are perceived to be "one of us" by their peers, can make especially significant contributions to a successful EHR implementation.

Belts: The final positions that George describes are called "belts." The four levels of belts (Master Black, Black, Green, and White) are thoroughly trained individuals who have a process view of the organization in addition to application expertise. Each belt level has a slightly different responsibility.

- *Master Black Belts:* These individuals provide internal expert consultation to Black Belts and their teams. They must be skilled leaders and expert resources. Master Black Belts provide the conduit to get best practices communicated with unit champions and the rest of the organization. Because most organizations do not have enough employees who possess these skills at the beginning of an EHR venture, it is common to use the experience of external consultants who bring knowledge from prior implementations. Eventually, the consultants will turn over their responsibilities to internal resources.

- *Black Belts:* Black Belts are responsible for delivering project value and benefits. They work with the line manager and unit champions, identify best practices, and act as mentors. They must be extensively trained in the system. Some organizations refer to this role as a "super-user" or "site specialist." In some cases, the super-users may become vendor certified in an application, and they might be part of a training team. Black Belts must be enthusiastic about the implementation and have strong technology skills. It is ideal to identify clinicians and other healthcare providers as super-users because they use the technology in the course of their everyday duties, understand the workflow of a unit, and can act as resources to colleagues.

- *Green Belts:* These individuals are team members who receive significant training and possess knowledge that is important to the project's success. Clinicians and members of the healthcare team who use the EHR on a daily basis fit this role.
- *White Belts:* These individuals have some understanding of the EHR, but may use only pieces of the application in their daily duties. Examples include medical records or laboratory staff, who need to access the EHR for "view only" purposes or to perform minimal data entry.

In summary, numerous roles and responsibilities must be accounted for in planning an EHR implementation. Identifying these roles and assigning team members to them early in the project will greatly enhance the chance of a successful outcome.

Training

Training is often placed near the bottom of an implementation project plan, when it actually deserves a prominent place prior to, during, and long after an EHR implementation. In fact, training never stops: It is not a one-time endeavor. When Amatayakul refers to training, her advice is to "train, train, and train" (Amatayakul, 2004, p. 19).

Unfortunately, training rarely gets the attention that it deserves, for the following reasons:

- **Healthcare training is expensive.** Clinicians are generally among the mostly highly paid members of a healthcare organization and, when they are released from patient care responsibilities to attend training, replacements may have to be hired to cover for them. Clinicians also use a greater proportion of the EHR functionality, so their training times are longer than those for other employee groups. It is common to require 20 or more hours of training during an implementation when integrating a full-featured EHR.
- **The amount of training required to achieve competency is often underestimated.** Vendors frequently advertise their systems as easy to learn—but these claims may not hold up in the classroom. Training entails more than knowing which button to click; it involves retraining to master new ways of performing numerous workflows.
- **Organizations focus their spending on the technology rather than on human resources.** By the time training begins in some organizations, expenditures may already be well beyond anticipated costs, and the training budget is an easy target for cost cutting. Administrators may base the number of hours they will fund based on financial constraints rather than the amount of time it takes clinicians to meet learning objectives.

The organization that skimps on training prior to an implementation will end up paying for that omission in other ways that may not be directly apparent in a training department's budget. If learners are not able to reach competency prior to the system's go-live date, they will generally require reduced schedules and patient loads for longer periods of time, and they will require more intensive, one-on-one, on-site post-implementation support. Although reduced schedules and on-site support are part of any implementation, they are very expensive support methods that, with proper planning and sufficient learner training opportunities, can be significantly reduced.

Technology-Based Training

Classroom-based, instructor-led training is the traditional approach for learning to use EHRs. Classroom instruction, although effective, can often be supplemented and, in some instances, replaced by technology-assisted instruction such as Web-based training (WBT). WBT has significant advantages in comparison to classroom-based training: (Ellis, Wagner, & Longmire, 1999):

- It addresses learning at the individual level.
- It can be designed for use anytime and anywhere.
- It can be designed to be learner driven at a pace that corresponds to an individual's learning style.
- It can be used at the trainee's job site, as time is available.
- It does not require additional physical space.
- It connects learners in diverse locations.
- It enables immediate implementation of the new learning.
- It facilitates seamless connection between training and performance support.

Leading large, multifacility, enterprise-wide WBT initiatives in which clinicians are able to quickly learn basic EHR functionality is possible, but it requires customized training to meet the needs of the various role-based groups. This author led an enterprise-wide WBT project that prepared thousands of learners for an EHR implementation. By using cutting-edge technologies, the course developers were able to assemble course content with such precision that a particular lesson could include, or exclude as needed, content at the task level. Because each task represented approximately 1.5 minutes of content, learners were offered only content that was relevant for their work. The WBT was supplemented by instructor-led training where clinicians could work in a simulated EHR environment, learn more about incorporating the EHR into their daily workflow, and integrate what they had learned. Although it is certainly expensive to develop, WBT should be considered as a training adjunct whenever large numbers of people with varying roles require training.

Learners should have ample opportunities to practice in a simulated EHR environment before working in a "live" system, where the simulation environment exactly parallels the job's workflow. This type of training provides an opportunity for trial-and-error learning, time to experiment with personalizing areas of the system if functionality permits, and development of speed in using the application. It also provides the clinician with an opportunity to see how end-to-end processes are handled in the system. Thus the creation and maintenance of a training environment with realistic-appearing clinical data is a valuable tool in implementing an EHR system.

A combination of online and face-to-face instruction is ideal when seeking to implement a new EHR system. This "blended" approach can enhance the learner experience and engagement, and can positively affect learner outcomes. It is also useful in providing enhanced opportunities to focus on the diffusion of innovation concepts that Rogers outlined.

THE FUTURE

The innovation and development of new technologies, and the diffusion of those technologies into healthcare environments, will most certainly improve the ability of clinicians to utilize CDSSs effectively and efficiently, and to apply the information to enhance a practice that is grounded in evidence. Wireless and mobile technologies such as tablet PCs, personal digital assistants (PDAs), and smart cell phone technologies will enhance both health data access and decision support tools. Patients, too, will increasingly become better informed as a result of the greater access to health-related information provided via the Internet, their online personal health records, and 24/7 communication opportunities with their care providers. With this knowledge, and by working in a partnership, both clinicians and their patients can anticipate better outcomes—one of the main goals for infusing technology into health care.

REFERENCES

AHIC Successor, Inc. (2008). AHIC Successor, Inc. announces board of directors. Retrieved October 14, 2008, from http://www.ahicsuccessor.org/hhs/ahic.nsf/newsroom.htm

Amatayakul, M. (2004). *Electronic health records: A practical guide for professionals and organizations* (2nd ed.). Chicago: American Health Information Management Association.

Amatayakul, M. (2007). *Electronic health records: A practical guide for professionals and organizations* (3rd ed.). Chicago: American Health Information Management Association.

American heritage dictionary. (2001). New York: Dell.

Balas, E. A., Weingarten, S., Garb, C., Blumenthal, D., Boren, S., & Brown, G. D. (2000, February 14). Improving preventive care by prompting physicians. *Archives of Internal Medicine, 160*(3), 301–308.

Barnsteiner, J., & Prevost, S. (2002). How to implement evidence-based practice: Some tried and true pointers. *Reflections on Nursing Leadership, 28*(2), 18–21.

Beck, E. (2004). *Analysis: Meeting the e-record challenge.* Retrieved November 30, 2008, from http://www.accessmylibrary.com/coms2/summary_0286–9040686_ITM

Brailer, D. (2004). *Health IT strategic framework preface.* Retrieved April 18, 2009, from http://www.hhs.gov/healthit/preface.html

Brailer, D., & Terasawa, E. (2003). *Use and adoption of computer-based patient records.* Retrieved April 18, 2009, from http://www.chcf.org/topics/view.cfm?itemID=21525

Bria, W. F. I. (2006). Applied medical informatics for the chest physician: Information you can USE! Part 2. *Chest, 129*(3), 777–782.

Bryan, C., & Boren, S. (2008). The use and effectiveness of electronic clinical decision support tools in the ambulatory/primary care setting: A systematic review of the literature. *Informatics in Primary Care, 16*(2), 79–91.

Connolly, C. (2009). Obama, lawmakers expanding health measures in stimulus plan. *Washington Post.* Retrieved April 18, 2009, from http://www.washingtonpost.com/wp-dyn/content/article/2008/12/12/AR2008121200003.html

Covell, D., Uman, G., & Manning, P. (1985). Information needs in office practice: Are they being met? *Annals of Internal Medicine, 103*(4), 596–599.

D'Alessandro, D. M., Kreiter, C. D., & Peterson, M. W. (2004). An evaluation of information-seeking behaviors of general pediatricians. *Pediatrics, 113*(1), 64–69.

Dawes, M., & Sampson, U. (2003). Knowledge management in clinical practice: A systematic review of information seeking behavior in physicians. *International Journal of Medical Informatics, 71*(1), 9–15.

Denekamp, Y. (2007, November). Clinical decision support systems for addressing information needs of physicians. *Israel Medical Association Journal, 9*(11), 771–776.

DesRoches, C., Campbell, E., Rao, S., Donelan, K., Ferris, T., Jha, A., et al. (2008). Electronic health records in ambulatory care: A national survey of physicians. *New England Journal of Medicine, 359*(1), 50–60.

Doncaster, B., & Hunter-Harvey, S. (2003). A macro-analytic perspective on e-learning: The context. In R. Geibert & S. Hunter-Harvey (Eds.), *Web-wise learning: Wisdom from the field* (pp. 23–46). Philadelphia: XLibris.

Ellis, A. L., Wagner, E. D., & Longmire, W. R. (1999). *Managing Web-based training.* Alexandria, VA: American Society for Training & Development.

Ely, J. W., Osheroff, J. A., Ebell, M. H., Chambliss, M. L., Vinson, D. C., & Stevermer, J. J. (2002). Obstacles to answering doctors' questions about patient care with evidence: Qualitative study. *British Medical Journal, 324*(7339), 710–716.

Ferris, N. (2009). *Obama ups the ante for national health IT.* Retrieved April 18, 2009, from http://govhealthit.com/Articles/2009/01/08/Obama-ups-the-ante-for-national-health-IT.aspx

Ford, E. W., Menachemi, N., & Phillkips, M. (2006). Predicting the adoption of electronic health records by physicians: When will health care be paperless? *Journal of the American Medical Association, 13*(1), 106–112.

Fox, S. (2008, August 26). *The engaged e-patient population* [podcast]. Retrieved April 18, 2009, from http://www.pewinternet.org/~/media/Files/Reports/2008/PIP_Health_Aug08.pdf.pdf

Garg, A. X., Adhikari, N. K., McDonald, H., Rosas-Arellano, M. P., Devereaux, P. J., Beyene, J., et al. (2005). Effects of computerized clinical decision support systems on practitioner performance and patient outcomes: A systematic review. *Journal of the American Medical Association, 293*(10), 1223–1238.

George, M. L. (2002). *Lean Six Sigma: Combining Six Sigma quality with Lean speed.* New York: McGraw-Hill.

González-González, A. I., Dawes, M., Sánchez-Mateos, J., Riesgo-Fuertes, R., Escortell-Mayor, E., Sanz-Cuesta, T., et al. (2007). Information needs and information-seeking behavior of primary care physicians. *Annals of Family Medicine, 5*(4), 345–352

Harris Interactive. (2007). *Harris Poll shows number of "cyberchondriacs"—adults who have ever gone online for health information—increases to an estimated 160 million nationwide.* Retrieved April 18, 2009, from http://www.harrisinteractive.com/harris_poll/index.asp?PID=792

Hayward, R. (n.d.). *Evidence-based information cycle.* Retrieved November 30, 2008, from http://www.cche.net/info.asp

HealthGrades. (2004). *In-hospital deaths from medical errors at 195,000 per year, HealthGrades' study finds.* Retrieved April 18, 2009, from http://www.healthgrades.com/AboutUs/index.cfm?fuseaction=mod&modtype=content&modact=Media_PressRelease_Detail&&press_id=135

HHS fact sheet. (2004). *HHS fact sheet: HIT report at a glance.* Retrieved April 18, 2009, from http://www.hhs.gov/news/press/2004pres/20040721.html

Hunter-Harvey, S., & Geibert, R. (2003). An organizational approach: Web development from a systems perspective. In R. Geibert & S. Hunter-Harvey (Eds.), *Web-wise learning: wisdom from the field* (pp. 19–22). Philadelphia: XLibris.

Hurwitz, S., Tornetta, P., & Wright, J. (2006). An AOA critical issue: How to read the literature to change your practice: An evidence-based medicine approach. *Journal of Bone & Joint Surgery, 88*(8), 1873–1879.

Institute of Medicine (IOM). (1999). *To err is human: Building a safer health system.* Washington, DC: National Academies Press.

Institute of Medicine (IOM). (2001). *Crossing the quality chasm: A new health system for the 21st century.* Washington, DC: National Academies Press.

Internet World Stats. (2008). *Internet usage and population in North America.* Retrieved October 26, 2008, from http://www.internetworldstats.com/stats14.htm

Jerome, R., Giuse, N., Rosenbloom, S. T., & Arbogast, P. (2008). Exploring clinician adoption of a novel evidence request feature in an electronic medical record system. *Journal of the Medical Library Association, 96*(1), 35–41.

Jha, A., Ferris, T., Donelan, K., DesRoches, C., Shields, A., Rosenbaum, S., et al. (2006). How common are electronic health records in the United States? A summary of the evidence. *Health Affairs, 25*(6), 496–507.

Kaiser Permanente (KP). (2008). *Kaiser Permanente has most hospitals in nation with inpatient electronic health records.* Retrieved December 1, 2008, from http://xnet.kp.org/newscenter/pressreleases/nat/nat_081021_inpatienthr.html

Kawamoto, K., Houlihan, C., Balas, E. A., & Lobach, D. (2005, March 14). Improving clinical practice using clinical decision support systems: A systematic review of trials to identify features critical to success. *British Medical Journal, 330*(7494), 765.

Liang, L. (2007). The gap between evidence and practice. *Health Affairs, 26*(2), 119–121.

Mark, D. B. (2008). Decision-making in clinical medicine. In A. S. Fauci, E. Braunwald, D. L. Kasper, S. L. Hauser, D. L. Longo, J. L. Jameson, et al. (Eds.), *Harrison's Principles of Internal Medicine* (17th ed., pp. 16–23). New York: McGraw-Hill.

McGlynn, E., Asch, S., Adams, J., Keesey, J., Hicks, J., DeCristofaro, A., et al. (2003). The quality of health care delivered to adults in the United States. *New England Journal of Medicine, 348*(26), 2635–2645.

Medical Records Institute. (2004). *Medical Records Institute's sixth annual survey of electronic health record trends and usage for 2004.* Retrieved April 18, 2009, from http://www.providersedge.com/ehdocs/ehr_articles/Survey_of_EHR_Trends_and_Usage_for_2004.pdf

Medical Records Institute. (2007). *2007 survey of electronic medical record trends & usage.* Retrieved November 30, 2008, from http://www.medrecinst.com/PressRoom/PressReleases.php?show=16#display.

Melnyk, B., & Fineout-Overholt, E. (2005). *Evidence-based practice in nursing & healthcare: A guide to best practice.* Philadelphia: Lippincott Williams & Wilkins.

Miller, R. H., Sim, L., & Newman, J. (2003). *Electronic medical records: Lessons from small physician practices.* Retrieved April 18, 2009, from http://www.chcf.org/documents/healthit/EMRLessonsSmallPhysicianPractices.pdf

National Library of Medicine. (2008). *Fact sheet: Medline.* Retrieved April 18, 2009, from http://www.nlm.nih.gov/pubs/factsheets/medline.html

ONC-Coordinated Federal Health. (2008). *The ONC-Coordinated Federal Health information technology strategic plan: 2008–2012.* Retrieved April 18, 2009, from http://www.hhs.gov/healthit/resources/HITStrategicPlan.pdf

Osheroff, J. A., Forsythe, D. E., Buchanan, B. G., Bankowitz, R. A., Blumenfeld, B. H., & Miller, R. A. (1991). Physician's information needs: Analysis of questions posed during clinical teaching. *Annals of Internal Medicine, 114*(7), 576–581.

Pryor, A. (1990). Development of decision support systems. *Journal of Clinical Monitoring and Computing, 7*(3), 137–146.

Rae, S., & O'Driscoll, T. (2004). Contextualized learning: Empowering education. *Chief Learning Officer, 3*(8), 18–23.

Randolph, A., Haynes, R. B., Wyatt, J., Cook, D., & Guyan, G. (2001). *How to use an article evaluating the clinical impact of a computer-based clinical decision support system.* Retrieved December 3, 2008, from http://www.cche.net/usersguides/computer.asp

Rogers, E. (2003). *Diffusion of innovations* (5th ed.). New York: Free Press.

Rosenberg, M. J. (2001). *E-learning: Strategies for delivering knowledge in the digital age.* New York: McGraw-Hill.

Sackett, D. L., Rosenberg, W. M., Gray, J. A., Haynes, R. B., & Richardson, W. S. (1996). Evidence based medicine: What it is and what it isn't. *British Medical Journal, 312*(7023), 71–72.

Scherger, J. (2006, June). Electronic health records coming of age. *Patient Care, 40*(6), 48–51.

Terry, A., Thorpe, C., Giles, G., Judith, B., Harris, S. B., Reid, G. J., et al. (2008, May). Implementing electronic health records: Key factors in primary care. *Canadian Family Physician, 54*(5), 730–736.

Walker, J., & Tingley, S. (2004) *Implementing an electronic health record system.* New York: Springer.

Wells, L. (2007). Role of information technology in evidence based medicine: Advantages and limitations. *Internet Journal of Healthcare Administration, 4*(2). Retrieved April 18, 2009, from http://www.ispub.com/journal/the_internet_journal_of_healthcare_administration/volume_4_number_2_20/article/role_of_information_technology_in_evidence_based_medicine_advantages_and_limitations.html

Wyatt, J. & Spiegelhalter, D. (1992). *Field trials of medical decision-aids: Potential problems and solutions,* 3–7. Retrieved June 14, 2009, from http://www.pubmedcentral.nih.gov/picrender.fcgi?artid=2247484&blobtype=pdf

Managing Variance Through an Evidence-Based Framework for Safe and Reliable Health Care

Kathy A. Scott

Health care in the United States depends on good people (from novice to expert) doing the right things (often despite evidence) at the right time (despite numerous interruptions and distractions). While the United States has the capacity to produce the greatest health care in the world, research clearly indicates that the healthcare industry has failed to do so with shocking regularity (Becher & Chassin, 2001). Healthcare errors represent the seventh leading cause of death in this country (Grube, 2001), resulting in 44,000 to 98,000 deaths per year, and costing the nation approximately $376 billion annually [Institute of Medicine (IOM), 1999]. The rate of misdiagnosis of patients experiencing a myocardial infarction in the emergency department is estimated to approach 20,000 to 80,000 cases per million (Merry & Brown, 2002). The estimated cost of non-fatal medical errors ranges from $17 billion to $19 billion each year (Rovner, 2000)—approximately $2500–$3500 per hospital bed/year for medication errors alone (Coile, 2001). Research also indicates that between 2.9% and 3.7% of all hospital admissions result in an injury from mismanagement (Benjamin, 2000), and 5.75% of hospitalized patients experience preventable adverse events (that is, an injury judged to be the result of an error or system design flaw) within two weeks following discharge (Forster, Murff, Peterson, Gandhi, & Bates, 2003).

High-reliability organizations (HROs) are complex systems that have a very different view of the organization and how it works—a view that is far removed from the traditional healthcare paradigm. HRO members collectively understand that uncertainty is irreducible, sources of harm are limitless, and human factors have a significant effect on outcomes. They share a common set of attributes and practices that make them much more safe and reliable than their non-HRO counterparts (Becher & Chassin, 2001; Weick & Sutcliffe, 2001).

This chapter explores and integrates the essence of evidence-based practice—best research, clinical expertise, and patient-focused values—and relates them to a high-reliability framework for managing process and outcome variability for safe patient care. Through strategies derived from an evidence-based, high-reliability framework, leaders are able to make better-informed decisions and effectively manage the organization in ways that decrease errors, promote employee retention, and improve patient outcomes.

RELIABILITY DEFINED

Reliability is the extent to which a system yields the same results on repeated trials. A highly reliable system is one that is error tolerant; it has consistent and positive results. A reliable healthcare system is not a product of everyone's hard work, best efforts, or good intentions. Rather, it is designed to ensure that every patient receives evidence-based and effective care every time, regardless of the time of day, day of the week, and participants' gender, expertise, ethnicity, and socioeconomic status.

Highly reliable practices and organizations are the result of individuals, teams, and systems that together (1) mitigate the effects of harmful variation/error, (2) prevent harm caused by variation/error, and/or (3) prevent the variation/error from happening in the first place. A framework is needed to view organizations in new ways that will help leaders actively prevent and/or manage the risks of active and latent failures at all levels of the organization.

HIGH-RISK AND COMPLEX HEALTHCARE SYSTEMS

Healthcare organizations have two uniquely defining characteristics: high risk and complexity. The more complex the system, the more likely it is that a random mix of events will combine to produce a mishap. Within a larger frame of reference, factors that produce small and subtle effects can have very large consequences. Seven characteristics of complex systems are identified from the literature (presented in **Table 7-1**), which make them highly accident/failure prone regardless of the intent of the leaders or members/actors.

Two complex system characteristics are identified by Perrow (1984), a researcher of accidents in high-risk industries, as being highly accident prone regardless of the intent of their leaders or members:

- *Interactive complexity:* A measure of the way in which parts are connected and interact. According to Perrow, complex interactions are unplanned, unexpected, and unfamiliar sequences that are either not visible or not immediately comprehensible.
- *Tight coupling:* Planned and unplanned interactions that occur quickly when delays in the process are not possible. There is little slack in the system, so precision must be there the first time or not at all.

Table 7-1 Seven Characteristics of Complex Systems That Lead to Breakdown and Failure

- Interactive complexity
- Tight coupling
- Conflicting goals
- Intransparence
- Fluid participation
- Dynamic nature, with complex delays
- Ignorance and mistaken assumptions

Sources: Perrow, 1984; Sagan, 1993; Dörner, 1996.

March, Cohen, and Olsen defined the presence of three general characteristics in complex organizations (Sagan, 1993) that are also reflective of healthcare organizations:

- *Conflicting goals:* There are inconsistent, conflicting, and differing goals at many different levels of the organization.
- *Intransparence:* Many aspects of the organization are not visible or are unclear. Organizational processes and influences are not well understood by the actors, planners, and decision makers, who often do not have direct access to information about the situation they are addressing.
- *Fluid participation:* The organizational participants are coming and going, with some paying attention and some not. Members of the decision-making groups are often uninformed, biased, or even uninterested actors.

Dietrich Dörner (1996), an internationally respected figure in the field of cognitive behavior and human error, identified the three previously mentioned characteristics as well as two additional properties of complex systems that lead to breakdown and failure:

- *Dynamic nature, with complex delays:* The system is always moving and changing on its own, whether the actors take it into account or not. Decisions have to be made before complete information is available, and it is difficult to determine where the whole system is heading over time. Many unrecognized system delays and side effects occur.
- *Ignorance and mistaken assumptions:* The organizational actors rely on and apply their past reality model (implicit and explicit) to situations, whether that model has been effective or ineffective in the past.

Healthcare organizations are at high risk in that error, failure, and breakdown can lead to loss of life or body function. Such organizations exhibit the seven evidence-based characteristics of complex systems. They are opaque, with many subsystems of specialists and services depending on one another for information. These subsystems are often not well understood by planners, leaders, or patient-care providers. In addition, healthcare systems are tightly coupled, requiring rapid decisions during unexpected situations where individuals and groups are unstable, personally threatened, or threatening to others.

Healthcare systems have many parts that are interdependent, in an environment where planned and unplanned interactions occur quickly and have serious consequences. In the operating room, for example, coronary bypass surgery requires the interaction of many team members with a variety of skill levels, communication styles, and abilities; use of high-tech equipment; coordination of processes; and timely precision with no second chances for many actions that affect the surgical procedure and experience. Imagine the immediate outcome of a distracted perfusion technician who forgets to prime the coronary artery tubing with saline prior to starting the case: The result would be a cardiac arrest from an air embolus within seconds. Likewise, even a short delay in the circulating RN's double check of the patient's surgical consent form at the time of surgery could result in the performance of the wrong surgical procedure for a patient due to tight coupling from the time in the operating room to the time of incision.

From a more administrative perspective, leadership decisions such as those related to human resources management, supply contracts and purchases, and productivity benchmarks exert a tremendous influence on organizational reliability and safety. A decision in the boardroom to purchase an inferior infusion pump can result in errors by the end user that are not understood, immediately visible, or comprehensible. Because of the complexity of the system, the decision maker may never have any understanding of his or her contribution to the harm that occurs.

Clinically, ignorance and mistaken hypotheses are evident when traditional medical and clinical practices continue even after research clearly identifies a better way that can improve outcomes. Practitioners are overloaded and desire to practice autonomously, often performing in ways that are most expedient and comfortable for them. Healthcare leaders have been reluctant to standardize care and practice based on the evidence because of political pressures and mistaken assumptions, such as the notion that diagnosis and treatment of disease require very specialized and individualized knowledge and experience.

Conflicting goals, ambiguous preferences, and conflicting interests often coexist in a state of uneasy tension in healthcare organizations. Leaders and other employees frequently take the easier path of generalization and political ease, paying only arbitrary attention to the details of the trade-offs, and hoping for the best. A study (Pronovost, Angus, Dorman, Robinson, Dremsizov, & Young, 2002) of intensive care units (ICUs) demonstrates how such conflicting goals can affect the quality of care delivered by healthcare organizations. When patients were managed or co-managed by physician intensivists, there were associated reductions in hospital mortality (30%) and ICU mortality (40%). These data suggest that more than 160,000 of the deaths that occur in U.S. ICUs annually could be avoided. Even so, it is estimated that only 10% of ICUs in the United States have implemented this type of staffing (Pronovost et al., 2002).

This evidence-based practice has become well known in the healthcare industry through the Leapfrog Group, a consortium of more than 160 companies and organizations (healthcare consumers) with a mission to improve the quality and affordability of health care in the United States. Nevertheless, political and professional interests—such as the desire of physicians to not relinquish any of their patient care privileges, control, or revenue in the ICU setting to the intensivist—are often placed ahead of patients' interests, resulting in higher mortality rates and injuries from errors.

The dual-minded organizational structure in healthcare organizations differs substantially from the structure found in other industries and contributes to the former's complexity. In the healthcare organization, the chief executive officer (CEO) receives delegated authority from the board and is responsible for managing the organization in conjunction with the senior management team. The medical staff constitutes a separate organizational structure that operates parallel to the administrative structure. Members of the medical staff are generally not paid employees of the hospital, yet they play a significant role in its success (Shi & Singh, 2001). Often the administrative and medical groups have different agendas, expectations, goals, and views of situations, as well as numerous competing interests and conflicts. The result is similar to a body with two heads, with each head having a different view of the world. Competing interests, hierarchical views, conflicts, and cultures that promote competition and avoidance are often the result—and represent a recipe for complexity and failure.

Conflicting and differing goals are evident within the nursing world as well, with tension arising from the presence of two competing "goods." Examples include the tension between standardization and individualized care; cost containment and specialized care; and care for the individual and care for the collective. Day-to-day decisions about diverting patients to other hospitals versus holding or admitting them when nurses believe their ability to provide safe patient care may be jeopardized are commonly encountered across the United States and exemplify the tension produced by the existence of two competing goals.

Another characteristic of healthcare organizations is fluid participation. These organizations have multiple member groups, whose voluntary turnover rates typically range from one-fifth to one-fourth of the groups annually, as well as physician-actors who have a separate leadership structure, great independence in their practice, and many conflicts of interest with the healthcare organization in which they provide services. Other contributors to fluid participation include 24/7 work schedules, and unexpected patient care situations that require immediate attention and divert the actors' time and limit their ability to participate in nonpatient care activities.

Through explicit recognition of the seven characteristics present in nonrational, high-risk, and complex healthcare organizations (interactive complexity, tight coupling, conflicting goals, intransparence, fluid participation, dynamic nature and complex delays, and ignorance and mistaken assumptions), new approaches will evolve that encourage a more realistic look at the antecedents and root causes of variance, practice breakdown, and organizational failures. The next section identifies many of the human tendencies when problem solving in complex situations that lead to variance, failures, and breakdown.

LEADERSHIP AND PROBLEM-SOLVING PITFALLS IN COMPLEX SYSTEMS

Dietrich Dörner, a researcher in the field of cognitive psychology, has extensively studied the nature of human thinking when dealing with complex problems. Using computer simulations at the University of Bambuerg, Dörner mapped out the strengths and weaknesses of human cognition when confronted with complex problem-solving environments. He identified "habits of thought that set failure in motion from the beginning" (1987, p. 11). Through the development of simulated complex situations for interactive problem solving that did not require any particular technical expertise, Dörner was able to observe and record the background of planning, decision making, and evaluation processes that were usually hidden. Dörner's research, combined with the findings of several other scholars, revealed six human tendencies when problem solving in complex situations. These tendencies are outlined in **Table 7-2**.

Difficulty Understanding Delays

The primary mistakes or errors made by almost all subjects during the simulated scenarios were insufficient consideration of processes in time and the tendency to think in terms of isolated cause-and-effect relationships. Each of these mistakes was related to the phenomenon of delays from the time of one's action to the consequences. Under time pressure, the participants had a tendency to apply overdoses of established measures (Dörner, 1996).

Table 7-2   Human Tendencies When Problem Solving in Complex Systems

- Difficulty understanding the consequences of delays with isolated cause-and-effect thinking
- Deterioration of planful thinking and disconfirming evidence
- Simplifying and economizing
- Preserving an optimistic view of oneself
- Focusing on the symptoms versus the fundamental issues
- Neglecting to reflect on the consequences of past decisions

Source: Dörner, 1987.

Deterioration of Planful Thinking

With repetitive failures, all participants in Dörner's study (1996) demonstrated a deterioration of "planful thinking." This was defined as a marked increase in willingness to bend the rules as failures were repeated; reductive hypotheses, which attributed all phenomena to a single cause; and confirmation biases that became more marked, with participants looking for evidence that confirmed their thinking rather than disconfirmed it (Reason, 1990).

In addition to difficulty with the phenomenon of delays (from the time of one's action to the consequences) and deterioration of planful thinking, four human failings were evident in the research of problem-solving tendencies in complex situations: the tendency to simplify and economize; the tendency to preserve an optimistic view of oneself; the tendency to focus on the symptoms versus the fundamental issues; and neglecting to reflect on the consequences of past decisions.

Tendency to Simplify

The tendency to economize or simplify when planning by not taking side effects and long-term repercussions into account is apparent when all effort goes toward treating the symptom(s) and not toward solving the underlying problem, because it is difficult and time-consuming to obtain the knowledge about all possible interactions with a particular system that led to the underlying problem (Weick & Sutcliffe, 2001). Humans prefer to develop and/or maintain a hypothesis rather than formulate a new one, ignoring information that does not conform to the existing hypothesis, and responding to the similarities (Dörner, 1996; Reason, 1990). Truth is commonly identified as being associated with comprehensibility and simplicity; what one does not understand is rejected as false (Gharajedaghi, 1999).

Delusional Optimism

A second reason for poor decision making in complex situations is the tendency to preserve an optimistic view about one's own abilities and accomplishments. Lovallo and Dahneman (2003)—a business scholar and a psychologist, respectively—referred to this tendency of executives as "delusional optimism." Research into human cognition has traced the phenomenon of being overly optimistic to many sources, with one of the most powerful being the tendency of individuals to exaggerate their own talents, believing they are above average in their endowment. The inclination to exaggerate one's talents is amplified by the tendency to misperceive the causes of, and degree of control over, certain events. Executives, especially, seem to be highly susceptible to these biases (Lovallo & Dahneman, 2003).

Dörner's research (1996) identified the tendency to preserve a positive view of oneself as an attribution failure that lies outside the realm of cognitive processes. In his studies, these preservation acts contributed significantly to shaping the direction and course of the participants' thought processes. Argyris's research (1991) observed that many professionals have difficulty learning from their errors because they so rarely experience them. He also noted that when professionals commit errors, they become defensive, screen out criticism, and push the blame on others. It was his view that their ability to learn shuts down precisely at the moment when they need it the most. This act of self-protection is essential—to a point—to maintain a minimum capacity to act (Dörner, 1996) but becomes a barrier without the injection of a healthy dose of realism (Lovallo & Dahneman, 2003).

Symptom Thinking Versus System Thinking

The third human tendency when dealing with complex situations is to focus on the wrong problems and goals, neglecting the fundamental issues and their long-term considerations and consequences. This "repair-service behavior" occurs when partial or interim goals capture the participant's attention and displace the primary goals (Dörner, 1996). Often the tasks that become the focus are those that the individual feels competent doing and challenged by, with the reward of gratification from achieving at least some success. These partial goals often have contradictory relationships with the primary goal, which are not always evident. This attention to "symptoms" leads to actions that inevitably replace one problem with another and engender a resulting vicious cycle.

Neglect to Reflect

Studies indicate that neither intelligence nor specialized experience or motivation differentiate the high performers from the low performers (Dörner, 1996;

Goleman, 1998; Senge, 1990). Instead, the difference in the two groups relates to the knowledge that individuals have about the use of their intellectual capabilities and skills. Successful individuals are capable of approaching problems in a variety of ways, learning as they go along.

Individuals who reflect on their own thinking and feeling and learn from their experiences demonstrate better problem-solving abilities. They are able to "make meaning" out of the experiences that they and others have in the world (Dixon, 1999) by recognizing their own underlying decision-making tendencies, emotional habits, assumptions, and unexpected side effects of earlier actions. This ability to make meaning requires an individual to pause and consider that there are relationships in the world that one cannot readily see, and to consider that one creates the world in which he or she lives through preferences of interpreting the world. Reflection with courage enhances an individual's ability to feel the dissonance that is experienced when one denies the validity of a situation, which can then be used to reconstruct new understanding of it.

LEADERSHIP'S VIEW: EFFECT ON RELIABILITY

A leader's view of the organization and how it works has a profound impact on the organization's reliability—that is, its ability to yield the same results on repeated trials. Therefore, a precursor to creating more highly reliable organizations is a "highly reliable" view of healthcare organizations. Today, a successive shift is occurring in the understanding of what the nature of organizations is and how they work across the country. Unfortunately, the healthcare industry is lagging in this understanding, which all too often results in decision making that detracts from its viability and reliability. This section describes three views of organizational leaders that influence outcome variance and reliability: the biological view, the sociocultural view, and the high-reliability view.

Biological View of Organizations

The biological (or "uni-minded") view is the dominant perspective found in many organizations today. This view emerged mainly in Germany and Great Britain and then spread to the United States. According to this perspective, an organization is a uni-minded living system, similar to the traditional Western view of the human body, with a purpose of its own—namely, survival. That purpose reflects the inherent vulnerability and unstable structure of open systems. To survive, according to conventional wisdom, biological beings have to grow. To grow, humans exploit their environment to achieve a positive metabolism. In organizational language, growth is the measure of success, and profit is the measure to achieve it (Gharajedaghi, 1999). This is very similar to a "marketplace" view, in which medical and healthcare institutions sell their services as commodities in the marketplace with a major goal of cost containment for survival purposes.

Sociocultural View of Organizations: A Precursor to High Reliability

A precursor to an HRO is the sociocultural ("multi-minded") view of organizations, which considers the organization to be a voluntary association of purposeful members who themselves manifest a choice of "both ends and means" (Gharajedaghi, 1999). This is a fundamentally different view of organizations than that taken by the biological model; it is purposeful because of its purposeful members who manifest choice. The members of a sociocultural organization are bonded together by one or more common objectives and collectively acceptable ways of pursuing them. The members share values that are embedded in their culture, and the culture serves as the cement that integrates the parts into a cohesive whole (Senge, 1990). Because the parts do have something to say about the organization of the whole, consensus is essential to the alignment of a sociocultural system (Gharajedaghi, 1999).

High-Reliability View of Organizations

HROs are high-risk systems that continuously operate under trying conditions and have fewer than their fair share of accidents. HROs share two essential characteristics: (1) they constantly confront the unexpected, and (2) they operate with remarkable consistency and effectiveness (Weick & Sutcliffe, 2001). HROs do not claim to be immune to catastrophes. Rather, they are distinguished by cultures of safety that include a collective view that recognizes their vulnerability to failure with a willingness to learn from trial-and-error means through devotion of time, attention, and effort to avoiding and/or minimizing variation and error. A common characteristic of HROs is that safety behaviors are collectively encouraged rather than discouraged (Klein, Bigley, & Roberts, 1995; Reason, 2000; Weick & Sutcliffe, 2001). A high-reliability view of organization perceives the members as the front-line protection against error and failure, who are supported by systems that are designed for failure prevention. HROs understand that uncertainty is irreducible and sources of harm are limitless. Therefore, they anticipate the worst and equip themselves to deal with the unexpected at all levels of the organization.

CULTURES OF DEVIANCE

Culture is "the set of shared attitudes, values, goals, and practices that characterize a company or corporation" (*Merriam-Webster's Collegiate Dictionary*, 2002). An organization's culture is often referred to as "the way things happen around here" or "the hidden rules that rule behavior." Within most healthcare organizations, there are social hierarchies or social stratifications that have a profound impact upon the relationships, communication practices, management of conflict, expectations for collaboration, displays of emotion, and patient care practices (Malloch & Porter-O'Grady, 2005).

Healthcare organizations, rather than having cultures that promote safety, are noted for having cultures of blame, which create incentives that have detrimental effects on safety (Becher & Chassin, 2001). A disaster from the nuclear industry in 1986 illustrates the negative effects of some cultures that have parallels to health-care culture. In the Chernobyl disaster, a Ukrainian atomic-energy plant in the (now former) Soviet Union exploded, destroying its concrete roof that weighed thousands of tons, and polluting the surrounding territory and all of Europe with radioactive particles. A key contributor to the event was the frequent violation of safety rules by the Chernobyl engineers (Dörner, 1996), or "normalization of deviance" (Fountain, 1999). Breaking safety rules had become the norm at that plant, a pattern that was continuously reinforced by no immediate negative consequences for failing to follow the rules as well as the positive consequences of acting more freely by getting rid of the encumbrances that rules imposed.

Healthcare cultures are rich with deviances that have become normalized. The medical profession, for example, has both formal and informal peer-review processes that often grant forgiveness for, deny, silence, discount, and/or cover up errors (Smith & Forster, 2000). The nursing profession often ignores poor clinical judgment and interpersonal skills of avoidance or aggression until a major event occurs. This nursing tendency to ignore is often related to lack of resources (nurses and/or managers), lack of standards for accountability, and lack of skills to hold one another accountable.

The IOM's report entitled *Keeping Patients Safe* (IOM, 2004) identifies three organizational elements that are critical for managing variation and promoting an effective safety culture: environmental structures and processes within the organization, the attitudes and perceptions of the workers, and the safety-related behaviors of individuals. Each element is addressed through a high-reliability framework in the following section.

MANAGING VARIANCE THROUGH A HIGH-RELIABILITY FRAMEWORK

HROs share a common set of ideas and practices that could serve as a framework for all healthcare organizations. More specifically, six evidence-based characteristics of HROs are applicable to healthcare leaders and organizations today: learning from feedback, effective teamwork, anticipating the unexpected, deferring to expertise, being extra-sensitive to operations, and reluctance to simplify. The acronym LEADER, as shown in **Table 7-3**, emphasizes the critical importance of purposeful and relentless leadership in creating HROs that minimize variation and promote positive outcomes. This work represents a fundamental change in thinking, rather than an incremental process of change. From this perspective, patient care breakdown and errors are seen primarily as a result of practitioners becoming overwhelmed by unsafe conditions rather than as the fault of a single individual who failed. This view, however, is balanced by a "fair and just culture," which seeks to compensate for human error rather than assign blame for mistakes, and requires accountability for reporting and learning, rather than perfection. It is balanced by sanctions for the few who knowingly violate the rules and disrupt the workplace.

Learn from Feedback

A paradox of organizational learning is that organizations can learn only through their individual members, yet they create systemic constraints that prevent their individual members from learning (Dixon, 1999). Some familiar organizational practices that limit learning are transferring poor-performing employees from one department to another rather than showing them out the door, implementing programs that implementers know will not solve the problem due to political or other pressures, softening (or neutralizing) bad news until it is not understood, concealing an unattractive program within an attractive one, and getting the agreement of principal players before a meeting while acting in the meeting as though no such agreement has been reached. The defensive routines that result from these accepted and often tacitly encouraged practices often lead to continued poor performance, unaddressed problems, and lack of learning (Dixon, 1999).

Sagan's research (1993) identified strong disincentives for exposing the serious failures that occurred at the National Aeronautics and Space

---

Table 7-3   Six Attributes of High-Reliability Organizations for Healthcare Leaders

L	Learn from feedback
E	Effective teamwork
A	Anticipate the unexpected
D	Defer to expertise
E	Extra-sensitive to operations
R	Reluctance to simplify

Source: Reprinted with permission from Scott, K. A. (2004). *Errors and failures in complex health-care systems: Individual, team, system, and cultural contributors.* Unpublished dissertation, Cincinnati, OH: The Union Institute & University.

Administration, which are applicable to the healthcare industry. These disincentives influenced the reporting of near misses by members, the beliefs of the members related to what was acceptable to report and record, and the public interpretation of events by senior leaders. Two sets of records (one for insiders and one for outsiders) were created, and careful instructions were given to the actors regarding which conversations could occur where and when. These activities veiled the actors' internal perceptions, obfuscated the recording and use of history, and hindered the organization's ability to learn from past mistakes. In fact, research has demonstrated that many organizations do, indeed, turn the experience of failure into a memory of success, which further obstructs their ability to learn from their failures.

Dörner's study (1996) identified the tendency of poor performers to act hastily and with reluctance to gather information when in complex situations. Organizations often perpetuate this tendency toward activity (acting eagerly) by rewarding swift action as if it were competence and by discouraging perceived "inaction" such as dialogue and reflection. Organizational psychologist Karl Weick identifies "action, tempered by reflection" as a critical component for organizational success when operating in the strange, chaotic, and unfamiliar (Coutu, 2003).

Another phenomenon that prevents learning is observed with "smart" people (such as healthcare professionals) who rarely experience, or who are unaware of experiencing, failure (Argyris, 1990). When they do commit errors, these individuals become defensive, screen out criticism, and place the blame on others. In Argyris's view, smart people's ability to learn shuts down just when they need it most.

HROs create cultures and structures that encourage members to report even small and inconsequential lapses swiftly to facilitate a rapid response for learning and correction. These organizations learn from their mistakes as a result of their openness to learn and their swift processing of data. Case studies demonstrate that people tend to be candid about the events surrounding a failure for a short period of time, and then they get their stories straight in ways that justify their actions and protect their reputations (Weick & Sutcliffe, 2001). In a book on military misfortunes, this truth is revealed: "on the actual day of battle naked truths may be picked up for the asking. But by the following morning they have already begun to get into their uniforms" (Cohen & Gooch, 1990, p. 44). Determining the root causes of errors and poor performance and identifying high-leverage interventions that will markedly improve performance require swift and nonjudgmental dialogue and action by organizational leadership.

Learning Strategies: Practical Application

Leadership Rounding

A formula borrowed from ecology states that for an organism to survive, its rate of learning must be equal to or greater than the rate of change in its environment. The formula is written $L > C$ (Dixon, 1999). One activity to help leaders learn and survive, called "leadership rounding," focuses on patient and environmental safety. When senior executives (such as the CEO, chief nursing officer, chief medical officer, or chief operating officer) visibly round with staff to explore the variations from safe patient practice, learning is greatly enhanced for all parties, and more effective strategies will result for minimizing variation and improving outcomes.

Ten basic steps for effective safety rounds are outlined in **Table 7-4** that promote feedback and learning. Leaders—equipped with the belief that vulnerability is inherent in the complex healthcare system and with a willingness to learn from the people performing the work—must pay particular attention to their words and body language during this process, and avoid reactions and rationalizations for current perceived failures, such as minimizing, denying, blaming, ignoring, or retaliation. The process begins and ends with nonjudgmental dialogue between leadership and staff to create and sustain the trust that is so critical to reporting and managing error/practice breakdown.

Debriefing

Learning from feedback also requires redesigned structures and/or processes that promote collaborative interaction and objective, forthright communication. The act of debriefing entails a constructive discussion of a team's activities quickly after a procedure or event is concluded (Leonard, Graham, & Taggart, 2004). When debriefing expectations and time are built into the day, individual, team, and organizational learning are enhanced. The focus is on promoting situational awareness, reinforcing and rewarding excellence, and identifying opportunities for improvement through dialogue inspired by the following questions: What went well? What would we do differently next time? What made this more difficult? What are the next steps to ensure that performance is improved?

Effective Teamwork

Teams often perform better than individuals. Teamwork is defined as "work done by several associates, with each doing a part but all subordinating personal prominence to the efficiency of the whole" (*Merriam-Webster's Collegiate Dictionary*, 2002). Teamwork matters in health care because most endeavors require groups to work together effectively, with failures to do so often having deadly effects. In the aviation industry (another complex and high-risk industry), more than two-thirds of the air crashes studied in one investigation involved human error, especially

Table 7-4   Patient Safety Rounds: 10-Step Process

1. Senior leader(s) schedule an appointment to round with staff in their department.
2. Ask staff to identify barriers to their practice that could potentially result in harm.
3. Ask employees to identify recent errors or "near misses."
4. Brainstorm perceived contributors (practitioner competence, team norms, and process design) to errors or "near misses" with employees.
5. Brainstorm actions necessary to prevent events from reoccurring.
6. Communicate the next steps in the process.
7. Meet with managers, prioritize issues, and create an action plan around key breakdown areas.
8. Assign responsibility and timelines for actions.
9. Track actions and changes.
10. Provide feedback regarding actions and outcomes to the original contributors.

failures in teamwork (Helmreich, 2003). Teams are of primary importance in preventing errors because individuals are imperfect in their skills, motivation, and cognition (Edmondson, 1996). Professional training has traditionally focused on technical, not interpersonal skills (Helmreich, 2003), and organizational systems are inevitably flawed (Edmondson, 1996; IOM, 2001; Leape, 1999).

Through the group-level phenomenon of synergy, unconscious processes of the group can manifest themselves in the individual group members' actions (Alderfer, 1987), creating either positive or negative outcomes collectively, which are quite different from the outcomes that would be obtained by simply adding up the contributions of the individual members working alone (Hackman, 1987; Weick, 1990). Teams in organizations can act as "self-correcting performance units" to counteract the ever-present potential for error (Benner, Hooper-Kyriakidis, & Stannard, 1999) as well as performance units that perpetuate errors and undesired outcomes (Weick, 1990). For instance, a study (Edmondson, 1996; Foushee, Lauber, Baetge, & Acomb, 1986) of fatigue on flight crew errors in the aviation industry found that crews who were fatigued after working several days together made significantly fewer errors than teams who were well rested but had not worked together. As expected, the fatigued individuals made more errors than their rested counterparts; nevertheless, as a team, the members of group who regularly worked together compensated for one another's shortcomings and overall made fewer errors than the rested team (Edmondson, 1996; Sexton, Thomas, & Helmreich, 2000).

Negative effects of the team can occur, however, when members of a work team communicate across tacit boundaries that are imposed by rank or identity group and that inhibit the transfer of valid data (Argyris, 1985; Edmondson, 1996). Nurses and physicians, for example, face group identity boundaries confounded with status differences that can affect within-team communication and patient safety.

Conflict is defined as "a clash or struggle that occurs when a real or perceived threat or difference exists in the desires, thoughts, attitudes, feelings, or behaviors of two or more parties" (Cox, 2003, p. 154). Human needs are at the center of all conflicts. People engage in conflict either because they have needs that they perceive as inconsistent with those of others, or because they have needs that are met by the conflict process itself (Mayer, 2000).

Group conflict refers to both intra- and inter-group conflict. Intra-group conflict occurs when disagreements or differences exist among members of a particular group or its subgroups; in contrast, differences and disagreements between two or more groups or their representatives are referred to as inter-group conflict (Cox, 2003, p. 155). In a survey of nurses employed in 13 different inpatient units, Cox found that intra-group conflict had direct negative effects on work satisfaction and team performance.

Research indicates that trust among members and a sense of group identity are essential conditions to a group's effectiveness (Druskat & Wolff, 2001). Trust is an important ingredient for fully optimizing any system. Without trust, members seek to protect their own immediate interests, to the detriment of the long-term effectiveness and well-being of the entire system (Deming, 1986). Teams and team members have values or principles that guide their behavior often without their awareness. They also have daily norms or actions at a more superficial level. When the team members share these values and actions collectively, they are able to develop a sense of group identity.

The social norms of a team may differ significantly from moral norms. On the one hand, social norms may require that team members support one another by hiding and/or minimizing what goes on within the team. Moral norms, on the other hand, could require blowing the whistle on what is considered unsafe practice, and may be viewed as "tattling" by another team member (Aroskar, 1985). Having greater commitment to the team than to the patient can result in actions and behaviors that feed the underlying problems in systems and allow them to continue; it can also result in harm to patients. Shared values and social norms that build trust, group identity, and group efficacy with "safety as the priority" are essential for creating cultures of safety.

Social hierarchies also have an effect on team conflict and collaboration. Healthcare organizations demonstrate unique social hierarchies. Because of the dominance of the professions of medicine (which goes considerably beyond the clinical realm) and management, the communication practices, conflict, collaboration, and displays of emotions are profoundly affected by these entities. The "professionalization" of management has contributed to the complexity of the healthcare organization and can lead to team ineffectiveness through its diversity of education, professional socialization that competes for professional dominance, and competition for finite resources (Clement, 2001). Conflict tends to escalate in diverse and stressful environments, leading to interdisciplinary and interdepartmental communication failures and conflict, which include dissatisfaction, disagreement, or unmet expectations. This diversity, however, can also lead to a better understanding of complex systems when multiple views contribute to a more comprehensive picture of the situation. Nevertheless, unless conflict utilization strategies deal with the underlying structures, they are often unsuccessful. This situation is akin to rearranging the deck chairs on the *Titanic:* While there is plenty of activity carried out by plenty of people, the fundamental problems are not addressed and the outcomes do not change.

Managers have a profound effect on intradepartmental team effectiveness through both their behavior and their relationships. Edmondson's (1996) research into the organizational factors that account for variance in drug error rates across hospital units suggested that detected error rates were a function of at least two influences: (1) actual errors made and (2) unit members' willingness to report errors. Higher error rates and interdisciplinary collaboration were reported in units where the nurse manager scored higher in direction setting, coaching, perceived unit performance outcomes, and quality relationships. This counterintuitive relationship to errors, however, suggests that a primary influence on detected error rates is the unit members' willingness to discuss mistakes openly. Such willingness may be influenced positively by leadership behavior that establishes a climate of openness and facilitates dialogue. By contrast, in units with authoritarian styles and climates, there is a significant decrease in willingness to collaborate across professions and report errors (Edmondson, 1996).

The medical profession has a significant effect on team collaboration in the hospital setting. Collaboration implies an interaction that is complementary, with input and responses from each participant allowing for synergistic building to promote patient care (Baggs, 1998). While collaborative practice is often talked about (mostly by nurses), research indicates that only 14% of physicians and 7% of nurses report actually using collaborative interdisciplinary problem-solving approaches. The most common modes used by both providers are competition and avoidance. The staff nurses' role in clinical decision making tends to be more supportive than collaborative, with physicians accepting nurses' input but handling final decision making (Forte, 1997). Many nurses do not want more responsibility than this level, however. Thus the obstacles to collaborative practice come from both the nursing and medical professions.

Teamwork Strategies: Practical Application
Briefings

The number one teamwork goal is to create an environment that promotes and rewards open communication and teamwork. Numerous strategies and much courage are needed to change the culture of the organization from hierarchical and autonomous practice to collaborative practice through a team approach. Therefore, strategies that bring people together around the core business of patient care are practical starting points.

A briefing is a structured type of interaction used to attain clear, timely, and effective communication (Leonard et al., 2004). When briefings are structured into the day and/or processes, critical information can be shared concisely and effectively, providing just-in-time information to monitor and correct situations. Examples of briefings include (1) "time-outs" before a surgical procedure, required by the Joint Commission, to double-check key risks associated with a surgical procedure such as patient identity and identification of the correct procedure, and (2) "time-outs" during a hectic day on a nursing unit to identify key risks and develop a plan to intervene and support quickly and effectively. In nursing units, briefings during shift changes, patient transfers, and hand-offs in general are critical to avoid information loss in the transition.

Physician–Nurse Interaction Tool

Nurses often feel unprepared to communicate information to physicians in a clear and concise fashion, especially in the middle of the night or when physicians have a tendency to act impatiently. The Institute for Healthcare Improvement recommends a tool for the purpose of improving physician–nurse interaction: the SBAR (situation, background, assessment, and recommendation) model. This template, outlined in **Table 7-5**, can be used to assist the nurse in his or her critical thinking by setting the expectations for communication of specific informational elements.

When used as the standard for communication, the SBAR model can be a very effective tool for the care team, as it helps the nurse to set expectations for gathering information before the conversation, critically think through the information, and provide clear recommendations for care that are relevant to the patient's current condition. Integration of this tool into the nursing curriculum, orientation, professional development, and case reviews is also an effective way to decrease variability in communication and enhance patient care management.

Anticipate the Unexpected

Human fallibility and errors have been found to be pervasive and foreseeable in numerous studies of large-scale disasters—for example, the nuclear power plant explosion at Chernobyl, the 1986 explosion of the Challenger space

Table 7-5   The SBAR Template for Nurse–Physician Communication

S	**Situation**	I am calling about: The patient's code status is: The problem I am calling about is: I have just assessed the patient personally: Vital signs are: I am concerned about the:
B	**Background**	The patient's mental status is: The skin is: The patient is not or is on oxygen.
A	**Assessment**	This is what I think the problem is: The problem seems to be: cardiac infection/neurologic/respiratory. I am not sure what the problem is, but the patient is deteriorating. The patient seems to be unstable and may get worse. We need to do something.
R	**Recommendation**	I suggest or request that you: Are any tests needed, such as: If a change in treatment is ordered, then ask about their next expectations for monitoring, calling, duration of symptoms.

Source: Adapted with permission from copyrighted material of Kaiser Foundation Health Plan, Inc., California Regions.

shuttle shortly after take-off, and the 1979 Three Mile Island nuclear meltdown. What was not pervasive, however, were well-developed systems, processes, and skills to detect and contain errors at their early stages.

A change of thinking is required if healthcare organizations are to become more resilient and move beyond prevention to include cure as a key practice goal. "To be resilient is to be mindful about errors that have already occurred and to correct them before they worsen and cause serious harm" (Weick & Sutcliffe, 2001, p. 67). Error and practice breakdown often occur when the unexpected is encountered. The skills related to noticing, coping, and correcting are very different from the skills needed for planning and anticipating—yet both sets of skills are clearly necessary.

Healthcare organizations often anticipate errors through the development of copious policies and procedures. Policies and procedures have their virtues, which include their ability to remove some uncertainty, promote interdepartmental coordination, provide a pretext for learning, protect individuals against blame, and discourage private informal modifications. However, a wholehearted commitment to anticipation is also dangerous (Wildavsky, 1991). Such a perspective presumes a level of simplicity and understanding that is impossible to achieve when dealing with complex situations. It gives people the illusion that they have things under control, and it can actually result in more complexity and opaqueness with each added policy or procedure.

This climate of anticipation in healthcare organizations consumes great quantities of resources and attention. Solutions to anticipated problems are created with the expectation that the group will actively retain them in their action repertoire and memory. The predesigned solutions are then considered to be available for accessing and application to any problem that arises.

One antidote to this obsession with planning is experiential learning. Experiential learning requires being open to having one's expectations refined, challenged, or disconfirmed by the unfolding situation. Patient care, for example, involves much uncertainty. When certainty is missing (as in situations that are ambiguous), somewhat undetermined, unexpected, or markedly different than one's preconceptions, thinking and judgment are required to act (Benner et al., 1999). Resilience comes through experiential learning during and following those times of uncertainty as well as through conceptual slack, or the willingness to question what is happening rather than simply feigning understanding.

The ability to anticipate the unexpected is enhanced through human factor and reliability science, which is the science of evidence-based design that takes into account human factors (such as fatigue, distractions, interruptions, cognitive shortcomings, and emotional tendencies) and applies system design principles for failure prevention, identification, and mitigation.

Anticipation: Practical Application

Healthcare organizations can enhance healthcare practitioners' ability to anticipate through adoption of evidence-based design and standardization. Healthcare environments are laden with individual-based preferences of practice, as well as numerous distractions and stressors that make it very difficult for practitioners to anticipate and focus on patient care (Scott, 2004). Rather than having a primary focus on retrospective attentional deficits, healthcare organizations can focus on clear expectations through evidence-based standardization. To expect everyone to remember everything is no longer realistic. When healthcare designers create systems that require standardization and adherence, such as required fields in electronic medical records, and when they integrate attentional tools, such as monitor alarms that communicate directly to the bedside nurse, the system becomes far easier to control and reliability is enhanced.

Concerted efforts must also be made to identify and minimize distractions and stressors in the environment. For example, designing areas for medication dispensing and review that are quiet and private, rather than being located in heavy traffic areas, greatly decreases the distractions that are so often the precursors to medication errors and enhances safe medication administration.

Leaders are responsible for intentional planning and implementation of evidence-based design strategies to maximize standardization, redundancy, and critical failure mode functions. They should also be driving forces behind the organization's monitoring of process compliance and results.

Defer to Expertise

HROs have mastered the ability to alter the typical patterns of deference as the tempo of operations changes and unexpected problems arise. Rather than status and rank determining who makes the decisions, expertise is the determining factor. An expert is the person(s) with the best knowledge of the current situation. Experts have a focus and understanding of the most salient issues, are able to recognize the unexpected, and develop new knowledge of the situation. In clinical scenarios, the person fitting this description is often the nurse at the bedside. He or she is focused on the patient and can identify and unravel the subtle changes in the patient's condition using tacit and conscious knowledge.

The patient and his or her significant others should also be considered experts; as such, they need to be integrated adequately into the systems we are striving to change (National Patient Safety Foundation's Patient and Family Advisory Council, 2003). Patients understand their bodies in ways that healthcare practitioners never will, and their participation in care, as well as the participation of their family members and significant others, is a critical factor in keeping patients safe. To build these partnerships, a fundamental shift in thinking is needed that moves healthcare organizations from being practitioner centered and toward being patient/family centered.

In the healthcare industry, multiple and rapid changes are approved at the executive level, often without the benefit of a clinical perspective. As a result, care delivery systems have sometimes been altered in ways that hinder or delay patient care (Benner et al., 1999). Many systems have gone through reengineering efforts whereby discrete functions, tasks, and goals have been identified and designed into the system, even as the broad integrative functions and knowledge work required for reliability and problem solving at the point of service were overlooked. System design approaches have often focused on efficiency and recurring problems, rather than the practices, contingencies, and reliability created by the front-line problem solvers (Benner et al., 1999).

By blending a hierarchical decision structure with a specialist decision structure at the unit and organizational levels, healthcare organizations are able to operationalize decision making by those with the experience and expertise. The decision makers migrate up and down the hierarchical structure, depending on the issue, accountability, responsibility, uniqueness of the problem, and environmental characteristics (Weick & Sutcliffe, 2001).

Deferring to Expertise: Practical Application
Critical Rescue Team

A critical rescue or rapid response team is a team created and trained to act as a self-correcting performance unit to counteract the ever-present potential for bad patient outcomes. Anyone can initiate the call to convene the on-call team for rapid convergence. The team quickly assembles to provide a second set of eyes, a second opinion, a focused dialogue, and/or direct assistance to the nurse and patient—whatever is needed. Triggers to initiate the team can range from staff uneasiness about a patient's condition to a change in the patient's heart rate, systolic blood pressure, respiratory rate, oxygenation, or level of consciousness. The goal is to intervene in the patient's decline early enough to turn the situation around, as evidenced by a decrease in cardiac arrests, ICU transfers, and patient mortality.

The team members are those providers with expertise in unstable patient conditions—that is, a critical care nurse, respiratory therapist, intensivist, and pharmacist—and expertise in interpersonal skills. It is essential that the team members be respectful and nonjudgmental when consulting, thereby positively supporting the clinicians and others involved in the situation. Fulfilling this role effectively requires clear expectations and training as well as feedback from those who utilize the services.

Evidence-Based Standards Through Shared Decision Making

Through the creation of structures that bring situational and content experts to the table to make decisions, evidence-based standards and practices can be developed and implemented for managing and leading nurses as well as for carrying out the clinical work of nursing. Many of the profession's current practices (both clinical and managerial) are based on tradition and are perpetuated without question. Structures are needed that bring the experts together in ways that enable them to voice their concerns as well as to understand and own the issues that they have the expertise to change. This understanding includes the necessity of seeing the connections to the whole organization and having the power to influence the system.

Behavioral, organizational, and reliability research has identified management practices that are consistently associated with successful implementation of change initiatives and achievement of safety in spite of high risk for error. The HRO framework is one such evidence-based management structure to guide nursing leaders' work. Through planned leadership and action, organizations can accomplish the changes required in nurses' work environments to minimize variability and improve patient safety.

Evidence-based nursing standards are needed to minimize the variation of practice. The development of standards focused on the key activities of direct-care nursing, for example, will enhance both patient-specific outcomes and the overall practice of nursing. Key nursing activities for organizations to focus on for standards development include monitoring of patient status (surveillance); physiologic/disease interventions; compensation for patient's loss of functioning; provision of emotional support; patient and family education; delegation and supervision; and communication, coordination, and integration of care.

Patients and Family Members as Experts

Several actions that have the potential to change the culture of healthcare organizations to become patient/family centered, rather than practitioner centered, have been identified by the National Patient Safety Foundation (2003):

- Teaching and encouraging effective communication skills for both patients/families and healthcare professionals
- Engaging leadership in promoting and training providers in open communication about medical errors (disclosure)
- Empowering hospital patient representatives to effectively advocate and facilitate communication for patients and families during and following practice breakdown and/or medical errors
- Establishing patient and family advisory councils to ensure a patient/family perspective is represented in all aspects of healthcare delivery

Realizing this change in thinking requires strong leadership at the unit and executive levels of the organization.

Extra-Sensitive to Operations

The term "operations" is defined as the performance of the practical work within the organization that produces the "output" of patient care. HROs elevate the value of day-to-day operations above the strategic planning and administrative functions. Prestige flows to the experts at the point of service, rather than primarily to the senior leaders and planners. HROs' hierarchies or bureaucracies do not promote dysfunction. Rather, they promote high interaction and communication flow to "enhance situational awareness" through connection of the big picture and current operations (Weick & Sutcliffe, 2001). This connection requires a more holistic view for planners and practitioners alike.

Sensitivity to operations requires paying attention to the subtle symptoms and elimination of "hopeful" thinking. Hoping a problem goes away when one is working in a high-risk environment is not conducive to reliable patient outcomes, nor is the human tendency to disconfirm evidence that does not fit within one's particular paradigm. Through a commitment to effective measures, timely interdisciplinary and interdepartmental dialogue, and active listening, organizational members' understanding of the complexities are deepened and enriched in ways that support early problem identification and early action.

Measures have a significant effect on the management of and behavior related to variability and reliability. Initiatives to reward employees for the best safety records, for example, often build in the incentive to withhold information about small accidents and near misses, resulting in an actual increase in unsafe activities. Likewise, measures of safety in healthcare organizations that are imposed by third parties can miss the mark and ultimately encourage behaviors that reinforce poor performance and errors, rather than reduce them. The logic of many third-party regulations is that the presence of certain qualifying criteria or processes will be correlated with safe and effective care. Unfortunately, this purported relationship is often a fallacy. For this reason, it is important for leaders to develop metrics to measure the most common practice breakdowns and failures; these measures should go beyond clinical process measures and include a balance of outcome metrics that are representative of the interrelatedness of the whole (i.e., productivity measures in parallel with clinical outcome measures).

Operations Sensitivity: Practical Application

Tests of Change

Available evidence shows that most public and private organizations can be significantly improved at an acceptable cost, but that often terrible mistakes are made when this move is attempted because history has not prepared the change agents for transformational challenges (Kotter, 1996). A "test of change" is defined as a small-scale iterative process of the plan–do–study–act (PDSA) cycle, with each cycle leading directly into the start of the next cycle. This process relies on experiential organizational learning, a type of learning process in which the organizational members who generate the data are involved in the interpretation and understand the context in which the test of change exists. When taking this approach, it is important that the new information generated through the iterative process is shared with the individuals involved and that the collective interpretation of the new information is acted upon by the group. The follow-up action serves both to test the interpretation and to generate new information to continue the learning (**Figure 7-1**).

Trigger Audits

The use of "triggers" to identify adverse events is an effective method for measuring the overall level of harm from medications and other high-risk events in healthcare organizations. "Trigger audits" are defined as retrospective reviews of patient records using high-risk triggers to identify possible adverse events, rather than simply depending on voluntary reporting and tracking of standard variances, practice breakdown, and errors.

The Institute for Healthcare Improvement (IHI), in partnership with Premier, Inc., has developed a trigger tool for measuring adverse drug events (ADEs). The tool, which is available on the IHI Web site (*http://www.ihi.org*), includes a list of known ADE triggers and instructions for measuring the number and degree of harmful medication events; it also provides instructions to measure ADEs per 1000 doses and the percentage of admissions with an ADE.

The concept of triggers goes beyond medication administration, however. Healthcare leaders and quality managers can identify triggers related to any risk process and conduct audits to determine the reliability of care in the organization. Triggers to inform nursing practice are many, as shown in **Table 7-6**.

Trigger audits are effective ways for healthcare leaders to identify contributors to events that can and do cause harm to patients, so that errors can be prevented, or at least mitigated when they are not prevented.

Figure 7-1   Test of change process.

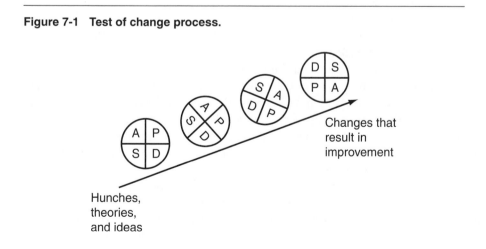

Changes that result in improvement

Hunches, theories, and ideas

Source: IHI, n. d. Reprinted with permission.

Table 7-6   Failure Mode Triggers for Evaluating Nursing Care

- Positive blood culture
- Patient fall
- Decubiti
- Restraint use
- Transfer to a higher level of care
- Respiratory arrest
- Narcan (naloxone) use
- Oversedation/hypotension
- Hospital-acquired pneumonia
- Unintentional extubation

Reluctance to Simplify

"Reluctance to simplify" has its roots in recognizing one's assumptions and expectations as well as in recognizing the human tendency to disconfirm evidence that does not meet one's expectations (Weick & Sutcliffe, 2001). The antidote to the simplification tendency is adoption of a mindful style of managing and practicing. Mindfulness preserves the individual's capability to see the significant meaning of weak signals and to give strong responses to weak signals versus the more intuitive act of responding only to the more obvious pitfalls and dangers.

Reluctance to simplify signals an understanding of the necessity of studying variability and deficiencies not in isolation, but as embedded in its system with many links and variables, or interdependencies, which are recognized by their effects on one another and on themselves (Dörner, 1987; Reason, 1990). Understanding interdependency requires new methods of inquiry that are distinct from analysis. Specifically, it requires systems thinking.

Analysis is a three-step process that first takes apart that which it seeks to understand. Next, it attempts to explain the behavior of the parts taken separately. Finally, it tries to aggregate understanding of the parts into an explanation of the whole. This linear view suggests a simple locus of responsibility: When things go wrong, there is an assumption that an individual, or individual agent, must be responsible (Senge, 1990).

In contrast, a systems-thinking approach uses a different process than analysis: It puts the system in the context of the larger environment of which it is a part and studies the role it plays on the larger whole (Gharajedaghi, 1999). Peter Senge (1990) identifies several generic structures, or archetypes, that embody the key to learning so that the structures in organizations can be seen that simplify the complexity of many management issues and resistance can be leveraged and overcome. These key structures often found in many feedback processes are (1) reinforcing feedback, (2) balancing feedback, and (3) delays.

Reinforcing feedback involves processes that amplify the situation, producing more movement in the same direction, such as financial incentives for goal attainment. Balancing feedback involves processes that stabilize a situation, thereby maintaining the status quo. Balancing processes are everywhere in complex systems, but are more difficult to see than reinforcing loops, especially when the system is plagued by delays. Balancing processes underlie all goal-oriented behavior, such as temperature regulation of the human body, or medication-error reduction. The balancing process maintains the status quo even when all participants want change. For example, when organizations create processes to decrease medication-administration errors, the actual training, monitoring, and information technology may either reinforce or accelerate error reduction. Conversely, some balancing processes seek to continue the status quo, such as cultures that blame and staffing practices. Rather than pushing harder to overcome resistance to change, artful leaders discern the source of the resistance by focusing directly on the implicit norms and power relationships in which the norms are embedded (Senge, 1990). In the medication example, the leader could identify barriers to open reporting and dialogue related to errors, such as sanctions and discipline, or reevaluate staffing based on medication administration volume.

In health care, there has been a strong movement toward simplification through standardization of the work via development of clinical protocols and care pathways. Reliable and standardized patient care, however, remains dependent upon an understanding of the complexity of the objective and subjective system within which it exists.

Resisting the Urge to Simplify: Practical Application
Incident Reviews
Healthcare leaders can understand the fundamental/root contributors to system and practice breakdown through conducting timely (within 24 hours) incident reviews that go beyond the root-cause analysis approach of problem solving to include a whole-systems thinking approach. Such an approach examines the more obvious objective behaviors, systems, and processes as well as the more subjective team dynamics, human interactions, underlying norms, values, and beliefs.

Table 7-7 presents selected items from an "error-event interview guide" that probes the objective and subjective contributors to an error-event that may have potentially resulted in harm to a patient. The guide is composed of 27 questions that explore key emotional intelligence skills identified through

Table 7-7   Selected Items from Scott's Error-Event Interview Guide

The Work Itself and an Overall Description of the Event

1. Tell me about your role and responsibilities in the organization.
2. Describe the event that happened on (date) from your perspective.
3. What explanation do you have for why the error occurred?

Culture

1. How would you describe the culture you currently work in, with "culture" defined as the norms and expectations of those whom you work with?
2. Is this culture you are describing unique to your area only, or is it found elsewhere in the organization?
3. What significant change or changes related to attitudes and/or behaviors would you recommend to hospital leadership that would promote a culture of patient safety?

Work Pressures (at the time of incident)

1. Describe your relationship with your immediate supervisor at the time of the incident.
2. Describe your relationship with the individual(s) you were communicating with around the time the incident occurred.
3. Describe your workload/assignment the day of the incident.

Emotional Self-Awareness

1. Describe your feelings before, during, and after the incident.

Emotional Expression

1. How do you feel when you are called upon to express an opinion?

Emotional Awareness of Others

1. Describe your perception of how the person you were interacting with was feeling at the time of your discussion.

Constructive Discontent

1. Describe how you usually handle difficult situations—that is, when you disagree with someone else about something important to you.
2. How did you handle disagreement with others in the time around the incident (if applicable)?

Trust Radius

3. What about on the day of the incident? Did you feel you could ask questions, disagree, provide input, problem-solve freely (if appropriate)?

Source: Adapted with permission from Scott, K. A. (2004). *Errors and failures in complex health-care systems: Individual, team, system, and cultural contributors.* Unpublished dissertation, Cincinnati, OH: The Union Institute & University.

research (Scott, 2004), using the emotional intelligence quotient map developed by Cooper and Sawaf (1996) and the HRO framework as a guide. It is critical to involve the individuals who contributed to an error-event in the interview process not only to obtain for their insights, but also to elicit their feedback and learning for future error mitigation and/or management.

Through partnering with risk managers and legal counsel, healthcare leaders must come to a consensus on the processes for candid assessment and disclosure of practice breakdown so that learning can occur throughout the organization. Through the development of a consistent approach using a structured plan that digs deep and unearths the fundamental problems, strategies can be leveraged for more effective results.

CONCLUSIONS

Healthcare organizations are complex, are encumbered with goals and information that are often ambiguous and uncertain, and must cope with an environment characterized by rapid changes that are communicated to and through many people during stressful times. The environment's uncertainty and complexity limit the attention and working memory of providers as well as their problem-solving abilities.

Healthcare organizations must become highly reliable if they are to regain the trust of the public, patients, and providers alike. The drive to create environments and structures that put patient safety first is a paradigmatic shift that will evolve through focused strategies derived from an evidence-based, reliability framework. Through approaching the work of patient care from a new place—a place that acknowledges human facilities, reexamines discarded information, monitors expectations through a reliability lens, and consciously removes ineffective thinking and replaces it with evidence-based systems thinking—the very foundation of health care will be transformed.

REFERENCES

Alderfer, C. (1987). An intergroup perspective on group dynamics. In J. W. Lorsch (Ed.), *Handbook of organizational behavior* (pp. 190–222). Englewood Cliffs, NJ: Prentice Hall.

Argyris, C. (1985). Interventions for improving leadership effectiveness. *Journal of Management Development, 4*(5), 30–50.

Argyris, C. (1990). *Overcoming organizational defenses.* Boston: Allyn & Bacon.

Argyris, C. (1991). Teaching smart people how to learn. *Harvard Business Review, 69*(3), 99–109.

Aroskar, M. (1985). Ethical relationships between nurses and physicians: Goals and realities—a nursing perspective. In A. Bishop & J. Scudder (Eds.), *Caring, curing, coping* (pp. 44–62). Tuscaloosa, AL: University of Alabama Press.

Baggs, J. G. (1998). Nurse–physician collaboration: The challenge of collaboration. In A. L. Suchman, R. J. Botelho, & P. Hinton-Walker (Eds.), *Partnerships in healthcare: Transforming relational process* (pp. 185–197). Rochester, NY: University of Rochester Press.

Becher, E., & Chassin, M. (2001). Improving quality, minimizing error: Making it happen. *Health Affairs, 20*(3), 68–81.

Benjamin, G. (2000). Addressing medical errors: The key to a safer health care system. *Physician Executive, 26*(2), 66–67.

Benner, P., Hooper-Kyriakidis, P., & Stannard, D. (1999). *Clinical wisdom and interventions in critical care.* Philadelphia: W. B. Saunders.

Clement, J. (2001). The leadership imperative: Managing conflict and resolving disputes creatively. *Seminars for Nurse Managers, 9*(4), 211–217.

Cohen, E., & Gooch, J. (1990). *Military misfortunes: The anatomy of failure in war.* New York: Vintage Books, Random House.

Coile, R. C., Jr. (2001). Quality pays: A case for improving clinical care and reducing medical errors. *Healthcare Trends, 46*(3), 156–160.

Cooper, R., & Sawaf, A. (1996). *Executive EQ: Emotional intelligence in leadership and organizations.* New York: Berkley/Penguin.

Coutu, D. (2003, April). Sense and reliability: A conversation with celebrated psychologist Karl E. Weick. *Harvard Business Review, 81*(4), 84–90.

Cox, K. (2003). The effects of intrapersonal, intragroup, and intergroup conflict on team performance effectiveness and work satisfaction. *Nursing Administration Quarterly, 27*(2), 153–163.

Deming, W. (1986). *Out of the crisis* (2nd ed.). Cambridge, MA: MIT Press.

Dixon, N. (1999). *The organizational learning cycle: How we can learn collectively* (2nd ed.). Cambridge, UK: Cambridge University Press.

Dörner, D. (1987). On the difficulties people have in dealing with complexity. In J. Rasmussen, K. Duncan, & J. Leplat (Eds.), *New technology and human errors* (pp. 63–83). London: Wiley.

Dörner, D. (1996). *The logic of failure: Recognizing and avoiding error in complex situations.* New York: Metropolitan Books.

Druskat, V., & Wolff, S. (2001, March). Building the emotional intelligence of groups. *Harvard Business Review, 79*(3), 80–90.

Edmondson, A. (1996, March). Learning from mistakes is easier said than done: Group and organizational influences on the detection and correction of human error. *Journal of Applied Behavioral Science, 32*(1), 5–28.

Forster, A., Murff, H., Peterson, J., Gandhi, T., & Bates, D. (2003). The incidence and severity of adverse events affecting patients after discharge from the hospital. *Annals of Internal Medicine, 138*(3), 161–167.

Forte, P. (1997). The high cost of conflict. *Nursing Economic$, 15*(3), 119–123.

Fountain, R. (1999). *The relationship of error-based experiential learning to organizational change: How and why what we learn may or may not change how we behave.* Unpublished doctoral dissertation, Cleveland, OH: Case-Western Reserve University.

Foushee, H., Lauber, J., Baetge, M., & Acomb, D. (1986). *Crew factors in flight operations III: The operational significance of exposure to short-haul air transport operations.* Technical Memorandum No. 88342. Moffett Field, CA: NASA–Ames Research Center.

Gharajedaghi, J. (1999). *Systems thinking: Managing chaos and complexity.* Woburn, MA: Butterworth-Heinemann.

Goleman, D. (1998). *Working with emotional intelligence.* New York: Bantam Books.

Grube, A. (2001). Learning from healthcare errors: Effective reporting systems. *Journal for Healthcare Quality, 23*(1), 25–29.

Hackman, J. (1987). The design of work teams. In J. W. Lorsch (Ed.), *Handbook of organizational behavior* (pp. 315–342). Englewood Cliffs, NJ: Prentice Hall.

Helmreich, R. (2003, October 3). Culture, threat, and error: Lessons from aviation. Paper presented at the 2003 Seventh Annual Magnet Conference, Houston, TX.

Institute for Healthcare Improvement (IHI). (n.d.). *Reliability: General.* Retrieved April 27, 2009, from http://www.ihi.org/IHI/Topics/Reliability/ReliabilityGeneral

Institute of Medicine (IOM). (1999). *To err is human: Building a safer health system.* Washington, DC: National Academies Press.

Institute of Medicine (IOM), Committee on Quality of Health Care in America. (2001). *Crossing the quality chasm: A new health system for the 21st century.* Washington, DC: National Academies Press.

Institute of Medicine (IOM), Committee on Quality of Health Care in America. (2004). *Keeping patients safe: Transforming the work environment of nurses.* Washington, DC: National Academies Press.

Klein, R., Bigley, G., & Roberts, K. (1995). Organizational culture in high reliability organizations: An extension. *Human Relations, 48*(7), 771–793.

Kotter, J. (1996). *Leading change.* Boston: Harvard Business School Press.

Leape, L. (1999). The causes and prevention of errors and adverse events in health care. *Image: Journal of Nursing Scholarship, 31*(3), 281–286.

Leonard, M., Graham, S., & Taggart, B. (2004). The human factor: Effective teamwork and communication in patient strategy. In M. Leonard, A. Frankel, T. Simmonds, & K. Vega (Eds.), *Achieving safe and reliable healthcare: Strategies and solutions* (pp. 37–64). Chicago: Health Administration Press.

Lovallo, D., & Dahneman, D. (2003, July). Delusions of success: How optimism undermines executives' decisions. *Harvard Business Review, 81*(7), 56–63.

Malloch, K., & Porter-O'Grady, T. (2005). *The quantum leader: Applications for the new world of work.* Sudbury, MA: Jones and Bartlett Publishers.

Mayer, B. (2000). *The dynamics of conflict resolution: A practitioner's guide.* San Francisco: Jossey-Bass.

Merriam-Webster's collegiate dictionary, 10th ed. (2002). Springfield, MA: Merriam-Webster.

Merry, M., & Brown, J. (2002). From a culture of safety to a culture of excellence: Quality science, human factors, and the future of healthcare quality. *Journal of Innovative Management, 7*(2), 29–46.

National Patient Safety Foundation's Patient and Family Advisory Council. (2003). *National agenda for action: Patients and families in patient safety: Nothing about me, without me.* North Adams, MA: National Patient Safety Foundation.

Perrow, C. (1984). *Normal accidents: Living with high risk technologies.* New York: Basic Books.

Pronovost, P., Angus, D., Dorman, T., Robinson, K., Dremsizov, T., & Young, T. (2002). Physician staffing patterns and clinical outcomes in critically ill patients: A systematic review. *Journal of the American Medical Association, 288*(17), 2151–2162.

Reason, J. (1990). *Human error.* New York: Cambridge University Press.

Reason, J. (2000, March). Human error: Models and management. *British Medical Journal, 320*(7237), 768–770.

Rovner, J. (2000). Washington wakes up to medical mistakes. *Business & Health, 18*(11), 19.

Sagan, S. (1993). *The limits of safety: Organizations, accidents, and nuclear weapons.* Princeton, NJ: Princeton University.

Scott, K. (2004). *Errors and failures in complex health-care systems: Individual, team, system and cultural contributors.* Unpublished dissertation, Cincinnati, OH: The Union Institute & University.

Senge, P. (1990). *The fifth discipline: The art and practice of the learning organization.* New York: Doubleday.

Sexton, J., Thomas, E., & Helmreich, R. (2000, March). Error, stress, and teamwork in medicine and aviation: Cross sectional surveys. *British Medical Journal, 320*(7237), 745–749.

Shi, L., & Singh, D. (2001). *Delivering health care in America: A systems approach.* Gaithersburg, MD: Aspen.

Smith, M., & Forster, H. (2000). Morally managing medical mistakes. *Cambridge Quarterly of Healthcare Ethics, 9*(1), 38–53.

Weick, K. (1990). The vulnerable system: An analysis of the Tenerife air disaster. *Journal of Management, 16*(3), 571–593.

Weick, K., & Sutcliffe, K. (2001). *Managing the unexpected: Assuring high performance in an age of complexity.* San Francisco: Jossey-Bass.

Wildavsky, A. (1991). *Searching for safety.* New Brunswick, NJ: Transaction.

CHAPTER 8

Partnership Economics: Creating Value Through Evidence-Based Workload Management

Tim Porter-O'Grady and Kathy Malloch

INTRODUCTION AND BACKGROUND

There is much concern these days regarding the availability and productivity of nursing resources. With nurses in short supply, interest is accelerating the effort to address the economics and resource implications of nursing in the healthcare system (Anderson, 2007; Horak, Welton, & Shortell, 2004; Institute of Medicine, 2004). Much has been written about the economic issues and effects of this nursing shortage as they relate to the drive for efficient, effective, and profitable healthcare organizations (Bolton, Aydin, & Donaldson, 2003; Buerhaus, 1991; Clarke, 2005; Stone et al., 2007).

While the supply and demand issues of nursing are certainly important, they become of general interest only when nurses are in short supply. When the supply issues are addressed and the nursing shortage no longer appears critical, nursing moves off the priority agenda of most healthcare leadership, descending down the ladder of operational or economic importance (Buerhaus, 1995). Because of this diminishing focus on nursing resources, many hospitals forget their core business—an omission that sometimes has even crippled their business and strategic viability (Hope, 2004).

Nursing has a colorful history of oppressed group dynamics (Ashley, 1976). Clearly, the fact that nursing historically has been a predominantly female profession in a subservient role has had a tremendous influence on the role, power, and position of nursing within the healthcare system. Two major barriers have affected the development of nursing. First—and most obvious—is the feminine predominance during the development of the profession. Second, the political and economic development of medicine as a social script, supported and encouraged by the servile role of nurses, has predominated in the development of the healthcare system (Butterworth, 1979). As a result, most nurses have been managed, controlled, and limited by the dominating lay management and medical system (Starr, 1984).

Simultaneously, as a largely masculine, medically dominated healthcare system emerged, the nursing resource silently, yet steadily, became central to the clinical and service efficacy of the system. Because of the need to have competently educated practitioners available to patients 24 hours a day, a growing commitment to the education, development, and impact of nursing created an insidious and central role for the nurse in the delivery of clinical services. Parallel to this important role, an equally insidious infrastructure has developed that is represented by tight control, significant and detailed regulation, and precisely defined parameters for clinical decision making, dependence on authority, and independence (Kalisch & Kalisch, 2003). While nurses have become increasingly well educated and advances in clinical practice have unfolded consistent with the increase in the complexity of clinical service, the challenges of control and influence remain.

Among such circumstances as inadequate resource planning, limited inclusion of nurses in strategic and policy decisions, financial and economic decisions made without nursing consultation, and external improvements in choice and opportunity for women, the shortage of nurses has regularly, and with increasing intensity, become ever more common in the healthcare system (Buerhaus & Needleman, 2000). It is at these times that the importance and central value of nursing become most visible to leaders in the healthcare and political arenas. Significant efforts are then made to increase the numbers, and recruitment of women (and some men) into the profession to address care needs occurs at a frenzied level. Nevertheless, very little is done to alter the power position, practice parameters, and long-term financial condition of nurses and nursing (including nursing educators), all of which have been indicated by nurses as central to their need for satisfaction and continuing interest in the profession (Traynor, 1999).

Together these factors challenge the economic, social, and political positions and conditions of nursing. Furthermore, they inform both general and specific responses to the issues of nursing finance, productivity, value, and sustainability (Moody, 2004). In fact, the issues of productivity often discussed at the management and leadership level in organizations tend to relate more to functional proficiency and basic competence determinations than they do to issues of positioning, politics, and practice (Whittmann-Price, 2004). Additionally, much of the language at the administrative level is frequently process and functionally oriented, focusing on issues of adequate numbers of nurses and appropriate levels of productivity (Eastaugh, 1998). The resulting costs in nurse dissatisfaction and job turnover are the clearest and most obvious indications of significant problems with these current functional and institutional approaches to addressing nursing resource issues (Waldman, Kelly, Arora, & Smith, 2004).

Different perceptions of the value of the nursing resource clearly must emerge in what are today challenging times for both nursing and health care.

Furthermore, the functional and institutional articulations about nurses' value and productivity should be reflected by increases in the economic and financial benefits made available to nurses. No longer can nursing be seen simply as a functional part of the cost of doing business within a hospital or healthcare system context. Nursing is not merely a support or budgeted functional resource that can be managed and accounted for in the same manner as materials management. While quantification of clinical care is certainly essential to managing financial and productivity concerns, taking a more evidence-based approach to determine this value and the subsequent financial representation of nurses' value must be a critical shift in focus. All too often, the reconfiguration of the financial equation in hospitals and health systems creates pressures to eliminate nursing work, which, in the end, does not result in improving either nurses' economic value or the financial circumstances of the entire organization. Because nursing is both critical and central to the functional work of the organization, eliminating its value through sometimes arbitrary and poorly delineated decision strategies threatens the viability of the organization as a whole and ultimately affects its sustainability.

Most hospitals and healthcare systems today are struggling with the issue of a nursing shortage that was created by decisions related to the nursing resource that were made nearly a decade ago. The hospital restructuring movement of the early 1990s led to reductions in the educated nursing work force, ultimately threatening the clinical viability of these organizations at precisely the same time that clinical interventions became more complex and intense. These so-called productivity decisions of the early to mid-1990s are now exacting an enormous toll on the nursing resources in healthcare systems (Barry-Walker, 2000; Weinberg & Suzanne, 2004). Further, the current economic downturn and failure of major financial institutions is negatively affecting the healthcare marketplace in ways once thought not possible. Deficits in state budgets are shrinking university capacity, lower employment rates are diminishing the use of disposable healthcare dollars, and the downturn in available resources continues apace. What is not certain is how the need for nursing care will be affected by these trends.

The historic lack of connection between the economic viability of the organization and its effects on the satisfaction and performance of its nursing resource is an untenable factor in the future consideration of the viability of healthcare organizations. Administrators and other leaders in the healthcare system can no longer make strategic and economic decisions without recognizing how those decisions will affect its primary resource: nursing.

Even in an evidence-based format, managerial decisions must reflect a balancing of the value equation—namely, the tension between service, resources, and outcomes (Malloch & Porter-O'Grady, 1999). This three-legged stool upon which clinical and performance viabilities are based becomes unbalanced when any one of the value factors is emphasized in a way that sacrifices its relationship to the other factors. Untenable and uncontrolled emphasis on providing service without consideration to issues of resource utilization creates an imbalance that ultimately diminishes service sustainability. Equally importantly, a focus on producing high levels of quality without efforts to develop the human or financial resources necessary to obtain and sustain that quality creates an imbalance. Uncontrolled and overriding focus on managing costs ultimately limits and threatens the organization's ability to provide adequate service or to ensure the high quality of that service. Again, the imbalance inherent in this situation is obvious.

The economic and financial sustainability of the organization depends on finding a continuous and dynamic balance between the three elements of the value equation, and keeping them in accord. To achieve this goal, productivity measurement must transcend its current constraints and evolve into a multifaceted model that reflects the complexity of the work of nursing. This level of understanding is much different than the simple and limited cost–benefit evaluation that compares work hours to budgeted units of service. Imagine the long-term impact that reactive cuts to the nursing resource create during an economic downturn, and the "turnaround" toll that is later exacted when these reduced numbers increase both risks and costs, alter the organization's market position, and raise recruitment and salary costs to untenable levels. Cutting out the core of a business does more than just alter the current balance sheet; it ultimately damages the sustainability of the business itself and positions it on a negative trajectory from which it may never fully recover.

Leadership must recognize the centrality of the nursing function if it is to sustain a balance in the value equation for the hospital or corporation. The nursing resource is not only the organization's largest human cost, but is also central to the successful clinical operation of the health system. The nurse is located at the intersection of the provision of all healthcare services. In fact, it is the nurse's role to coordinate, integrate, and facilitate all of the clinical functions related to the delivery of patient care. Empirical evidence of the critical value of "intersection management"—that is, interdisciplinary coordination—is needed, however.

Fulfilling the role of intersection management clearly places the nurse in a critical position with regard to the financial and service viability of the organization. In addition, elements of high levels of quality in the delivery of clinical service are influenced and often coordinated by nursing professionals. Nurses are the physician's "eyes and ears"—a role in which they evaluate the patient's condition, response, and progress in a timely fashion. Therefore, in a high-level interface, the nurse has a direct and powerful impact on the clinical and service viability of the organization. Through this direct relationship, the nurse controls the financial variables that ultimately affect the economic viability of the organization as a whole (Finkler & Graf, 2001).

Organizations that recognize and build management, operational, and financial support systems for professional nursing functions in the organization actively contribute to both their service and financial variability. Administrators often argue that nursing should not be valued in a broader framework like other clinical disciplines. They forget that all other clinical disciplines value nursing by virtue of the nurses' coordination and integrative roles, which influence their clinical actions and relationships both with one another and with patients. Ultimately, no specific role has greater importance than any other in healthcare delivery. It is vital to recognize nursing's central role, however, as nurses integrate all of the work of other disciplines with regard to the patients' progress along their healing continuum. This realization is the key to the clinical success of the entire health organization (While, Forbes, Ullman, Lewis, Mathes, & Grifiths, 2004).

At the same time, it is crucial for nursing professionals to recognize that there must be a clear delineation of specific measures of value. In an evidence-based world, the nursing profession needs to explicitly enumerate and articulate its value in sufficiently objective terms so that real value can be identified and measured. Historically, the problem with nursing care delivery has been the difficulty in defining and scientifically evaluating evidence of clinical practice at the level of performance, in a way that yields specifically delineated outcomes (Duffy, 2004). The failure to clearly tie practice elements and activities to specifically defined outcomes makes it exceptionally difficult to identify any unique and specified value for nursing practice. While this task is admittedly extremely difficult because of the need to account for the coordinative and integrative relationships and activities that characterize nursing practice, it is no longer acceptable to omit that step: Nurses cannot claim value on one hand and provide little definitive evidence of that value on the other hand.

Reframing nursing within the context of the value equation calls for the profession to critically delineate both its clinical foundations and supporting financial demands. Viable clinical practice requires that a clear foundation for that practice be elucidated and accepted. Within an evidence-based context, a collective effort to establish clinical best practices calls for the consideration of several factors:

- Clearly delineated service-based protocols and practices that reflect broader best practice standards
- A professionally designed, service-specific best practices framework that incorporates generic standards into specific performance standards

- A specifically defined tie between clinical tasks, best practices, and the payment formats within which they are financed
- A real-time process that articulates clinical performance and the costs of that performance within payment parameters for those clinical processes
- An infrastructure within which nursing practice is evaluated according to the context of both clinical quality and financial enumerators
- The societal mandate for nursing services based on reliable nursing knowledge
- Variance documentation as a vehicle to improve the management of resources

What is implied in building a formal process is a commitment to both the healthcare management system and the nursing clinical system, so that the relationship between clinical practice, performance outcomes, and the payment structure is clearly delineated (Wannisky, Centers for Medicare & Medicaid Services, & U.S. General Accounting Office, 2003). All of these factors are critical for creating a sustainable and viable relationship between the value of nursing practice, the quality of clinical outcomes, and the cost and payment factors associated with obtaining them. Recently, nursing organizations have aggressively encouraged the Centers for Medicare and Medicaid Services (CMS) to consider modifying the Medicare cost report requirements to separate out nursing costs and hours of care, thereby allowing construction of a nursing cost-to-charge ratio within existing routine and intensive care cost centers (Welton, Fischer, Degrace, & Zone-Smith, 2006; Welton, Zone-Smith, & Fischer, 2006). This pay-for-performance approach offers an exciting and data-rich means of determining the place and value of nursing resources in overall patient care.

The goals of this work are to improve the overall payment accuracy and create a better understanding of how nursing care hours and costs are allocated to individual patients and by diagnosis-related group (DRG) within and across hospitals; to identify hospital nursing performance; and to inform policy makers about the state of inpatient nursing care in the United States. Given that many hospitals do not track patient-level data that would enable them to identify case-level differences in nursing intensity, the first phase of this work will focus on nursing summary data rather than attempt to extract individual patient data.

In addition to creating this value foundation, the profession itself must become aware of the need for a deeper understanding of the value elements of clinical practice. Too many nurses ignore the need to balance clinical performance against resource availability and quality outcomes. Because of the history of nursing and its predominant focus on clinical process, rather than specific identification with clinical outcome, many nurses have become addicted to process (Hughes & American Nurses Association, 1958). In fact, for many nurses, the process has become ritual, routine, and intellectually mindless. Further, experience itself has become a mantra, even though in most cases experience tends to be a limitation: The more experience one has, the more one is inculcated in the values that experience provides (Smith, 2002). *Competent* practice is *changing* practice. As technology enhancements and innovations continually challenge the foundations of clinical practice, it is the very fluidity, flexibility, and mobility of clinical practice that ensures its continuing viability and efficacy. In this set of circumstances, nurses who continually value specific performance experience may actually limit their availability and exposure to the considerable demands for flexibility and changing practice in increasingly shorter periods of time. This blind dependence and valuing of experience over innovation and education must be overcome if meaningful value is to be found and defined (Corey, 2001).

This new focus provides a great opportunity for building a framework that supports economically and financially viable evidence-based practice. The direct connection between evidence and payment must be established to lay out a clear, direct path between nursing activity, productivity, and value. Ultimately, there must be a direct relationship between which services are paid for in health care and how much of that payment relates specifically to nursing-driven activities. The difficult aspect of this equation lies in determining the value of those activities that are predominantly coordinating and integrating processes. Because this coordination and integration account for the majority of professional nursing activity (in terms of value), it is clearly important to provide a financial definition for it (Rubin, Plovnick, & Fry, 1975).

At the same time, it may be less important that individual costing and value determination processes are applied to the specific coordinative and integrative activities of the nursing professional. In fact, it might be wiser to determine the role and functional contribution made within the integrated plan of clinical activities for each patient. Such a process makes it easier to determine the aggregated costs of service and, ultimately, break out the individual costs contributed by each discipline. In any given clinical circumstance, this percentage of contribution will be different. When the data are collected and analyzed, the normative distribution of time and service will emerge, thereby enabling the percentage of cost allocation associated with that distribution to be normalized.

While nursing must clearly delineate its own specific functions and activities, the importance attached to those functions and activities is not gained unilaterally. The value of enumerating specific professional clinical function finds form only when those data are collected and integrated with the clinical activities of other associated disciplines within the context of DRGs. However, integration of the data first requires a clear determination of the component contribution. It is here where nursing's work is recognized as most important. In fact, it is at the level of component contribution that each discipline has specific work. Each discipline must meet five specific performance expectations before clinical integration can result in financial valuing.

1. A specific determination of professionally delineated task and performance expectations that define the unique contributions of the discipline
2. A clear enumeration of the gross cost factors associated with the human resource and functional elements of the work of the discipline
3. A clear indication of the discipline's specific and unique contribution to the clinical outcome expectations within specified patient populations
4. An ability to clearly articulate, in language that is understood and agreed upon by other disciplines, the specific performance contributions of each discipline
5. A willingness and ability to engage in dialogue and intersect with other disciplines to build an aggregated clinical framework for specific protocols and clinical processes that best represent the contribution of each discipline to the needs of specific patient populations

Nursing will have an especially difficult time in meeting the obligations of discipline-specific definitions. The challenges for nursing derive from its historical commitment to the process and its lack of a clearly defined relationship to clinical outcomes. The more valuable activity for nursing in undertaking this process will be to assess the time commitments related to coordinating, integrating, and facilitating the clinical work of all the disciplines, and then assign a specific value to that time and effort. Important to this process, which will put nursing farther along the road to adoption of an evidence-based format, is attention to the following factors:

- Establishing a clear value for the nonfunctional clinical activities related to nursing performance
- Enumerating the type and character of coordinative and integrative activities fundamental to the role of the nurse
- Locating and articulating the value of nursing performance in the identified nonfunctional processes with the intersection management activities associated with nursing
- Specifically identifying those particular clinical practice standards and professional performance characteristics against which value can be established, so the outcomes indicated by them can be more clearly defined
- Distinguishing between the generic standards of practice that address activities of the profession as a whole and those clinical standards that are specific to services, procedures, or patients
- Creating a method (formula) for determining costs and value related specifically to the clinical and coordinative activities undertaken at the point of service that reflects the standard of practice identified there

Each of these initiatives is essential for nursing (and every discipline) and accounts for one part of the drive to identify nurses' technical, relational, and coordinative functions in the course of delivering patient care. Included in this process should be those team-based activities and expectations that also incorporate issues of time and relationship influencing patient outcomes and that ultimately affect the financial value assigned to this process. Attaching financial value to the various roles and functions is the last stage of the preliminary activities of ascertaining units of value. When the discipline-specific contributions can be identified and the specific values more clearly enumerated, the aggregation and analysis of that information can provide a clear service value within a particular patient population or DRG.

To clearly delineate value, it is crucial to utilize the prevailing methodology, which uses payment factors as a part of value determination. Perhaps the most obvious unit of value is the DRG, the predominant value unit that is used for payment in healthcare organizations. Evidence-based practice processes driving the formulation of protocols, standards, or best practices should be designed in such a way that they fit the DRG format for payment. Simply because this format is already well defined, the DRG alignment approach to clinical valuing would be useful. Of course, nothing in evidence-based practice would *require* a DRG-based process to be the sole viable approach. No matter which approach is ultimately identified and used, it must be consistent, be reducible to financial value, integrate and link the contributions of the healthcare disciplines, and be useful as an evaluative and comparative mechanism. In addition, it should provide an opportunity to evaluate the criteria, performance, and impact of medical practice.

CREATING AN ENVIRONMENT FOR PRACTICE

In addition to establishing simple and direct values for nursing, it is equally important to recognize the value in creating a relevant environment and climate for the practice of nursing. Evidence-based practice does not unfold in isolation of the context for practice. As health care shifts in radical ways, the environment and contextual framework for practice are shifting as well. Creating a healing environment for the patient in a fast-paced, short-term, highly technical frame of reference also calls for the creation of a work environment that makes it possible for nurses and other professionals to successfully render care in a different model for patient service (Institute of Medicine, Committee on Quality of Health Care in America, & NetLibrary, 2001).

This goodness-of-fit issue between the built (or physical) environment and practice is as critical to the success of practice as clarity around the elements and the protocol are for care delivery. Gone are the days when environmental design included utilities and services at one end of a very long hallway, with patients needing care at the opposite end of this same hall. Also gone are the cold, sterile, and colorless environments that did not lend support to their impact on the healing process (Ulrich, Quan, Zimring, Joseph, & Choudhary, 2004).

Environments are now a critical element of the care dynamic itself—not only for patients, but also for providers. Creating a management and leadership environment characterized by engagement, openness, and valuing of the clinical provider is a key aspect of creating an appropriate supporting structure. Other elements related to the creation of a positive work environment and increased productivity relate to the building, structural format, color, inclusion of nature, and peaceful aesthetics. All of these factors help create a viable milieu within which to work (Ulrich et al., 2004).

The conditions of stress embedded in clinical work during a highly transforming time and equally fast-paced clinical environment have a tremendous impact on retention and turnover in clinical practice (Eberhardt, Szigeti, & University of North Dakota, 1990). Clearly, a cost–benefit analysis and review of the relationship between personal satisfaction in the exercise of clinical work and the structural environment within which it unfolds are important corollaries to supporting evidence with regard to the influence of environment. Nevertheless, simply factoring in the fatigue and support issues associated with environment and the practitioner is not sufficient to address the financial and economic concerns (King & Hinds, 2003). The Center for Health Design's Pebble Project Model goes beyond this level to address issues including the desirability of the environment for the patient, the market value of a healing environment to the community, and the fiscal impact of reducing length of stay, care intensity, and patient need. According to this model, creating a physical environment that facilitates healing is important as other influences on cost (Berry, Parker, Coile, Hamilton, O'Neill, & Sadler, 2004).

Furthermore, when measuring productivity and resource use, the contextual circumstances must be included in the value determination. Historical work studies and other resource measurements in nursing and clinical practice have provided ample evidence dealing with the impact of environment, structure, and support systems as it relates to the generation of clinical costs and the distribution of a clinician's time (Rice, 2000). Finding a balance between these variables, determining the financial specifics and considerations related to their effects, and incorporating these factors into the variable cost determination is an important methodology for ensuring the full consideration of resource use and all associated costs.

Yet another concern with regard to economic and financial value is the need for further refinements of data that lead to an increased understanding of the relationship between environment and provider risk, clinical error, and personal health and safety (Child, Institute of Medicine, Board on Health Care Services, Committee on the Work Environment for Nurses and Patient Safety, & NetLibrary, 2004). Certainly, a host of considerations must be taken into account in regard to the work environment and its impact on risk and safety from both providers' and patients' perspectives. These issues also exert a powerful effect on the cost of providing service as well as the ability to create an environment that establishes a marketable relationship between the organization and those whom it serves. Much evidence supports the existence of a close relationship between environmental issues of safety and clinical error rates. As a consequence, fiscal and service leaders should be able to make a clear distinction of the costs associated with these environmental and structural factors. Also, these factors should be incorporated into any of the data analysis related to productivity and work value determinations.

At a minimum, the environmental considerations are critical to establish evidence of the environment's influence on clinical practice as well as economics and health service costs. In building a contextual evidence-based framework for these environmental influences, the following issues should be considered:

- Identification of specific healing, comfort, and patient satisfaction considerations related to the physical environment and structural context for care
- Delineation of the structural and organizational (delivery system) considerations affecting clinical practice and specific elements of workflow
- Enumeration of the impact of physical plant, environment, and structures on provider attitudes, satisfaction, and turnover rates
- Determination of the impact of environment and structure on issues of clinical error, patient safety, and circumstances of care
- Incorporation of structural and environmental considerations in productivity measures and formulas associated with appropriate resource use and service time values

Development of an evidence-based framework to determine optimal productivity, patient–staff ratios, clinical assignments, and provider categories is now fundamental to efforts to accurately determine value and its effects on quality and cost (Harrington & Estes, 2004). Indeed, the accuracy of the financial data pertaining to the clinical relationship between patient and provider is now an essential construct of an appropriate, meaningful, and sustainable delivery of clinical services. Failing to include these environmental and structural considerations in the determination of productivity and clinical care not only contributes to a lack of cost control, but also facilitates the inappropriate and possibly expensive use of unevaluated human resources.

BUILDING AN EVIDENCE-BASED FRAMEWORK

Many workload management systems are now attempting to address the management and control of nursing resources. The attempt to objectively validate the distribution of staff based on the needs of care is clearly a critical measurement when defining the appropriate use of the clinical resource. Even so, simply looking at nursing actions and activities without reflecting on the wider number of variables cannot accurately or adequately establish the evidence of their value, nor can it build a frame of reference upon which value determination can be sustained. In fact, most workload management systems for nursing have not accurately and adequately incorporated the financial and economic values of nurses' contributions from the perspective of process, structure, or outcome. Many workload management systems measure only process (time and motion) (American Nurses Association [ANA], 2000).

It is clear that to ensure effective resource management, workload systems must be transformed into evidence-based systems and reflect a prevailing and sustaining reality (ANA, 2008). At a minimum, the following should be accomplished:

- Clearly delineate the foundations, standards, and protocols for clinical practice that relate to specific populations, DRGs, or other generally acceptable methods of patient service measurement and payment
- Link and integrate workload systems within an interdisciplinary set of standards or protocols that provide a comprehensive delineation of clinical service to the patient
- Incorporate issues of levels of expectations for clinical competence, differentiation between levels of provider, and clearly delineated performance expectations for specific patient populations or DRGs
- Obtain a more clear and strident incorporation of the structural and environmental cost factors associated with delivery of care
- Include the organizational and operational variables affecting the structure and process of care, especially those factors of the administrative infrastructure that affect the cost of delineating service
- Connect the financial, accounting, and budgeting processes of the organization to workload management and resource allocation within the context of specific clinical protocols or DRGs
- Develop, refine, and maintain a clinical resource information infrastructure for real-time data related to acuity, patient demand, resource allocation, clinical standards or protocols, structural and environmental considerations, and a continuous and effective reporting mechanism
- Be able to adjust staffing and resource allocation related to specific clinical standards, protocols, or DRG delineations in real time as the patient's condition requires

For an effective evidence-based workload management framework to unfold, these issues must be specifically and clearly addressed. Furthermore, an integrated regional and national approach must begin to emerge in relationship to the specific appropriate measures, protocols, and standards that are applied as well as the structural and environmental considerations that are included in a workload/resource management model.

From an evidence-based practice perspective, what may be helpful when more clearly articulating nursing's value within an economic framework is the joining of interdisciplinary activities under the rubric of an integrated clinical standard of practice. Using an objective payment-related structure (such as the DRG) can provide a contextual framework within which all of the various clinical disciplines can identify their contributions to the frame of reference for specific patient care protocols or processes. It is this linkage and integration among the disciplines that will create the composite framework for value determination. The evidence of impact on patient outcome, the viability of clinical process, and the cost framework that supports clinical practice can be more clearly elucidated when the disciplines speak the same language and use a common framework. Until that time, however, focusing on effective nursing workload management and creating an integrated structure for valuing that work will be critical first steps toward valuing nursing practice, establishing its relationship to financial and payment concerns, and providing a baseline with which nursing resource value can be connected across the interdisciplinary healthcare network.

A MODEL FOR THE FUTURE

Given the complexity and inadequacies of the current measurement systems for the work of nursing caregivers, healthcare leaders are duly challenged to create more appropriate systems. The purpose of creating a new clinical productivity model is not to more accurately represent the work of nursing as we now know it, but rather to create a new mindset that moves leaders from expecting adequate numbers of nurses to focusing on achieving adequate patient care outcomes within the existing healthcare structure and resources. Six strategies are essential steps in the creation of a more contemporary model:

- Reframing the measurement of healthcare services
- Describing the work of nursing
- Quantifying the work of nursing in an economic model that is linked to patient outcomes
- Embedding the new measures within existing systems
- Evaluating performance in an aggregated model
- Managing the variance or system feedback to ensure system sustainability

Reframe the Measurement of Healthcare Services

New models that embrace and reflect the reality of nursing patient-care services, focusing on the holistic and dynamic human condition with associated scientific, societal, and economic factors, will improve the ability of leaders to manage resources from an evidence-based perspective. In this model, the first consideration is to reconcile the separation of nursing science and nurse caring. Nursing science, which is easily represented within the economic and clinical aspects of health care, and the socially valued and essential caring dimension of nursing, which is not as easily quantified, must be inexorably linked and integrated into the economic system.

The first and most difficult step for healthcare leaders is not only to admit that the current system is not working, but also to have the courage to do something about it. Patient care services continue to evolve in a technologically savvy and humanistic environment, even as the measurement of these services remains embedded in basic linear principles of "cause and effect" based on the industrial manufacturing model. The work of nursing is ill suited for the assembly-line "widget" model for several specific reasons: the nonlinear work of nursing; the frequent overlapping of tasks or multitasking; interruptions from providers, families, and other patients in need of care; and the unpredictable patient priorities for pain, elimination, and nutrition. These realities of patient care require a model that embraces all of these challenges. A new model that views and measures the work of patient care as an aggregated whole rather than as a series of disconnected tasks better represents the work of nursing in a much simpler way.

This new model also must integrate the achievement of clinical outcomes resulting from the services provided, the number of hours of care for the service, and the level of provider required to achieve these outcomes. Further, the effects of this integration are reflected in the patient care value equation in which resources, outcomes, and value are examined and evaluated, forming the philosophical foundation for a new, aggregated productivity model.

Leaders will necessarily need to modify expectations as they shift their focus from the number of hours or the quantity of work to an aggregation of resources used, resulting outcomes, and perceived value obtained. The clinical productivity model is necessarily different for nonclinical areas that do not experience the interruptions, family needs, and unpredictable patient needs for elimination, food, and comfort. Issues of multitasking are common to all employees. A new model must also include expectations for accessing real-time data using computerized systems to guide processes of care and providing information to support process modifications in a timely manner to ensure optimal patient safety. Common definitions specific to workload management are listed in **Table 8-1**.

Table 8-1   Common Definitions of Nursing Workload Management

Term	Definition
Labor productivity	A measure of output divided by input; the number of units of production per hour of workload (Meyers & Stewart, 2002).
Nursing productivity (traditional definition)	Ratio of output (patient-care hours per patient-day) to input (paid salary and benefit dollars) (O'Brien-Pallas et al., 2004).
Nursing work	Includes attention to the full range of human experiences and responses to health and illness without restriction to a problem-focused orientation; integration of objective data with knowledge gained from an understanding of the patient or group's subjective experience; application of scientific knowledge to the processes of diagnosis and treatment; and provision of a caring relationship that facilitates health and healing (ANA, 2003).
Patient care workload	Number of patients assigned to one nurse in a specific time frame (i.e., 6 patients assigned to 1 nurse for this shift).
Staffing variance	Number of hours required for care that differs from those available hours of staff.
Value	Relative worth or importance (*Merriam-Webster's Collegiate Dictionary*, 2002).
Work	Effort or exertion directed to produce or accomplish something (*Merriam-Webster's Collegiate Dictionary*, 2002).
Workload	The amount of work that a machine, employee, or group of employees can be or is expected to perform (*Merriam-Webster's Collegiate Dictionary*, 2002).

Describe the Work of Nursing

The second consideration of the model is the work of nursing, which is described by many nurses as "providing quality nursing care"—a general and qualitative description of the service that has no quantification. Others who do not understand the work of nursing may wonder if nursing is necessary given this vague and subjective description. Recent publications (Aiken, Clark, Cheung, Sloane, & Silber, 2003; Aiken, Clark, Sloane, Sochalski, & Silber., 2002; Buerhaus, Donelan, Ulrich, Norman, DesRoches, & Dittus 2007; Kane, Shamliyan, Mueller, Duval, & Wilt, 2007; Lang, Hodge, & Olson, 2004; Needleman et al., 2002; Savitz, Jones, & Bernard, 2005; Tourangeau, Cranley, & Jeffs, 2006; Upenieks, Akhavan, Kotlerman, Esser, & Ngo, 2007; White, 2006) have shown that better outcomes resulted from provision of nursing care, whereas poor outcomes and patient deaths resulted from the lack of nurses.

What is also lacking is the linkage between identified and specific interventions of the nurse and the health of people. The work of nursing requires objective descriptions to embed it in current healthcare measurement structures, and to link these services provided with value-based outcomes that do, indeed, affect the quality of health. The description also requires recognition and integration of a societal mandate for nursing, the professional scope of practice, and the economic realities of the marketplace. A qualitative, descriptive overview of the work of nursing must include more than tasks that are easily observed and quantified, such as procedures and administration of medications.

Examination of nursing from the opposite side of the outcome—namely, from the time before nursing occurred or in the absence of nursing as it is now known—is both illustrative and enlightening to assist in the description of nursing. When nursing is absent, it is not merely medications that are not administered and dressings that are not changed; much more occurs. What is lost is subtle at first, and then overwhelmingly thunderous. Patients are not monitored regularly for condition changes; failure to rescue is common and emergency codes occur; condition changes are not communicated to physicians; care is not coordinated; patient knowledge is not improved; and measures of preventable conditions, such as pressure ulcers, urinary tract infections, pneumonia, and length of stay, all increase.

In general, the core dimensions of the work of nursing are both physical and cognitive (Squires, 2004). These dimensions include the following components:

- Skill performance/task management that represents the technical work of nursing. Examples include patient assessment, medication administration, intravenous access and line management, pain management, safety or restraint management, and interpretation of vital signs. Note that the focus and information needed for productivity management systems are the specific interventions of the nurse rather than a description of the patient's condition. For example, identifying a "combative patient" as work to be done does not provide objective and measurable information for a clinical productivity system. In contrast, identifying the "application of restraints and assessment every 15 minutes" provides the required information for a valid productivity system.

- Monitoring progress and oversight of patient conditions. These tasks include acting as the eyes and ears of physicians to prevent or manage crises.
- Evidence from the intersection management or interdisciplinary coordination of work of nursing. These responsibilities include creating and modifying plans of care in a timely manner based on patient conditions, prioritizing through analysis and synthesis of information, and coordinating the work of all disciplines caring for the patient. The work of nursing is distinct, but necessarily embedded in an interconnected multidisciplinary model. Advocating for the patient is an integral component of interdisciplinary coordination.
- Information management. This component includes knowing not only what to communicate, but also to whom and when to communicate. It incorporates patient and family education as well as information management among members of the caregiver team.
- Leadership behaviors specific to the delegation and supervision of work processes. These behaviors include skilled performance management of other staff and precepting new nurses.
- Relationship management, including monitoring and modifying behaviors and personalities of team members. Nurses are deeply entrenched in daily processes of relationship management with all patient-care team members (e.g., physicians, nurses, managers, allied health personnel, and unlicensed assistive personnel). Experience and collective wisdom emerge from team members who work together effectively.

Eliminate Non-Value-Added Work

In addition to describing the work of nursing, it is important to identify the current work of nursing that does not improve patient outcomes or provide value to the equation of care. Necessarily, the work of nursing must be integrated into the value equation in which resources and outcomes are essential elements. Providing a service merely because one is competent to perform a procedure is unacceptable when it does not add any measurable value to the health status of the patient. The work of nursing is about providing appropriate goal-oriented services rather than providing as many services as possible, irrespective of the cost and outcomes. Wise choices—rather than rich choices—for care that take into account fiscal implications, appropriateness of nursing care specific to outcomes, and goodness of fit, service quality, and patient impact are needed. Unfortunately, the elimination of non-value-added work may be as difficult and challenging as it is to describe the work of nursing.

In Hill-Rom's study of acute care organizations, approximately 85% of nurses' time was spent on direct and indirect activities that did not move the patient along the care path (Lanser, 2001). Murphy (2003) reported that wasteful work—including excessive documentation requirements, inefficient shift-to-shift or departmental reports, and searching for colleagues, supplies, and equipment—consumed 35% of hospital employees' time. These significant percentages of non-value-added work are cause for both concern and further study. The challenge in identifying the truly valued work is coupled with the reality that evidence is lacking to support some interventions that may, indeed, positively affect patient outcomes.

To be sure, nurses find it quite difficult to give up any of their current nursing work because all work is believed to be valuable and appropriate. In fact, the phenomenon of not being able to give up work that is believed valued is not unique to nursing. In a *Harvard Business Review* article, Johnson (2002) noted that time is always the scarcest commodity—no one ever has enough—and that quality of work suffers as a result of this lack of time.

Another explanation for this phenomenon offered by Johnson is thought provoking. The following hypothetical situation was posed to hundreds of managers, with most of them believing they already lacked the time to do their jobs properly:

> A supervisor asks an employee if he or she is interested in taking on a special project. The project is of strategic importance and will provide major growth opportunities. The offer has one catch, however: The assignment is part-time and requires one day per week, which would require the individual to do the current job in four days rather than five days.

Ninety-nine percent of the managers took on the assignment. These managers admitted that if the motivation was powerful enough, they could eliminate or do in much less time eight to ten hours of activities each week without negative consequences.

Would the same thing occur if nurses were given the opportunity to participate in creating a new clinical service? Could nurses in such a scenario evaluate the value of their work more critically? Would giving up work actually yield untold benefits for nursing?

To begin the challenging process of eliminating non-value-added work, nurses must examine the specific nursing work that has been identified on the basis of core dimensions, professional standards, and nurse practice acts. Asking questions such as "Do we need this work at all?" or "Is some work duplicative or redundant?," nurses should create multiple lists of tasks to be completed and things not to do anymore. Systematically and rigorously identifying and eliminating those activities that are extraneous to achieving goals will further contribute to organizational effectiveness. At the same time, eliminating interventions or work that has uncertain value without careful examination is inappropriate and can negatively affect outcomes. Structured and rigorous methods are necessary to ensure continuing improvement in credible identification of nursing work that is based on principles of evidence-based practice. This effort must incorporate the best research, clinical expertise, and values of the individual members of the profession.

Non-value-added work includes both direct and indirect nursing work as well as work resulting from system inefficiencies. The following examples identify tasks that do not provide value to patient outcomes:

- Provision of patient education to those patients who are historically noncompliant. It is unrealistic to expect that an 80-year-old diabetic patient will become enlightened and change his or her behaviors. Extensive reviews and presentation of information in these situations serve only to complete checklists and provide inappropriate feelings of accomplishment. Brief, meaningful encounters with known noncompliant patients are necessary to check for new interest, however. In the value equation, unrealistic interventions render the equation out of balance given the lack of outcomes and overuse of scarce resources associated with these efforts.
- Frequency of vital signs. When a patient has consistent and stable vital signs, is it still necessary to repeat these measures every four hours, especially since caregivers are present who can monitor the patient?
- Telemetry monitoring. Is all telemetry monitoring value based? Is the intervention of telemetry monitoring linked to improvements in the patient's status and effective use of available resources?
- Searching for equipment. Does this task promote the patient's movement along the healing continuum?
- Searching for supplies. Is this an appropriate task for nurses?
- Passing out meal trays. Is this the best use of a nurse's time? Should someone from another division handle this task?
- Searching for other providers and colleagues. Is this an appropriate task for nurses?
- Replenishing procedure carts; monitoring levels in supply rooms. Do these activities directly affect the patient?
- Searching for information and reference manuals. Can this task be managed differently?

Improvements that focus on the elimination of non-value-added work and increase productivity include computerized electronic health records, technology for communication, pocket reference guides, personal digital assistants, and pocket-sized hand sanitizer packets. Elimination of non-value-added work provides more time for nurses to comfort and talk with patients, develop and update plans of care, and provide patient and family education—all types of work that are typically foregone when time is scarce.

Standardized Language

Another expectation is the use of standardized language, which requires that the interventions of nursing must be specified and described with sufficient clarity that another researcher or practitioner can replicate the action. Standardized language comprises terminology and communication styles that can be used in all settings by all clinicians, is grounded in clinical practice and research, is functionally appropriate for computerized clinical documentation systems that need to simplify the exchange, and makes it easier to manage and integrate clinical data into the electronic health record. The language must allow for the measurement of patient, family, and community healthcare interventions and outcomes (Moorhead, Johnson, & Maas, 2004).

Expected Nursing Outcomes

The evidence supporting a relationship between caregiver performance, patient outcomes, and financial performance is strong (Aiken, Clark, Cheung, Sloane, & Silber, 2003; Aiken, Smith, & Lake, 1994; Blegen & Vaughn, 1998; Cho et al., 2003; McCue, Mark, & Harless, 2003). Evidence supporting the relationships between variables in the organizational structure and patient outcomes has been also identified. Unfortunately, the intervening specific work processes that produce those outcomes have not been clearly articulated, nor are they embedded in the analysis of these relationships.

Once the work of nursing is described, its linkage to patient outcomes and available resources must be established. The value equation in which clinical practice, performance outcomes, and the available payment structure are examined serves as a template to assess the overall value of the nursing work. Desirable outcomes of nursing interventions include achievement of clinical goals, improvement in the ability to manage one's own health, and a safe environment as measured by the absence of adverse outcomes. Examples of outcomes specific to nursing that affect not only the patient, but also the conditions that influence a patient's health, include the following:

- Increased ability to provide self-care
- Improved mobility
- Improved stress management and coping skills
- Improved knowledge of clinical condition
- Improved knowledge of healthy behaviors specific to nutrition and mobility
- Improved parenting skills
- Community health/well-being
- Improved knowledge of behaviors for safety specific to health care

Historically, healthcare leaders have believed that it is impossible to objectively quantify the clinical, social, and caring work of nursing in an aggregate manner, while simultaneously obtaining objective and reliable data. However, the process of quantifying and enumerating the work of nursing must be embraced if we are to develop valid and reliable information that will serve to increase the visibility and value of nursing within the healthcare environment. This effort will, in turn, provide credibility within the financial sectors of health care. Responding to this challenge is required for the advancement of the profession.

Computerized Nursing Information

The ability to readily access information using powerful software, which incorporates easy data input capabilities, necessarily improves the consistent and standardized collection and measurement of patient information. Systems to support documentation of interventions, achievement of patient goals, the time and skill mix of caregivers required to achieve those goals, and examination of the relationship of these variables are essential. This documentation provides critical information that links the economic viability of the organization with resources, outcomes, and value-based service; the satisfaction levels of nursing personnel; and the performance of nursing using evidence-based interventions.

Context in Which Nursing Work Occurs

As discussed in Chapter 4, the work environment—that is, the conditions in which nursing care is provided—significantly influences patient outcomes. Information specific to the location, physical environment, organizational culture, operational structure, technology, and availability of support services is necessary to determine those conditions in which nursing interventions are (or are not) effective. Pinkerton and Rivers (2001), for example, identified 64 variables that affect nurse staffing needs, including variables specific to interdepartmental interactions, intradepartmental interactions, the care environment, professional competency, physicians, and the external environment.

The high level of complexity of nursing work requires appropriate systems to assess and integrate measures of the multiple variables, including actual nurse-work hours and context variables for a credible clinical productivity system. Five major variables contribute to the complexity of system processes and the achievement of desired outcomes: the physical environment, the organizational culture, the operational structure, technology, and support systems. **Table 8-2** summarizes the six categories of context variables, which are discussed in detail next.

Table 8-2   Aggregated Productivity Measurements of Context Variables

Physical Environment	Organizational Culture	Operational Structure	Technology	Systems	Support
Single-bed rooms	Shared leadership	Point-of-care decision making	Electronic health record, fully interfaced programs	Messenger	
Noise control	Physician–nurse collaboration	Expert resources: hospitalists/advanced practice nurses		Computerized physician order entry	Transportation
Hand-washing dispensers	Values of respect, accountability, and healing	Decentralized pharmacists	Clinical documentation	Pharmacy	
Patient lift system	Bilingual/multilingual associates	Adequate staffing	Electronic medication administration record		
Medication preparation rooms	Community partnership	Management tools to evaluate work processes and outcomes	Scanning system		
Family space					
Ergonomic workstations		Patient classification system			
Adequate lighting and ventilation					

Physical Environment   A range of design characteristics—such as single versus double rooms, reduced noise, improved lighting, better ventilation, more ergonomic designs, workplaces that better support tasks, and improved layout—can be used to reduce errors, reduce stress, improve sleep, reduce pain and drugs, and improve other outcomes. Compelling scientific evidence from more than 600 studies amply demonstrates that design affects both staff and clinical outcomes (Ulrich et al., 2004). When the design supports clinical practice processes, patient healing in a stress-minimizing environment and worker productivity should increase dramatically.

Organizational Culture   Commitment to behaviors and values that support and expect shared leadership, nurse–physician collaboration, therapeutic relationships, and visible accountability for these behaviors positively affects caregiver work processes. Evidence continues to emerge supporting the relationships between behaviors and values of healing, and respect and accountability, with more efficient and effective processes (Neuhauser, 2002).

Operational Structure   The structure of the organization—namely, its decision-making processes, types of caregivers, skill mix percentages, and availability of expert resources such as hospitalists and advanced practice nurses—clearly actualizes the mission and vision of the organization as well as supports the desired organizational culture and work of caregivers. Unit-based management tools to examine patient care quality, processes, outcomes, and costs are also essential operational tools that support first-time, effective decision making in a timely manner.

Technology   The challenges of time and distance are disappearing with the advent of computer-enabled healthcare delivery and information systems that have been reconfigured to be available virtually everywhere (Ligon & Das, 2004). The availability of electronic, computerized, and integrated systems for patient care is believed to decrease the use of labor resources and increase the quality of organizational outcomes. Consideration must be given to the impact of the electronic health record, computerized physician order entry, physiologic monitoring, electronic medication administration records, scanning capabilities, and integration (or lack of integration) of these systems when determining the productivity measure. Wide variations in the availability of technology may be found not only among organizations, but also among departments within a particular organization.

Support Systems   The presence of support systems for clinical caregivers directly affects the ability of nurses to perform the work of nursing. These support systems include the availability of pharmacy, housekeeping, transportation, and messenger services on a 24/7 basis. The lack of or partial availability of support resources historically has resulted in nurses adding nonclinical tasks to their workload, which in turn decreases their clinical productivity.

Quantify the Work of Nursing in an Economic Model

The third step in creating a model for the future is to quantify the value-based work of nursing identified in the second step of the process. In addition, this quantification must consider the impact of the five contextual variables—that is, the physical environment, organizational culture, operational structure, technology, and support systems. The purpose of quantification is to develop information to extend the current productivity system that identifies the direct link between the evidence-based work of caregivers, patient outcomes, and payment. Necessarily, this effort requires quantification of (1) the specific work and (2) the link or relationship of the work to the achievement of desired patient outcomes. The health status of the patient must be affected positively to justify the resource expenditure.

The historical adequacy of the overarching position of medicine and its specific measures of procedural-based coding and billing have precluded the need for more accurate clinical productivity measures for nursing that are quantifiable, credible, and useful. Unfortunately, development of appropriate measures for nursing work tend to garner attention only during times of nursing shortage and nursing dissatisfaction.

Organizations today may struggle to control costs through cost reductions associated with the poorly defined work of nursing, yet the need for competently educated practitioners remains significant. Despite the increases in nursing education and the increasing complexity of nursing work, clarity in the work of nursing and appropriate workload measures have not emerged to achieve the desired recognition of the value of nursing work in the marketplace. Because it is poorly defined and described, nursing work is difficult to measure and evaluate, which too often results in uncertain patient outcomes. When attempts are made to decrease or increase nursing resources for work that is poorly defined, the effects of these measures on patient outcomes is uncertain as well. While it is believed that less nursing care results in poor patient outcomes, such conclusions are not universally supported. The lack of evidence identifying the specific interventions of nursing and their implications for patient outcomes must be addressed. Tallying simple hours of care, without delineating the actual work performed, will not produce data that can be confidently correlated to patient outcomes, whether those outcomes are positive or negative. Describing the work of nursing from an evidence-based perspective is the first step in the process; the second step, integrating these principles into practice, is evolutionary and ongoing.

Nurses' monitoring, integrating, and evaluating roles need to be captured adequately in a more appropriate clinical productivity system. The summative list of tasks based on the manufacturing model of work has not traditionally encompassed these processes. Clear and quantifiable information is needed that identifies the specific amount of nursing work performed by a specific level of caregiver, and the resulting quantifiable patient outcomes.

Aggregating Care for Quantification

The historical inadequacy of summative task workload calculations can be improved upon by using an aggregated or comprehensive workload unit approach to measure patient care; the latter approach better represents the essence of the work of nursing. The comprehensive unit of service (CUS) captures the nonlinear nature of nursing practice, the routine multitasking, and frequent interruptions. A CUS is developed using expert opinion or expert panel methodology for determining workload time and skill mix standards. Specifically, a panel of experts—individuals with a great deal of experience and the ability to estimate time in their area of expertise—identifies the time requirements. This consensus approach uses professional judgment to assess staff, which provides a flexible means of evaluation that is focused on a critical review of nursing practice, staffing, and the utilization of both supply and demand information (Dunn, Norby, Cournoyer, Hudec, O'Donnell, & Snider, 1995). Service work and one-of-a-kind jobs make setting time standards with more traditional techniques cost-prohibitive. Even though some workers never do the same thing twice, goals are still needed.

An expert is necessary to estimate the aspects of every job and to maintain a log of estimations. The "best estimation" technique is a low-cost, fast, and initially acceptable way of quantifying information using estimation and self-reporting techniques. The "expert opinion" technique attempts to remedy the criticism of the inability of the work sampling technique to capture professional judgment required in health care (Dunn et al., 1995). Because sampling can easily become biased and does not always reflect current conditions, it is considered reliable only if the results obtained approximate the results generated by experts.

In health care, the expert panel approach has been used to create a CUS as the foundational workload unit of measure for the Expert Nurse–Patient Classification System (Malloch & Conovoloff, 1999). Experienced nurses create workload standards from a comprehensive perspective of the work performed; expert nurses compile the nurse interventions provided to a patient for an entire shift or event, and identify the time required to provide this care as a unit rather than as summation of tasks. This approach integrates the multitasking processes employed by nurses and avoids the risk of double counting any tasks.

Typically, the expert panel consists of nurses who practice in clinical, educational, research, and administrative roles, such as experienced staff nurses, clinical nurse specialists, nurse managers, and associate nurse executives. The members of this panel collaborate to estimate the amount of time and level of caregiver (skill mix) required to provide the total care in the CUS.

Consider the following care situation representing one shift of patient care. The patient is totally dependent on others for physical care, has difficulty communicating, is unable to identify pain, and is hemodynamically unstable; also, the patient's Spanish-speaking family is having difficulty with the current full code status. An expert panel of nurses reviewed these care needs and determined the appropriate skill mix and hours of care needed as the standard for this type of care (**Table 8-3**); a total of 4.5 hours of care in a 12-hour shift was identified as being necessary.

Standardized Patient Classification Systems

Quantifying the work of nursing using a standardized approach to patient acuity is the foundation for a valid and reliable patient classification system, another important element of an evidence-based workload management system. The patient classification used by an organization must reflect the major clinical intervention categories applicable to all clinical specialties. At a minimum, categories specific to the technical work of nursing, monitoring activities, interdisciplinary coordination, communication, and leadership must be represented.

The nonreducible CUS, rather than the single task, when used as the unit of workload measurement better represents the work of nursing. The consistency in the description and quantification of caregiver interventions using the CUS serve as the foundational unit for constructing a valid and reliable clinical productivity management system. Further, computerization of the collection and management of these data reduces the variability and subjectivity in patient classification systems, which have historically been fraught with inconsistency and mistrust.

Multidisciplinary Units of Service

Extension of the nursing patient classification system to include all disciplines providing care further enhances the robustness of a clinical productivity system. The ideal workload management system is one in which the unit of service is multidisciplinary and patient specific for a defined period of time. All disciplines providing services are integrated and considered as a "multidisciplinary comprehensive unit of service" (MCUS). The work of each discipline can be identified on the basis of interventions and associated contributions to patient outcomes. The MCUS represents the integrated, interwoven

Table 8-3 Comprehensive Unit of Service: Complex Medical Patient

Category	Patient Needs	Caregiver Interventions
Cognitive status	Responds to name by opening eyes—no verbalization other than garbled phrases.	Assess and monitor cognitive status q 2 h.
Self-care	Totally dependent.	Provide total ADLs, hygiene and mobility; requires 2 persons.
Emotional/social/ spiritual	Minimal social interaction.	Provide emotional support q 6–8 h.
Comfort/pain management	Assess—but no indication of pain.	Assess and monitor non-self-reporting patient at least q 6–8 h.
Family information	Niece/spouse and others. Spanish-speaking, frequent visits.	Family conference re: code status. Requires q 4–6 h reinforcement of realistic expectations; support through interpreter at least q 2 h.
Treatments and interventions	Hemodynamically unstable (mod.); respiratory failure; full code.	Dialysis, medications—IVP & IVPB q 2 h. Monitor ventilator status q 15 min. Titrate 3 drips; provide tracheotomy care.
Interdisciplinary coordination/ patient teaching and documentation	Change in code status.	Frequent communication with 4 services.
Transition needs	Patient not meeting goals.	Plan for family conference. Modify care plan.
Expert time estimation	**Total hours (12-hour shift) = 4.5 h**	**RN = 2.5 h** **LPN/LVN = 0.5 h** **NA = 1.5 h**

contributions of associated disciplines such as physical therapy, respiratory therapy, and social services.

An example of a MCUS is provided in **Table 8-4**, which illustrates the quantification of patient care for all contributing disciplines within a defined period of time. In this exemplar, the interventions of social workers and respiratory and physical therapists are integrated into workflow and processes along with the registered nurse (RN), licensed practical nurse (LPN), and nursing assistants. Using the expert panel method, experts determined that a total of 6.5 hours of care for all six disciplines was necessary. The appropriate percentage of the six disciplines is also identified in **Table 8-4**.

New Approach to Clinical Productivity

In a study on hospital nurse productivity, Eastaugh (2002) analyzed the impact of the current trend toward using nurse extenders or unlicensed personnel. Data from 37 hospitals using primary nursing staffs, all-RN staffs, and team nursing were compared. The study concluded that the tradition of 100% RN primary care nursing must be abandoned, given that it was the least productive and not affordable with the current funding limitations. A significant omission noted in this analysis, however, was that there was no mention or analysis of output or the patient outcomes specific to each delivery model. While the use of RNs' hours was the highest in the all-RN delivery model, more information is needed before such a broad conclusion can be drawn with confidence. It is possible that this model might prove the most economical over the long term if it truly reduces the incidence of nosocomial infections, patient falls, and medication errors.

Historically, the measurement of productivity has compared the resources used to the resources budgeted or hours used for each patient unit of service, without considering the specific work performed to achieve the results. Knowing which outcomes resulted from which work performed by which category of caregiver is critical if the profession is to effectively articulate its value and contribution to the health of individuals. Understanding the important relationships between specific work processes and integrating them into the productivity measurement systems of organizations will require new knowledge, new mental models, and commitment to staffing on the basis of evidence or trend data created from best practices.

Unfortunately, this approach and limited analysis have been used in most organizations to measure nurse productivity and to make decisions specific to the allocation of staffing resources. The hours used are typically compared to patient units of service without considering the actual output, which is an essential component of a productivity measure. These traditional productivity measures of "hours used per patient-day" represent a limited analysis and do

Table 8-4 Multidisciplinary Comprehensive Unit of Service: Complex Medical Patient

Category	Patient Needs	Caregiver Interventions
Cognitive status	Responds to name by opening eyes—no verbalization other than garbled phrases.	Assess and monitor cognitive status q 2 h.
Self-care	Totally dependent.	Provide total ADLs, hygiene, and mobility; requires 2 persons. Physical therapist assistance with range of motion.
Emotional/social/ spiritual	Minimal social interaction.	Provide emotional support q 6–8 h.
Comfort/pain	Assess—but no indication of pain.	Assess and monitor non-self-reporting patient at least q 6–8 h.
Family information	Niece/spouse and others. Spanish-speaking, frequent visits.	Family conference re: code status.
		Requires q 4–6 hour reinforcement of realistic expectations; support through interpreter at least q 2 h.
Treatments and interventions	Hemodynamically unstable (mod.); respiratory failure; full code.	Dialysis, medications—IVP and IVPB q 2 h. Monitor ventilator status q 15 min. Titrate 3 drips; provide tracheotomy care; respiratory therapy, management of ventilator.
Interdisciplinary coordination/ patient teaching and documentation	Change in code status.	Frequent communication with 4 services.
		Social worker communication for 1 h.
Transition needs	Patient not meeting goals.	Plan for family conference. Modify care plan.
Expert time estimation	**Total hours (12-hour shift) = 6.5 h**	**RN = 2.5 h Social worker = 1.25 h** **LPN = 0.5 h Physical therapist = 0.25 h** **NA = 1.5 h Respiratory therapist = 0.50 h**

not reflect the notion of theoretical productivity, which calls for the greatest output for the least input (Drucker, 1990).

Measurements that are limited to comparisons of total hours worked per patient-day and projected budgeted hours can only serve the financial analyst's purposes. Such comparisons provide no information specific to the level of patient acuity, provision of appropriate interventions, achievement of clinical outcomes, and absence of adverse outcomes—all of which require a framework for productivity measurement based on principles that integrate values of effectiveness, utility, and cost. Productivity measurement that reflects and supports the position and complex production involved in the practice of nursing, rather than the functional efficiency comparison of hours worked to hours budgeted, is needed. Metrics that reflect the output of care as compared to the input of providers, and adjusted for environmental factors, provide a more accurate representation of nursing productivity.

Embed the Framework for Aggregated, Adjusted Productivity Measurement Within Existing Systems

The fourth consideration addresses the need for an aggregated productivity measurement that encompasses a combination of inputs and outputs, and that is expressed and examined in a matrix format rather than as a single productivity ratio calculated by comparing output to input. Current measurement and payment systems, while cumbersome and outdated, can serve as vehicles to create improved systems. Any consideration for modifications to existing systems should emphasize the need to improve the value of data and their utility to the healthcare system. Consistency of definitions, attribution of value to work processes specific to the mission of the organization and patient clinical status, and reimbursement specific to value rather than procedures performed should also drive any modifications.

The current metric of hours per patient-day identifies how long it took for the care to be delivered, but not what was done; it is an incomplete representation of the work of nursing (simplicity) that does not incorporate structural and environment considerations in productivity measures. Relative value unit (RVU) measures attempt to recognize the degree of patient care variation based on a median unit but are limited by the description of the value of 1.0 unit. The limited accuracy and completeness of describing the 1.0 RVU continues to be problematic, because descriptors for all categories of the core work of nursing are not included in this system.

The purpose of modifying current processes and measures is not to devalue the historical clinical productivity measurement, but rather to extend the existing productivity system to quantify the relationship between patient care services, value, and payment, and to adjust for those variables that influence the work of nursing. The Medicare payment system, International Classification of Diseases (ICD) codes, and other accepted billing and reimbursement models can be strengthened with additional principles and parameters.

To be sure, this work may prove challenging. Reengineering anything is a risk that requires knowledge of not only the desired state of improvement, but also the failures that one desires to correct. Successes provide confidence that something right is occurring, but not necessarily *why* it is right. Failures provide unquestionable proof that we have done something wrong. Creating new models for healthcare clinical labor productivity requires knowledge of the best features of effective existing processes and failures that have negatively influenced outcomes (**Table 8-5**).

Evaluate the Results

The fifth consideration is evaluation. As previously noted, the financial representation of nursing's throughput or interventions is best determined using the value equation consisting of a combination of quality, cost-effectiveness, and service. The value equation now serves as the vital unifier and clarifying link between service and cost (Malloch & Porter-O'Grady, 1999). All care providers must now be cognizant of the relationship between what they do, what it costs, and what is achieved as a result of having done it. Of course, the challenge remains to determine a good number for clinical productivity. Is there a single metric that is robust enough to reflect clinical productivity? If so, what is the number?

The continuing dilemma faced by healthcare organizations—the need to have adequate RN surveillance, yet remain cost-effective—begs the question as to what the ideal number of nurses per patient and the mix of caregivers should be for a given group of patients. Inadequate numbers of RNs lead to "failure to rescue" situations, and total RN staffing is not required for all types of patient care. The answer lies somewhere in between.

While adequate numbers of nurses are essential to avoid "failure to rescue" situations, specific patient information is needed to determine safe staffing. To be sure, as long as patients vary, the ratio of patients assigned to nurses will vary. But appropriate staffing encompasses more than the right number or ratio of nurses: It entails the right nurse doing the right things during the time available. Staffing ratios in which nurses are performing clerical services, finding equipment, and engaging in low-skill clinical activities seriously undermine the perceptions of staffing adequacy. To date, the ideal ratio of nurses to patients has not been identified; rather, a range of numbers of patients has been hypothesized for specific clinical areas (Curtin, 2003).

One hundred percent productivity requires homogeneity—that is, patients with the same disease, patients arriving at the same rate, providers equal in

Table 8-5   Clinical Productivity Evaluation Matrix

Input: Caregiver Hours of Care/Skill Mix	Input: Caregiver Actual Interventions	Required Hours of Care: Patient Acuity/Variance	Context: Variables/Adjustments	Output: Patient Clinical Outcomes	Output: Patient Safety Outcomes
RN	Assess and monitor	Plus or minus 5% comparing actual to patient classification needs.	Physical environment	Respiratory stability	Falls
LPN	Administer medications		Organizational culture	Knowledge of disease	Medication errors
NA	Insert IV line		Operational structure	Minimal medications	Nosocomial infections
Critical thinking	Patient education		Technology	Patient satisfaction	Medical errors
Certification	Assess and monitor		Support systems		
Advanced practice nurses	Family education and support				
Technicians	Coordinate care				
	Document care				

their ability to provide patient care, and families with the same level of knowledge and understanding. The most reasonable approach for operational decision making is longitudinal monitoring of productivity by organizational units combined with indicators of quality of patient care (O'Brien-Pallas et al., 2004). This care must be described, documented, and measured using a standardized patient classification system to support decisions that will support safe patient care. O'Brien-Pallas and colleagues identified 85% (± 5%) as the optimal nursing unit productivity, with 93% as the maximum productivity because 7% of the shift is made up of mandatory breaks.

Data analysis of nursing work using the best available evidence is an expected standard of practice. Several methods of economic evaluation may be considered for this purpose. Each method is based on specific goals (Stone, Curran, & Bakken, 2002) and includes the following:

- *Cost minimization:* Costs are compared between alternatives only. Equal effects are assumed. No outcomes are measured.
- *Cost-effectiveness:* Consequences are measured in the same units between alternatives. Outcomes are measured using ratios such as expenditures/outcome or dollars/life-year gained.
- *Cost utility:* Effects include both quantity and quality measures. Measures are dollars of quality of life-years gained.
- *Cost benefit:* Effects are measured as a single dollar measure. Measures are in dollars gained.
- *Cost consequences:* Costs and effects are listed separately. Effects between alternatives may have different measures. Expenditures and a separate list of outcomes are measured.

Each of these evaluation methods offers a different lens through which to view the work of nursing. Ultimately, a combination of several methods is likely to better represent nursing work based on the intended goals and resources.

Variance Management

The sixth and final consideration in the clinical productivity model of the future is variance management. The most significant information produced from any system is that specific to the variances—that is, the differences between the desired outcome and the actual outcome. Seldom is there a perfect match between what is desired and what actually results. The resulting variance between needs and resources reflects the reality of balancing the workload processes with the inherent expectations for reducing, eliminating, or managing these differences. It is this variance that provides the data from which to manage, monitor, and improve system performance. Merely counting and documenting the desired and actual outcomes does not provide any value for the system in outcome management. Instead, ensuring the accountability of the articulation and reporting of variance management is an essential unifying link in the process. Efforts to produce high levels of quality without devoting human or financial resources to those efforts is irrational and doomed to eliminate (destroy) the system. Effective evaluation processes lay the foundation for safe and timely management of the variance between what is desired and what actually occurs.

Leaders are continually challenged to consider variations in the known natural clinical variances of disease, levels of severity, patients' responses to treatment, variability in workflow due to random arrivals of patients, and inherent variability of clinicians in regard to their knowledge, critical thinking, prioritizing, and communication skills. According to Long (2002), the goal is to eliminate "artificial variance"—that is, clinical errors, medication errors, lack of knowledge, inappropriate scheduling, and scheduling based on staff needs rather than patient needs. Leaders should focus on managing the natural variation or the uncertain occurrence of care needs by patients, both predicted and unpredicted, and the inherent professional differences in ability.

"System variances" result in high and low levels of workload, characterized by frequent internal diversions of patients to other units, backups in the post-anesthesia care unit, external diversions from the emergency department, staff overload, and increased length of stay as a consequence of system gridlock. When a system variance is identified, the following management practices are appropriate:

- Delineate protocols and link their required interventions to desired outcomes.
- Create a framework to examine performance standards.
- Define the linkage between interventions, best practice, and payment formats.
- Continue to monitor, evaluate, and adjust for gaps in desired linkages needed for value (cost–service–quality).

A "staffing variance" occurs when there is a difference between the identified patient care needs and the resources available to meet those needs. Given that there will always be discrepancies between needs and available staff, and given that nurses will continue to accept responsibility for providing safe, competent care, development of strategies to manage this type of variance is essential. When a staffing variance is identified and efforts to obtain additional staff are exhausted, consider the following 10 strategies:

1. *Take a teamwork approach:* Commit to working as a team to address the gap. Planned variance management from a team perspective is proactive

and stress minimizing. In contrast, individual variance management is impulsive, reactive, and highly stressful.

2. *Prioritize:* Identify specific patient care issues that require immediate attention and those that can be safely left until later in the shift or for the next shift.
3. *Manage decision making:* As a team, determine how work will be organized or reorganized, and then assign work for the shift based on the type of staff available and patient needs. Decide which aspects of care can be eliminated or safely assigned to others.
4. *Delegate and supervise:* Delegate work to the appropriate caregivers and supervise accordingly to ensure that the work is being performed as required.
5. *Control workflow to the unit:* Reroute admissions if possible and appropriate.
6. *Communicate:* Arrange for a short, mid-shift report to assess how well all team members are managing the workload, and reassign and reprioritize tasks as needed. Communicate how breaks and lunches will be organized.
7. *Plan:* Once the team is organized, have each team member do a quick walkabout to assess those clients identified as high-priority.
8. *Evaluate:* If circumstances require modification of a patient's plan of care, inform the patient about these changes and provide clear, factual information about the care the patient can expect.
9. *Document:* Complete a variance report that identifies the specific patient care concerns. Clearly describe the safety concerns. Provide examples of care that could not be completed or situations in which the timing of prescribed interventions was delayed.
10. *Communicate:* Share the variance management data with stakeholders and develop plans to minimize future gaps.

Obstacles to a New Productivity Management System

Despite the clear and convincing theoretical rationale for system change, the obstacles to making the needed transformation happen cannot be ignored or taken lightly. Creating a new model for productivity measurement and management requires support, passion, and resources. For many healthcare leaders, the process involved in making a significant system change is far too complex to embrace. Many leaders will struggle with any modification of the current system under the misguided notion that the system is functional and provides the appropriate information to make decisions supportive of quality patient care outcomes. The control and influence of the existing powerful organizational infrastructure over nursing resource allocation, coupled with the inability of nursing to articulate its specific work and outcomes achieved within the existing productivity framework, are imposing obstacles that many may find difficult to challenge.

Simplicity

The simplicity of ratio calculations for two variables has overshadowed the benefits (including greater accuracy) that might be realized with the use of multiple data values. Overcoming the deeply entrenched tradition of ratio- or grid-based staffing models to create evidence-based processes that recognize and address the daily variations of patient care needs and staff availability requires courage and commitment to the creation of a better system. The obvious simplicity of these historical calculations is antithetical to the real goal of quality patient care. To overcome this resistance, increasing numbers of organizations are selecting computerized database management systems to provide more sophisticated, more complex, and timelier data that can be used to develop the next generation of productivity measurements. The reality is that it is difficult to use resources effectively without such systems and evaluations.

The "moral dilemmas" associated with variance management—namely, prioritizing work and/or delaying nursing work—are difficult to accept. These concerns, coupled with the historical nursing emphasis on the social mandate for care and the public's positive perception of their work, mean that nurses are often reluctant as individuals to not attempt to do as much as possible. The long-embedded nursing behaviors of oppression, the ongoing dominance of the medical model, and a fluctuating supply of nurses have discouraged nurses from challenging the system. Not only are new models of productivity needed, but new skills for nurses are required so that they can understand and practice in an environment based on evidence and value.

SUMMARY

A new clinical productivity system will serve to decrease or minimize current practices specific to the management of nursing resources, which ultimately affect the viability of the organization providing healthcare services. Altering the response to nurse resource shortages in a manner that advances the economic, social, and political state of nursing requires new thinking. Efforts to increase or decrease the number and skills of nurses can be sustained only through development of evidence that specifically supports the structure, processes, and expected outcomes of nursing. If no such evidence is forthcoming, the cyclical shortages will continue, with resulting frustration and expectations for their future recurrence. According to Gilenas and Loh (2004), there is not a lack of knowledge linking the existing work force and quality; rather, there is a performance gap because of the lack of execution. Using an evidence-based approach to clinical productivity management presents nursing with a significant but essential challenge, a challenge that today's nurses are well suited to address.

REFERENCES

Aiken, L. H., Clark, S. P., Cheung, R. B., Sloane, D. M., & Silber, J. H. (2003). Education levels of hospital nurses and patient mortality. *Journal of the American Medical Association, 290*(12), 1–8.

Aiken, L. H., Clark, S. P., Sloane, D. M., Sochalski, J., & Silber, J. H. (2002). Hospital nurse staffing and patient mortality, nurse burnout, and job dissatisfaction. *Journal of the American Medical Association, 288*(16), 1987–1993.

Aiken, L. H., Smith, H. L., & Lake, E. T. (1994). Lower Medicare mortality among a set of hospitals known for good nursing care. *Medical Care, 32*(8), 771–787.

American Nurses Association (ANA). (2000). *Nurse staffing and patient outcomes in the inpatient hospital setting.* Washington, DC: Author.

American Nurses Association (ANA). (2003). *Nursing's social policy statement* (2nd ed.). Washington, DC: Author.

American Nurses Association (ANA). (2008). *Safe staffing saves lives.* Retrieved January 26, 2009, from http://www.safestaffingsaveslives.org/default.aspx

Anderson, S. (2007, September). Deadly consequences: The hidden impact of America's nursing shortage. *National Foundation for American Policy: NFAP policy brief.* Retrieved April 27, 2009, from http://www.nfap.com/pdf/0709deadlyconsequences.pdf

Ashley, J. A. (1976). *Hospitals, paternalism, and the role of the nurse.* New York: Teachers College Press.

Barry-Walker, J. (2000). The impact of assistance redesign on staff, patients, and financial outcomes. *Journal of Nursing Administration, 30*(2), 77–89.

Berry, L., Parker, D., Coile, R., Hamilton, D. K., O'Neill, D., & Sadler, B. (2004). *Can better buildings improve care and increase your financial returns?* Chicago: Frontiers of Health Services Management.

Blegen, M. A., & Vaughn, T. (1998). A multisite study of nurse staffing and patient occurrences. *Nursing Economic$, 16*(4), 196–203.

Bolton, L. B., Aydin, C. E., & Donaldson, N. (2003). Nurse staffing and patient perceptions of nursing care. *Journal of Nursing Administration, 33*(11), 607–614.

Buerhaus, P. (1991). Dynamic shortage of registered nurses. *Nursing Economic$, 9*(5), 317–328.

Buerhaus, P. (1995). Economics and reform: Forces affecting nurse staffing. *Nursing Policy Forum, 1*(2), 8–14.

Buerhaus, P. I., Donelan, K., Ulrich, B. T., Norman, L., DesRoches, C., & Dittus, R. (2007, May/June). Impact of the nurse shortage on hospital patient care: Comparative perspectives. *Health Affairs, 26*(3), 853–862

Buerhaus, P., & Needleman, J. (2000). Policy implication of research on nurse staffing and quality of care. *Policy, Politics & Nursing Practice, 1*(1), 5–16.

Butterworth, V. (1979). *Girls in white.* Independence, MO: Herald.

Child, A. P., Institute of Medicine, Board on Health Care Services, Committee on the Work Environment for Nurses and Patient Safety, & NetLibrary. (2004). *Keeping patients safe: Transforming the work environment of nurses.* Washington, DC: National Academies Press.

Cho, S. H., Ketefian, S., Barkauskas, V. H., & Smith, D. G. (2003). The effect of nurse staffing on adverse events, morbidity, mortality, and medical costs. *Nursing Research, 52*(2), 71–79.

Clarke, S. P. (2005). The policy implications of staffing-outcomes research. *Journal of Nursing Administration, 35*(1), 17–19.

Corey, M. (2001). *Groups: Process and practice.* London: Wadsworth.

Curtin, L. L. (2003, September). An integrated analysis of nurse staffing and related variables: Effects on patient outcomes. *Online Journal of Issues in Nursing, 8*(3), 5.

Drucker, P. (1990). *Managing the nonprofit organization.* New York: Harper Collins.

Duffy, W. (2004). Representing our value. *AORN Journal, 80*(2), 197–200.

Dunn, M. G., Norby, R., Cournoyer, P., Hudec, S., O'Donnell, J., & Snider, M. D. (1995). Expert panel method for nurse staffing and resource management. *Journal of Nursing Administration, 25*(10), 61–67.

Eastaugh, S. R. (1998). *Health care finance: Cost, productivity, & strategic design.* Sudbury, MA: Jones and Bartlett Publishers.

Eastaugh, S. R. (2002). Hospital nurse productivity. *Journal of Health Care Finance, 29*(1), 14–22.

Eberhardt, B. J., Szigeti, E., & University of North Dakota, Bureau of Business and Economic Research. (1990). *Predictors of nursing staff turnover intentions in North Dakota nursing homes: Implications for management practice.* Grand Forks, ND: University of North Dakota Press.

Finkler, S., & Graf, C. (2001). *Budgeting concepts for nurse managers.* New York: W. B. Saunders.

Gilenas, L., & Loh, D. Y. (2004). The effect of workforce issues on patient safety. *Nursing Economic$, 22*(5), 266–272, 279.

Harrington, C., & Estes, C. L. (2004). *Health policy: Crisis and reform in the U.S. health care delivery system* (4th ed.). Sudbury, MA: Jones and Bartlett Publishers.

Hope, H. (2004). Working conditions of the nursing workforce: Excerpts from a policy roundtable at academy house 2003 annual research meeting. *Health Service Research, 39*(3), 445–455.

Horak, B., Welton, W., & Shortell, S. (2004). Crossing the quality chasm: Implications for health services administration education. *Journal of Health Administration Education, 21*(1), 15–38.

Hughes, E. C., & American Nurses Association. (1958). *Twenty thousand nurses tell their story: A report on studies of nursing functions sponsored by the American Nurses Association.* Philadelphia: Lippincott.

Institute of Medicine (IOM), Committee on Quality of Health Care in America, & NetLibrary. (2001). *Crossing the quality chasm: A new health system for the 21st century.* Washington, DC: National Academies Press.

Institute of Medicine (IOM), Committee on the Work Environment for Nurses and Patient Safety, & Netlibrary. (2004). *Keeping patients safe: Transforming the work environment for nurses.* Washington, DC: National Academies Press.

Johnson, C. (2002). How busy are you? *Harvard Business Review, 80*(10), 132.

Kalisch, P., & Kalisch, B. (2003). *American nursing: A history*. Philadelphia: Lippincott Williams & Wilkins.

Kane, R. L., Shamliyan, T. A., Mueller, C., Duval, S., & Wilt, T. J. (2007). The association of registered nurse staffing levels and patient outcomes: Systematic review and meta-analysis. *Medical Care, 45*(12), 1195–1204.

King, C. R., & Hinds, P. S. (2003). *Quality of life: From nursing and patient perspectives: Theory, research, practice* (2nd ed.). Sudbury, MA: Jones and Bartlett Publishers.

Lang, T. A., Hodge, M., & Olson, V. (2004). Nurse–patient ratios: A systematic review on the effects of nurse staffing on patient, nurse employee and hospital outcomes. *Journal of Nursing Administration, 34*(7–8), 326–337.

Lanser, E. G. (2001). Leveraging your nursing resources. *Healthcare Executive, 80*(10), 50–51.

Ligon, K., & Das, E. (2004, October). The benefits of automated nursing documentation. *Nurse Leader, 2*(5), 29–31.

Long, M. C. (2002). *Translating the principles of variability management into reality: One physician's perspective*. Boston: Boston University, School of Management, Executive Learning.

Malloch, K., & Conovoloff, A. J. (1999). Patient classification systems, part 1: The third generation. *Journal of Nursing Administration, 29*(7/8), 49–56.

Malloch, K., & Porter-O'Grady, T. (1999). Partnership economics: Nursing's challenge in a quantum age. *Nursing Economic$, 17*(6), 299–307.

McCue, M., Mark, B. A., & Harless, D. W. (2003). Nurse staffing, quality, and financial performance. *Journal of Health Care Finance, 29*(4), 54–76.

Merriam-Webster's collegiate dictionary, 11th ed. (2002). Springfield, MA: Merriam-Webster.

Meyers, F. E., & Stewart, J. R. (2002). *Motion and time study for lean manufacturing* (3rd ed.). Upper Saddle River, NJ: Prentice Hall.

Moody, R. (2004). Nurse productivity measures for the 21st-century. *Healthcare Management Review, 29*(2), 98–106.

Moorhead, S., Johnson, M., & Maas, M. (2004). *Nursing outcomes classification (NOC)* (3rd ed.). St. Louis, MO: C. V. Mosby.

Murphy, M. (2003). *Research brief: Eliminating wasteful work in hospitals improves margin, quality, and culture*. Washington, DC: Murphy Leadership Institute.

Needleman, J., Buerhaus, P., Mattke, S., et al. (2002). Nurse-staffing levels and the quality of care in hospitals. *New England Journal of Medicine, 346*(22), 1715–1722.

Neuhauser, P. C. (2002). Building a high-retention culture in healthcare: Fifteen ways to get good people to stay. *Journal of Nursing Administration, 32*(9), 470–478.

O'Brien-Pallas, L., Thomson, D., Hall, L. M., Pink, G., Kerr, M., Wang, S., et al. (2004). Evidence-based standards for measuring nurse staffing and performance. Retrieved April 28, 2009, from http://www.chsrf.ca/final_research/ogc/pdf/obrien_e.pdf

Pinkerton, S., & Rivers, R. (2001). Factors influencing staffing needs. *Nursing Economic$, 19*(5), 236–237.

Rice, V. H. (2000). *Handbook of stress, coping, and health: Implications for nursing research, theory, and practice*. Thousand Oaks, CA: Sage.

Rubin, I. M., Plovnick, M. S., & Fry, R. E. (1975). *Improving the coordination of care: A program for health team development*. Cambridge, MA: Ballinger.

Savitz, L. A., Jones, C. B., & Bernard, S. (2005). Quality indicators sensitive to nurse staffing in acute care settings. In K. Henriksen, J. B. Battles, E. S. Marks, & D. Lewin, *Advances in patient safety: From research to implementation* (pp. 375–385). Rockville, MD: Agency for healthcare Research and Quality.

Smith, J. (2002). Analysis of differences in entry-level or and practice by educational preparation. *Journal of Nursing Education, 41*(11), 491–495.

Squires, A. (2004). A dimensional analysis of role enactment of acute care nurses. *Journal of Nursing Scholarship, 36*(3), 272–278.

Starr, P. (1984). *Social transformation of American medicine: The rise of a sovereign profession in the making of the vast industry*. New York: Basic Books.

Stone, P. W., Curran, C. R., & Bakken, S. (2002). Economic evidence for evidence-based practice. *Journal of Nursing Scholarship, 34*(3), 277–282.

Stone, P. W., Mooney-Kane, C., Larson, E. L., Horan, T., Glance, L. G., Zwanziger, J., et al. (2007). Nurse working conditions and patient safety outcomes. *Medical Care, 45*(6), 571–578.

Tourangeau, A. E., Cranley, L. A., & Jeffs, L. (2006). Impact of nursing on hospital patient mortality: A focused review and related policy implications. *Quality and Safety in Health Care, 15*(1), 4–8.

Traynor, M. (1999). *Managerialism and nursing: Beyond oppression and profession*. London: Rutledge Press.

Ulrich, R., Quan, X., Zimring, C., Joseph, A., & Choudhary, R. (2004). *The role of the physical environment in the hospital of the 21st century: A once-in-a-lifetime opportunity*. Concord, CA: Center for Health Design.

Upenieks, V. V., Akhavan, J., Kotlerman, J., Esser, J., & Ngo, M. J. (2007). Value-added care: A new way of assessing nursing staffing ratios and workload variability. *Journal of Nursing Administration, 37*(5), 243–252.

Waldman, J., Kelly, F., Arora, S., & Smith, H. (2004). The shocking cost of turnover in healthcare. *Healthcare Management Review, 29*(1), 2–7.

Wannisky, K. E., Centers for Medicare and Medicaid Services, & U.S. General Accounting Office. (2003). *Department of Health and Human Services, Centers for Medicare and Medicaid Services Medicare Program: Prospective payment system and consolidated billing for skilled nursing facilities—update*. Retrieved March 30, 2005, from http://purl.access.gpo.gov/GPO/LPS37825

Weinberg, D. B., & Suzanne, G. (2004). *Code green: Money-driven hospitals and the dismantling of nursing (The culture and politics of healthcare work)*. Ithaca, NY: Cornell University Press.

Welton, J. M., Fischer, M. H., Degrace, S., & Zone-Smith, L. (2006). Hospital nursing costs, billing and reimbursement. *Nursing Economic$, 24*(5), 227, 239–245, 262.

Welton, J. M., Zone-Smith, L., & Fischer, M. H. (2006). Adjustment of inpatient care reimbursement for nursing intensity. *Policy, Politics, & Nursing Practice, 7*(4), 270–280.

While, A., Forbes, A., Ullman, R., Lewis, S., Mathes, L., & Grifiths, P. (2004). Good practices that address continuity during transition from child to adult care: Synthesis of the evidence. *Childcare Health and Development, 30*(5), 439–452.

White, K. M. (2006). Policy spotlight: Staffing plans and ratios. *Nursing Management, 37*(4), 18–22, 24.

Whittmann-Price, R. (2004). Emancipation in decision-making in women's health. *Journal of Advanced Nursing, 47*(4), 437–445.

CHAPTER 9

Evidence-Based Practice and Health Policy: A Match or a Mismatch?

Susan R. Cooper, Virginia Trotter Betts, Karen Butler, and Jill Gentry

The emergence of evidence-based practice (EBP) as a popular process to promote informed healthcare delivery over the course of the past two decades has prompted health professionals, policy makers, and the public to seriously consider whether health policy should and could be informed by clinical EBP. It has been suggested that evidence-based health policy would then be a next step and that policy makers should perhaps join this clinical bandwagon. Of course, such a move toward evidence-based health policy as a "best practice" will force policy makers to face some of the very same challenges, competing agendas, and shifting priorities that are present in the move to EBP as a clinical norm. This chapter explores the relationship between EBP and health policy, and identifies some of the challenges, pro and con arguments, potential outcomes, and difficulties in drawing EBP closer to health policy.

To understand the relationship between EBP and health policy, it is important to define some terminology. *Policy* is a purposeful plan of action aimed toward solving a problem or issue of concern in the public or private sector (Sudduth, 1999). It is both an entity and a process.

As an entity, policy may be viewed as the "standing decisions" of an organization (Eulau & Prewitt, 1973) and often refers to goals, programs, and proposals (Milstead, 1999). Policy can be an action or nonaction, and is made in different venues, including the legislative, judicial, and executive arenas, as well as within organizations both large and small. Policy is often the outcome of a complex labyrinth of decisions that develop over time as a result of competing agendas and necessary compromise.

Policy is a process when its stages are viewed over time. For governmental policy making, these stages include agenda setting, legislation, and subsequent rule making, program implementation, and program evaluation. The process involves a series of activities that brings an issue or problem to the government and results in direct action by the government to address the problem (Milio, 1989). Governmental policy making occurs in a political environment (i.e., decisions about who gets what, when they get it, and how much they get), within a context of power and influence, negotiation, and bargaining (Lasswell, 1958). Public policy directs problems to the government for a response (Jones, 1984) and is generally developed by a governmental body or agency. The use of evidence is also applicable to policy making that occurs in the private sector and on an individualized level—that is, policy within healthcare settings, professional organizations, a specific patient population by diagnosis, or all the citizens in a country (DePalma, 2004).

Health policy directly addresses health problems (Milstead, 1999). It is generally classified using the determinants of health over which it is possible to have influence; these arenas include the physical, biological, or social environment or healthcare services (Muir Gray, 2001). There are two major reasons for formulating health policy: (1) to change the way in which healthcare services are funded, organized, or held accountable (healthcare policies); and (2) to improve health through changes in the physical, biological, or social environments (health or public health policies) (Muir Gray, 2001). Healthcare policies aim to improve efficiency, quality, accountability, or acceptability. Health or public health policies can also affect both the incidence and prevalence of disease (Muir Gray, 2001).

While there is little disagreement that clinical decisions for an individual should be based on the best available evidence, policy makers often face the challenge of dealing with competing definitions of evidence in the healthcare field for policy purposes. Does the best evidence come only from randomized controlled trials or can the evidence come from observational studies? Certainly, even within healthcare clinical interactions, there is disagreement about what constitutes the best available evidence and what qualifies as EBP.

EBP has evolved over the past two decades as an outgrowth of the rapid expansion of science and knowledge as well as the introduction of innovative technology that increases the availability of research findings and the development of enhanced research methodologies. As these advances have been used to inform and support new practices, clinical decision making has increasingly been based on research. This is the premise of evidence-based health care (Muir Gray, 2001). Yet, others have defined EBP through other lenses, and those definitions are variable and not always straightforward (Jennings & Loan, 2001).

The original definition pertaining specifically to evidence-based medicine (EBM) came from the predominately Canadian-formed Evidence-Based Medicine Working Group (EBMWG):

Evidence-based medicine de-emphasizes intuition, unsystematic clinical experience, and pathophysiologic rationale as sufficient grounds for clinical decision making and stresses the examination of evidence from clinical research (EBMWG, 1992, p. 2420).

This definition emphasizes clinical research while assigning less value to intuition and the clinical experience of health professionals. For their part, Rosenberg and Donald (1995) defined EBM as "the process of systematically finding, appraising and using contemporaneous research findings as the basis for clinical decisions" (p. 1222).

Sackett and colleagues (whose work is cited in many of the chapters in this text) expanded these definitions to include the "conscientious, explicit, and judicious use of current best evidence in making decisions about the care of individual patients" (Sackett, Rosenberg, Muir Gray, Haynes, & Richardson, 1996, p. 71). These authors went on to say that EBP involves using individual clinical expertise along with the best available external clinical evidence from systematic research. This definition is important for nurses, in that it allows for clinical expertise as a building block of evidence while still emphasizing randomized controlled trials in the hierarchy of evidence (Jennings & Loan, 2001).

Definitions of EBP are found in nursing literature as well, all of which emphasize evidence from research as a part of the fundamental definition. Gerrish and Clayton's (1998) definition of EBP highlights the use of research findings primarily from clinical trials or other types of experimental designs to evaluate nursing interventions. Stevens and Paugh (1999) seem to agree, proposing the following definition: "Evidence-based nursing [is] practice that relies on information generated from results of scientific research" (p. 155).

Goode and Piedalue (1999) expanded upon this definition to include other forms of evidence, such as pathophysiology, quality improvement and risk data, standards of care, infection control data, cost-effectiveness analysis, and benchmarking data. Perhaps the most significant differential in their definition was the addition of patient preference and nursing clinical expertise as forms of evidence to be used in the decision-making process. Accordingly, Ingersoll (2000) included the use of theory and research and acknowledged the value of the individual's needs and preferences in the delivery of evidence-based care.

Despite the varying definitions of EBP, all are intended to be used as models for establishing best practice. However, this inconsistency of definition, even in the familiar clinical context for which it was intended (i.e., the kind of evidence allowed, the value or weight of the evidence, and/or how that evidence should be utilized in decision making), creates enormous difficulty for policy makers: They may or (usually) may not have any experience in health care or research, and are being asked to consider and apply EBP in the policy context.

LEVELING OR GRADING THE EVIDENCE

In addition to the multiplicity of definitions of evidence and various opinions about what constitutes best evidence, many published schemas are available that can be used to grade evidence. The Agency for Healthcare Research and Quality (AHRQ) supported the publication of a guide to systems used to rate the strength of scientific evidence (West et al., 2002). The authors of this AHRQ study examined 121 systems designed to rate the strength of scientific evidence. The goals of this project were to "describe systems used to rate the strength of scientific evidence, including evaluating the quality of individual articles that make up a body of evidence on a specific scientific question in health care, and to provide some guidance as to 'best practices' in this field today" (p. 1).

Central to the discussion of evidence, of course, is the concept of quality. Methodological quality has been defined as "the extent to which all aspects of a study's design and conduct can be shown to protect against systemic bias, non-systemic bias, and inferential error" (Lohr & Carey, 1999, as cited in West et al., 2002, p. 1). Gaps were identified in the AHRQ study in rating quality, strength of evidence, and application of grading schemas to "less traditional" bodies of evidence such as observational studies. Thus these gaps may be of particular importance to nurses who are interested in defining evidence.

It is clear from the summary in the AHRQ publication that no single schema is currently available (or likely to become available in the near future) that can be used to grade evidence across all types of scholarly work. In addition, the evidence-gathering process will differ from clinician to clinician, and from researcher to researcher. These facts alone illustrate the problems inherent in trying to determine exactly what evidence is and how it might be best applied in the policy-making process.

OBSTACLES IN THE SEARCH FOR EVIDENCE

Even if policy makers were determined to use evidence as the basis for their decisions in healthcare policy development, they would encounter formidable stumbling blocks along the way. Muir Gray (2001) identifies these blocks as "gaps" and has suggested actions that can be taken to overcome them. Gaps identified include those related to relevance, publication, hunting, and quality.

Relevance Gap

The relevance gap equates to the lack of high-quality data, especially in certain conditions or situations. According to Muir Gray, the research agenda frequently depends on investment in research and development, yet there are many areas without sufficient investments. The absence of high-quality data in a particular area of health does not make decision making impossible, but instead requires the use of the best available evidence using a well-researched published grading schema (Muir Gray, 2001).

Publication Gap

The publication gap exists because, although the main source of evidence is in the published literature, not all evidence is published in scientific journals (Muir Gray, 2001). The following reasons have been cited to explain this gap:

- Researchers who fail to write up and submit their findings for publication
- Researchers who do not complete their work and submit those findings for publication due to negative research results (submission bias)
- Reluctance on the part of proprietary companies, such as pharmaceutical companies, to publish information that may not show their products in the most advantageous light
- Biased editors who are more prone to publish positive rather than negative results (publication bias)
- The influence of language—positive findings are more likely to be published in English-language journals and negative findings in other-language journals (language bias)

Searching for unpublished data if time allows, or at least conducting a thorough systematic review, and having a conscious awareness of the phenomenon of positive biases when critiquing/utilizing research articles (Muir Gray, 2001), are publication gap-reducing suggestions.

Hunting Gap

The hunting gap refers to difficulties in finding published research due to the limitations of current electronic databases (Muir Gray, 2001). These limitations include limited database coverage and inadequate indexing of articles. Use of the Cochrane Library and improved search strategies, for example, can minimize the impact of this gap.

Quality Gap

The quality gap addresses the need for critical appraisal of evidence (Muir Gray, 2001). Abstracts can be misleading in that they tend to be written with a bias toward highlighting the positive findings within a paper. In the search for evidence, it is essential to critique abstracts carefully—looking for structure and carefully appraising the methods section—before accepting the results as good-quality evidence. It is also important to be aware of sources of bias within research, and to critique the study design and presentation of results carefully.

The integrity and quality of an EBP as a policy fundamental is critical because an adopted policy has broad and far-reaching implications for health-care delivery. For this reason, to suggest or promote an EBP that has serious quality flaws as clinical evidence can lead to serious consequences for the researcher, organization, or policy maker, as well as for health delivery in general.

Evidence-based health policy may be viewed as the interface between evidence-based health care and public policy analysis (Lin, 2003). An evidence-based policy process should be guided by the collection of valid and reliable data, with policy makers then following a process of determining the problem, developing a plan to address the problem, judging the feasibility of the plan, guiding the implementation of the plan, and finally providing evidence from evaluation on which to base any needed future revisions (DePalma, 2002). Unfortunately, all too often policy is shaped by the interplay of political and philosophical differences. One must also recognize that policy making is rarely a perfectly linear or systematic process. Conversely, focusing on evidence in policy making may allow those involved in the process a way to agree on a solution that is acceptable to all (DePalma, 2002). Attending to the policy problem by exploring the evidence related to both the problem and its optional solutions may serve to reframe the debate, shifting it away from entrenched philosophies and toward application of scientific findings as new ways to move forward, thereby nurturing sound, reasoned solutions.

A CONCEPTUAL MODEL OF THE POLICY PROCESS: THE KINGDON MODEL

Researchers have developed a variety of models of agenda setting and policy formulation (Baumgartner & Jones, 1993; Cobb & Elder, 1983; Kingdon, 1995), while political scientists have developed theoretical modeling of policy design (Hedge & Mok, 1987). Ingraham (1987) noted the lack of one design, theory, or model in policy design. Because of its applicability to health care, we have chosen the Kingdon Model for discussion in this chapter. This model is designed to answer two public policy questions: (1) How do issues get on the political agenda? and (2) Once they are there, how are alternative solutions derived? (Milstead, 1999). The Kingdon Model looks at both participants and processes involved in policy making.

Policy participants can be interested parties either inside or outside of government and may include disparate players—for example, elected officials and their staff, political parties, special-interest groups, professional organizations, and corporations. At a federal level, Kingdon ranks members of Congress second only to the President (the administration) in importance in agenda setting. He notes that members of Congress get involved in developing policy for the following reasons: to meet their constituents' needs, to enhance their own political reputations with regard to ability and power, and to develop good policy to solve problems in which they are interested. According to Kingdon's model, elected officials are more important to agenda setting, whereas their staff members are more important to generating alternative solutions to policy problems. Kingdon asserts that special-interest groups are more likely to block—rather than promote—a policy agenda item.

Kingdon's processes are conceived as three streams: problem streams, policy streams, and political streams.

- The problem stream includes ideas that get on an agenda if there are indicators of a problem or if there is inequity in the distribution of resources between groups of constituents.
- In the policy stream, officials push certain initiatives because of electoral reasons (from their party or their district) and because of their belief in the worth of the initiative. In the policy stream, five criteria must be met for proposals to survive: (1) technical feasibility, (2) value acceptability within the policy community, (3) a cost that is acceptable or at least tolerable, (4) anticipated agreement from constituents, and (5) a reasonable chance that other elected decision makers will be receptive to the initiative (Kingdon, 1995).
- The political stream consists of elements such as upcoming elections, partisan distribution, ideological concerns in the policy-making body, and popular "mood" related to the problem or specific initiative.

For agenda setting to occur, there must be a coupling of streams during a critical time when a window of opportunity appears. According to Kingdon, "Policy windows open infrequently, and do not stay open long" (p. 166). Windows of opportunity can open either because new problems have been brought to elected officials' attention or because changes have occurred in the political stream, such as the election of a new administration or partisan power shifts after an election. Kingdon believes that the source of an idea is not as important as how it is nurtured: "[T]he key to understanding policy change is not where the idea came from but what made it take hold and grow" (p. 76). Kingdon's model is dynamic: "A problem is recognized, a solution is available, the political climate makes the time right for change, and the constraints do not prohibit action" (p. 93).

THE POLITICS OF EVIDENCE-BASED HEALTH POLICY

Policy making at the state and federal levels is first and foremost a political process. Politics may be defined as "the process of influencing the allocation of scarce resources" (Mason, Leavitt, & Chaffee, 2002, p. 9). Relatively few policy makers at the state and federal levels have professional experience in the healthcare arena. For these decision makers, their views are framed by their personal experiences with the healthcare system or by anecdotal stories heard from their constituents. Policy makers must balance competing agendas, claims, and spheres of influence when making policy decisions. Specifically, decisions may be influenced by politicians, party politics, campaign strategies, lobbyists, consumer groups, industries, media, and public opinion.

Evidence about the merits of a solution is but one aspect to be considered in the policy process. Policy makers must also integrate values, cost, resources, and benefits (Muir Gray, 2001; Sturm, 2002) at a population level. Muir Gray acknowledges that "the clinician has to take into account the condition and values of the individual patient; that the policymaker has to take into account not only best current knowledge but also the needs of the populations, the values, the resources available, and the opportunity costs of the decision" (2001, p. 371). Policy decisions are difficult, and the dynamics are more layered and complex than those found in clinical care. Difficulty in reaching resolution on the "right" policy often results from a conflict between differing realms of influence, such as ethical, social, cultural, economic, and electoral concerns and considerations (Black, 2001). Even given the strength of the evidence, policies may be made that run contrary to the evidence base.

Two such oppositional health policy examples come to mind. In 1988, the Office of Technology Assessment released a report documenting strong fiscal and clinical evidence that, in less than a year, a $1.00 investment in prenatal care, including maternal nutrition, returned $3.38 that might otherwise be spent on care of low-birth-weight babies in neonatal intensive care. The 100th Congress appeared oblivious to these numbers and limited federal funding for pregnant women in the Women, Infants, and Children (WIC) supplemental nutrition program. That same Congress, again presented with even more data (evidence) on the value of good nutrition for growth and development in children, voted to count catsup as a green or yellow vegetable in the public school food supplement programs.

What do these examples say? Surely their message is that much more is valued in policy than facts, data, evidence, or even just "the right thing to do." Ideology, economics, debate over the size and role of government, and winners and losers are just a few of the factors that may influence policy decisions and products.

Obstacles Faced by Policy Makers

Just like clinicians, policy makers are presented with a number of challenges when trying to formulate health policy using EBP, including the multiple definitions of evidence, the difficulty of searching for evidence, the complexities of evaluating or grading the evidence, and the myriad nuances of the policy process. Policy makers and their overworked staffs are challenged to understand the often subtle nuances in the criteria and to equate or compare levels of evidence from one schema to another. Therefore, it is incumbent upon those parties wishing to influence the policy decision-making process, such as health professionals, to conduct the search for evidence, present the evidence in an easy-to-understand format and a completely honest and transparent manner, and look for ways to have evidence become a high priority on the political agenda.

Lin (2003) suggests that policy results as a response to a perceived need or problem that is contingent upon the context in which the perceived need or problem occurs. Thus EBP is made relevant in policy when the problem and its solutions—quality of care, technology dispersion, cost of care, and so on—provide the context.

The questions that are generated as a result of the policy-making process are inherently different from the questions that may be asked and answered as part of a clinical randomized controlled trial (RCT). Large numbers of persons are directly or indirectly affected by policy decisions at the state and federal levels. The general population represents a heterogeneous group and does not fit into a trial model of efficacy even under ideal circumstances.

Policy makers are not likely to be experts at evaluating evidence per se. Haynes (1999) promotes three questions to be utilized to evaluate healthcare interventions (based on the work of A. Cochrane, a British epidemiologist):

- Can it work?
- Does it work?
- Is it worth it?

The question "Can it work?" addresses efficacy, or the extent to which the intervention does more good than harm under ideal circumstances. "Does it work?" focuses on effectiveness, or the extent to which the intervention works under usual or common circumstances. Answering the question "Is it worth it?" measures the outcomes of the intervention compared to the resources consumed (Haynes, 1999). The policy picture becomes cloudy when the answer to "Can it work?" conflicts with the answer to "Is it worth it?" At this point in the balancing act, the policy maker is most susceptible to the other spheres of policy-shaping influences, including economics, politics, philosophies, and values.

Atkins, Siegel, and Slutsky (2005) have offered a framework for evaluation by policy makers when the evidence is in dispute to assist policy makers in separating questions and concerns over the evidence from the other spheres or influence. Their framework consists of the following questions:

- What is the ultimate goal, and how does the intervention achieve those ends?
- How good is the evidence that the intervention can improve outcomes?
- How good is the evidence that the intervention will work in my setting?
- How do the potential benefits compare with the possible harms or costs of the intervention?
- What constitutes "good enough" evidence for a policy decision?
- Which other considerations are relevant to policy decisions?

INTENDED AND UNINTENDED CONSEQUENCES

Policy makers work toward creating policy that will effect a set of intended outcomes. The intended outcomes of EBP in health policy development are meritorious and much needed. EBP should be able to tell good science from bad, improve quality of care, decrease the costs of care, make technology diffusion both rational and rapid, and embrace multidisciplinary and systematic approaches to solving complex care problems. Together, these are both the promises of EBP and their intended outcomes.

Of course, many unintended consequences also occur in health policy. We have come to recognize that EBP may raise further examples of the unintended consequences of policy decisions. Thus, unintended results can negate positive outcomes of the evidence-based policy, complicating far-ranging treatment preferences among medical professionals and payment issues within insurance coverage. Several factors may contribute to this phenomenon, including inconsistent evidence from RCTs, lack of evidence from RCTs, and cost considerations. Despite their best intentions to predict and control the effect of any policy, it is difficult for decision makers to foresee all possible consequences of that policy. These unintended consequences can have dramatic repercussions for the availability of services and procedures throughout the system.

A notable example of policy and the law of unintended consequences involved the implementation of the Health Insurance Portability and Accountability Act of 1996 (HIPAA). Portability of insurance as one moves from job to job, privacy of medical information, and accountability of the healthcare system were all well-intentioned goals of the policy makers who enacted HIPAA. However, unintended consequences abounded with the implementation of the Administrative Simplification Compliance Act of 2001 (ASCA). ASCA has provisions for administrative simplification rules aimed at streamlining administrative processes of care through the implementation of transaction standards, privacy standards, and security standards. Unfortunately, the reality is that these simplification rules are anything but simple.

As an example, the privacy regulations require all healthcare entities—including providers, health plans, and health data clearinghouses—to protect all patient information and to release the minimum information necessary only after obtaining the appropriate patient consent. The span of these regulations extended far beyond electronic medical information (as originally intended) to include oral and written communication and records as well. There is disagreement about the resulting balance between the rights of patients to privacy and the rights of the health professionals to use the information to improve their care of the patients (Langner, 2001). Healthcare providers and entities have been faced with innumerable challenges associated with HIPAA implementation, such as increasing costs of healthcare business processes; increased documentation requirements related to release of information; increased staffing needs, such as the need to hire institutional privacy officers; training and education of all levels of staff; and health service delivery delays as a result of difficulties that arise as clinical information is shared between providers when conflicting understandings of "the minimum information necessary" arise. Challenges also exist when communications with families must occur. These are but a few examples of areas where the balance between patient rights and the challenges of complying with the regulations conflict. Few—if any—providers, health facilities, health plans, or business associates have been free from the unintended consequences of HIPAA.

In theory, all healthcare policies should be derived from the settled results of unflawed clinical trials. These trials, in turn, should tell us whether a particular drug, procedure, or service is effective among the target audience and is superior or inferior to all other treatment choices. Of course, the reality is far more complicated. Similar clinical trials can yield vastly different results. The trials might show benefits among certain participants, but be unable to identify future users who might benefit from the product or service. Such was the case for implantable cardioverter defibrillators (ICD): Studies could not conclusively determine which persons at risk would benefit from an ICD (Hlatky, Sanders, & Owens, 2005). Because of these inconsistencies, the healthcare industry disagreed on the effectiveness of the procedure, although it did help a significant number of persons in the trial. As a result, insurance coverage on this procedure was restricted to only those persons with a certain kind of medical history (Hlatky et al., 2005). This EBP example illustrates how the differences among trials can change reimbursement and insurance coverage for procedures and, therefore, the accessibility of those procedures to the public.

The reliance on evidence-based policies can negatively affect important interventions that lack sufficient trials and data to prove their effectiveness and value. RCTs can take several years to complete, and multiple trials may be required to have enough data to satisfy standards of grading. Emerging technologies and practices in many fields are moving at a much faster pace, and it is impossible for researchers to keep up with the development of these new services. Thus, if reimbursement or insurance coverage is based only on the accepted EBP, many new treatments could be stalled for several years until sufficient evidence is available that supports their use, and some promising practices may never be fleshed out. Furthermore, there are not enough EBPs to cover all available treatments in every specialty of care.

For example, mental health care organizations in the United States have established only six nationally recognized EBPs. The scope of these six practices in no way meets the needs of the field, the illnesses, or the many valid treatment possibilities. Therefore, any policy making that would limit reimbursement to only those services based on EBPs could have serious consequences for persons who might otherwise benefit from the services that are considered "promising" or "best," but have not been fully vetted as evidence based.

Finally, EBPs are not classified as such based solely on their effectiveness and available data. Financial considerations can deter or promote certain healthcare policies over others. To return to the ICD example, insurance coverage was restricted not only because of the inconsistent trial results, but also because of the high cost of the procedure in conjunction with the significant number of persons at risk (Hlatky et al., 2005). For payers, the potential cost of covering this procedure is enormous.

Drug formularies can also be affected by policy decisions based on finances. Although the intent of a drug formulary is to lower the cost of drug therapies, it could prove difficult if not impossible to add newer and often more expensive drugs to the formulary, even when the more expensive drug is a more effective treatment. EBP could be an enormous plus in some situations (i.e., when comparing an expensive drug regimen with rehospitalization costs), yet getting to that point will require a long, arduous trip that requires navigation of both the EBP issues and the vagaries of health policy development. As a consequence, consumers may receive lower-quality care while waiting for either EBP or promising "breakthrough" practices to be developed further and inform health policy.

CONCLUSION

The use of EBP in health policy has a long way to go. Just because EBP may be "the way of the now and the future" in the delivery of clinical health care, it is not certain that EBP is "the way" in health policy development. Actually, considering the complexities and uncertainties of the state of the "science" of EBP as described throughout this text, it is likely that many policy makers will remain on the sidelines rather than explicitly calling for EBP to inform health policy.

REFERENCES

Atkins, D., Siegel, J., & Slutsky, J. (2005). Making policy when the evidence is in dispute. *Health Affairs, 24*(1), 102–113.

Baumgartner, F. R., & Jones, B. D. (1993). *Agendas and instability in American politics.* Chicago: University of Chicago Press.

Black, N. (2001). Evidence-based policy: Proceed with care. *British Medical Journal, 323*(7307), 275–279.

Cobb, R. W., & Elder, C. D. (1983). *Participation in America: The dynamics of agenda-building* (2nd ed.). Baltimore: Johns Hopkins University Press.

DePalma, J. A. (2002). Proposing an evidence-based policy process. *Nursing Administration Quarterly, 26*(4), 55–61.

DePalma, J. A. (2004). Health policy and research: Evidence-based decision making. *Home Health Care Management and Practice, 16*(5), 405–407.

Eulau, H., & Prewitt, K. (1973). *Labyrinths of democracy.* Indianapolis, IN: Bobbs-Merrill.

Evidence-Based Medicine Working Group (EBMWG). (1992). Evidence-based medicine: A new approach to teaching the practice of medicine. *Journal of the American Medical Association, 268*(17), 2420–2425.

Gerrish, K., & Clayton, J. (1998). Improving clinical effectiveness through an evidence-based approach: Meeting the challenge for nursing in the United Kingdom. *Nursing Administration Quarterly, 22*(4), 55–65.

Goode, C. J., & Piedalue, F. (1999). Evidence-based clinical practice. *Journal of Nursing Administration, 29*(6), 15–21.

Haynes, B. (1999). Can it work? Does it work? Is it worth it? *British Medical Journal, 319*(7211), 652–653.

Hedge, D. M., & Mok, J. W. (1987). The nature of policy studies: A content analysis of policy journal articles. *Policy Studies Journal, 16*(1), 49–62.

Hlatky, M. A., Sanders, G. D., & Owens, D. K. (2005). Evidence-based medicine and policy: The case of the implantable cardioverter defibrillator. *Health Affairs, 24*(1), 42–51.

Ingersoll, G. L. (2000). Evidence-based nursing: What it is and what it isn't [editorial]. *Nursing Outlook, 48*(4), 151–152.

Ingraham, P. W. (1987). Toward more systematic consideration of policy design. *Policy Studies Journal, 15*(4), 611–628.

Jennings, B. M., & Loan, L. A. (2001). Misconceptions among nurses about evidence-based practice. *Journal of Nursing Scholarship, 33*(2), 121–127.

Jones, C. O. (1984). *An introduction to the study of public policy* (2nd ed.). Monterey, CA: Brooks-Cole.

Kingdon, J. W. (1995). *Agendas, alternatives and public policies.* New York: Harper Collins.

Langner, B. (2001). Unintended consequences: An inherent risk in public policy development. *Journal of Professional Nursing, 17*(2), 69–70.

Lasswell, H. D. (1958). *Politics: Who gets what, when, how.* New York: Meridian Books.

Lin, V. (2003). Competing rationalities: Evidence-based health policy? In V. Lin & B. Gibson (Eds.), *Evidence-based health policy: problems and possibilities* (p. 3–17). South Melbourne, Victoria, Australia: Oxford University Press.

Lohr, K. N., & Carey, T. S. (1999). Assessing the "best evidence": Issues in grading the quality of studies for systematic reviews. *Joint Commission Journal of Quality Improvement, 25*(9), 470–479.

Mason, D., Leavitt, J. K., & Chaffee, M. W. (2002). Policy and politics: A framework for action. In D. Mason, J. K. Leavitt, & M. W. Chaffee (Eds.), *Policy and politics in nursing and health care* (p. 1–18). St. Louis, MO: W. B. Saunders.

Milio, N. (1989). Developing nursing leadership in health policy. *Journal of Professional Nursing, 5*(6), 315–321.

Milstead, J. A. (Ed.). (1999). Advanced practice nurses and public policy, naturally. In *Health policy and politics* (p. 1–41). Gaithersburg, MD: Aspen.

Muir Gray, J. A. (2001). *Evidence-based health care: How to make health policy and management decisions* (2nd ed.). London: Churchill Livingstone.

Rosenberg, W., & Donald, A. (1995). Evidence-based medicine: An approach to clinical problem-solving. *British Medical Journal, 310*(6987), 1122–1126.

Sackett, D. L., Rosenberg, W. M. C., Muir Gray, J. A., Haynes, R. B., & Richardson, W. S. (1996). Evidence-based medicine: What it is and what it isn't [editorial]. *British Medical Journal, 312*(7023), 71–72.

Stevens, K. R., & Paugh, J. A. (1999). Evidence-based practice and perioperative nursing. *Seminars in Perioperative Nursing, 8*(3), 155–159.

Sturm, R. (2002). Evidence-based health policy versus evidence-based medicine. *Psychiatric Services, 53*(12), 1499.

Sudduth, A. L. (1999). Policy evaluation. In J. A. Milstead (Ed.), *Health policy and politics* (pp. 219–256). Gaithersburg, MD: Aspen.

West, S., King, V., Carey, T. S., Lohr, K. N., McKoy N., Sutton, S. F., & Lux, L. (2002). *Systems to rate the strength of scientific evidence.* Evidence Report/Technology Assessment No. 47. (Prepared by the Research Triangle Institute-University of North Carolina Evidence-Based Practice Center under Contract No. 290–97–0011.) AHRQ Publication No. 02-E016. Rockville, MD: Agency for Healthcare Research and Quality.

CHAPTER 10

Creating Nursing System Excellence Through the Forces of Magnetism

Amy Steinbinder and Elaine Scherer

Magnet Organizations will serve as the fount of knowledge and expertise for the delivery of nursing care globally. They will be solidly grounded in core Magnet principles, flexible, and constantly striving for discovery and innovation. They will lead the reformation of health care; the discipline of nursing; and care of the patient, family, and community (ANCC, 2008a).

INTRODUCTION

In 2008, the Magnet™ Commission took a very, strong courageous stand in declaring its belief in the future of Magnet Organizations and the nursing profession. The Magnet program has come a long way since 1991, when the American Nurses Credentialing Center (ANCC) introduced the Magnet Hospital Recognition Program for Excellence in Nursing Services, which included the initial Forces of Magnetism (FOM) (**Table 10-1**). The American Nurses Association's (ANA) Standards for Organized Nursing Services was used as the framework of the program (ANA, 1991). Many program changes have occurred since 1991 based on research, evidence-based practice (EBP), and consensus opinions of experts and other recognized authorities, including the International Organization for Standardization. Since its inception, the Magnet Recognition Program has awarded the Magnet designation to more than 310 organizations; the latest listing can be found on the Magnet program Web site (*www.nursecredentialing.org*; ANCC, 2008a).

The Magnet Recognition Program has been highly visible over the past 14 years. Not only is the Magnet designation known and desired by nursing leaders and nursing staffs, but it is also a highly prized goal of hospital chief executive officers (CEOs) and healthcare system leaders, who see it as a way to attract physicians, develop market excellence, and recruit clinical staff.

Table 10-1   Fourteen Forces of Magnetism

Force of Magnetism	Expectations of the Magnet Environment[*]
Quality of nursing leadership	Nurse leaders are knowledgeable, strong, visionary risk takers. They advocate and support staff and patients. Their philosophy is clear and well articulated, and guides the day-to-day operations of the nursing services.
Organizational structure	The structure is characterized as flat and decentralized. Shared decision making is functioning and productive. The structure is dynamic and responsive to change. Nursing is present and actively involved in organizational committees. The chief nursing officer (CNO) reports to the organization's chief executive officer (CEO), and executive-level nursing leaders serve at the executive level of the organization.
Management style	A participative management style is pervasive and staff feedback is encouraged, valued, and used by leaders in decision making. Nursing leaders are visible and accessible, and they communicate effectively with staff.
Personnel policies and programs	Salaries and benefits are competitive. Staffing and scheduling systems are flexible and creative. Evidence-based staffing based on acuity is expected. Staff nurses are involved in creating personnel policies and programs that support professional nursing practice, work/life balance, and delivery of quality care.
Professional models of care	Care models give nurses responsibility and authority to provide patient care. In addition, nurses are accountable for coordinating care and ensuring that continuity of care is provided across the continuum. Patients' unique needs are addressed to achieve desired outcomes.
Quality of care	Staff nurses perceive that the care provided is of high quality. Positive patient outcomes are achieved. Patient safety, ethical practice, research, and evidence-based practice are included.

Quality improvement	Structures and processes are in place to measure quality and improve care and service to patients. Staff nurses actively participate in improvement activities and gain knowledge in the process.
Consultation and resources	Experts including advance practice nurses are available to staff. Nurses are encouraged to participate in professional organizations.
Autonomy	They are expected to use independent judgment in providing appropriate care for patients. An interdisciplinary approach to care is expected, and nursing care is consistent with professional standards and scope of practice.
Community and the healthcare organization	A strong community presence is maintained, and outreach programs are offered that benefit the community.
Nurses as teachers	Nurses incorporate teaching in their practice, which includes patient education and precepting/ mentoring new graduates and students as well as experienced nurse colleagues.
Image of nursing	Nursing services are perceived as essential by other members of the healthcare team. Nurses are integral to care and are recognized as vital contributors to care delivery.
Interdisciplinary relationships	Collaborative relationships and mutual respect are evident throughout the organization as all members of the healthcare team contribute to achieving clinical outcomes.
Professional development	Education is a high priority and includes orientation, in-service programs, continuing education, formal education, and career development. Clinical and leadership competencies are valued, and nurses have the opportunity to obtain national specialty certifications as well as participate in clinical career advancement programs.

*As defined by the Expert Panel for 2005 Magnet Application Manual.

Likewise, elected officials and the public are becoming aware of the significance of the Magnet designation:

- As part of the Nurse Reinvestment Act, then-Senator Hillary Clinton helped create grants to assist more hospitals to achieve the Magnet designation (2001).
- In January 2006, Laura Marquez of ABC News told the public on *Good Morning America* that prospective patients and their loved ones can try to protect themselves by selecting a Magnet hospital and referred viewers to the Magnet Web site (*http://abcnews.go.com/WNT/Health/story?id=1529546*).
- The then-Governor of Vermont, Howard Dean, M.D., recognized Southwestern Vermont Medical Center's Magnet achievement when it became the forty-seventh nursing service to achieve the designation (*www.svhealthcare.org*).
- The *Wall Street Journal* published an article to help patients make informed choices when they have the opportunity to select a hospital; one of the recommendations was to choose a Magnet-designated hospital because it would have better outcomes and fewer deaths (Kleinman, 2008).
- *Reader's Digest* recommended that patients "would be foolish" not to check into a Magnet hospital if one was located nearby (Pekkanen, 2003, p. 91).
- A Continuing Education Unit (CEU) offering in May 2007 calls Magnet recognition "The Nobel Prize for Nursing practice" (Trofino, 2007).

The 14 FOM have been well researched over the last 20 years and continue to be subject to major scrutiny. A major change occurred in 2004 when the ANCC Commission on Magnet completed a thorough evaluation of the application procedures and restructured the process around the FOM (ANCC, 2004). This led to a major program evaluation in 2005, bringing 22 highly interrelated major recommendations to the leadership of the Magnet Program. The recommendations covered eight areas: (1) appraiser qualifications, selection, training, and developments; (2) compensation of appraisers; (3) the team constellation; (4) the appraisal process; (5) site visits and document review; (6) commission size and members; (7) new product development; and (8) use of technology for information and training (Triolo, Scherer, & Floyd, 2006). Additional recommendations made were to balance the scoring of the FOM among process, structure, and outcome, and to create a dynamic model for the FOM.

Data from 147 facilities, rated by two to four appraisers, were subjected to factor analysis, cluster analysis, and multidimensional scaling. These analyses revealed 7 clusters of evidence that represented where Magnet had been. The 14 FOM and the 7 clusters were then integrated into a new model to guide the future of Magnet principles and the future of the nursing profession (Wolf, Triolo, & Reid-Ponte, 2008). This major philosophical change will greatly impact both the ailing U.S. healthcare system and a nursing profession in which shortages are projected to continue far into the future.

The courageous leadership of the Magnet Commission has significantly strengthened the program and positioned its designees to design the future of health care and set the standards for excellence in nursing for years to come.

OVERVIEW

For this chapter, two primary sources of information were used to provide evidence demonstrating the relationship of Magnet designation to system excellence. First, ten chief nurse officers (CNOs) of Magnet-designated organizations who served as Magnet program implementation and/or redesignation experts were selected to be interviewed once again by the co-authors (**Table 10-2**). Sixty percent of the original CNOs interviewed in 2004 have since moved on to other leadership opportunities—supporting Havens, Thompson, and Jones' findings that 62% anticipated making a job change in less than five years (2008). These CNOs candidly discussed their hospitals' continuing journeys and provided specific examples of programs that led to Magnet redesignation. (All facilities had been redesignated at least once by the time of the interviews.)

Second, a literature search was performed, which produced evidence consistent with many of the findings gleaned from the CNOs' interviews. The 14 FOM identified in the original Magnet study were discussed, as were their relationships to the "Eight Essentials of Magnetism" identified by Kramer as the elements necessary to support high-quality patient care from staff nurses' perspectives (Kramer & Schmalenberg, 2002). While none of the CNOs interviewed had undergone the redesignation experience under the criteria in the 2008 manual, their initial perceptions of and plans regarding implementation of the new Magnet Model were also discussed. Interviewer stories and insights were highlighted with each FOM.

The demographic characteristics of the interviewed CNOs and their organizations are described in this chapter. Each FOM is discussed, and pertinent literature supporting the force and its relationship to outcomes of organizational performance is included. Any evidence linking the FOM to one or more Essentials of Magnetism is identified as well. Finally, comments provided by the interviewed CNOs are included to illustrate the relationship of actual practice to research findings.

Table 10-2   Study Sources: Chief Nursing Officers, Hospital Affiliations, Original Designation Dates of Facility Designation, and Redesignation History

CNO, Credentials, and Title	Hospital Affiliation and Location	Magnet Initial (I) Designation and (R) Redesignation Dates
Rebecca Burke, RN, MS Senior Vice President for Patient Care Services/ Chief Nursing Officer	Miriam Hospital Providence, Rhode Island	I: January 1998 R: 2002, 2006
*Lore Bogolin, RN, MSN Vice President/Chief Nursing Officer (new to role as of December 2005; Director of Medical–Surgical Nursing, 2004)	Delnor Community Hospital Geneva, Illinois	I: February 2004 R: 2008
*Karlene Kerfoot, PhD, RN, CNAA, FAAN Vice President/Chief Clinical Officer (new to role as of 2007; external to organization prior to that year)	Aurora Health Care Metro Region: St. Luke's Medical Center, St. Luke's South Shore, Aurora Sinai Medical Center, West Allis Memorial Hospital, Aurora Medical Center Washington County, Wisconsin	I: January 2001 R: 2005
Val Gokenbach, DM, RN, RWJF Vice President/Chief Nurse Executive	William Beaumont Hospital Royal Oak, Michigan	I: January 2004 R: 2008
*Lorie Wild, PhD, RN, NEA-BC Chief Nursing Officer/ Senior Associate Administrator, Patient Care Services, University of Washington Medical Center Assistant Dean, University of Washington School of Nursing	University of Washington Medical Center Seattle, Washington	I: May 1994 R: 1998, 2002, 2006

Craig Luzinski, MS, RN Vice President of Patient Care Services/Chief Nurse Executive	Poudre Valley Health System Fort Collins, Colorado	I: June 2000 R: 2004 (scheduled site visit, January 2009)
Deb Mals, RN, MS, NEA-BC Chief Nursing Officer/ Vice President of Operations	Miami Valley Hospital Dayton, Ohio	I: June 2004 R: 2008
*Kim Sharkey, RN, MBA, NEA-BC Vice President for Medicine/ Chief Nursing Officer (new to role as of 2006; several positions over previous 27 years)	St. Joseph's Hospital Atlanta, Georgia	I: 1995 R: 2000, 2004 (scheduled site visit, January 2009)
*Katherine Riley, MSN, RN, CNA, BC Vice President of Nursing Services/Chief Nursing Officer	Southwestern Vermont Medical Center Bennington, Vermont	I: 2002 R: 2006

*New CNO since 2004.

CHIEF NURSING OFFICER INTERVIEWS

The interviewed CNOs described their journeys toward achieving and then sustaining the prestigious Magnet designation. CNOs initially were chosen based on the type of facility, the length of time the facility had been designated as a Magnet organization, and the geographic location of the hospital. Four of the CNOs were from large urban, academic-affiliated hospitals (**Table 10-3**). One individual was the CNO of a five-hospital system. One of the hospitals was a large tertiary care teaching facility in an urban setting. The remaining four facilities were community-based organizations. Four of the CNOs were in community hospitals, and one CNO was in a rural hospital. All the facilities have now redesignated at least once (**Table 10-4**), and one facility (the University of Washington Medical Center [UWMC]) has been redesignated a third time. Unfortunately, the CNO of one of the large, tertiary care hospitals in the eastern part of the United States, which was first designated more than 10 years ago, was unable to participate in this current interview process.

Fifty percent of the six individuals who were in their CNO role at the time of original designation currently remained in that position. Three CNOs who were not in the CNO role at the time of original designation were working in

Table 10-3   Type of Hospital

	Tertiary/ Academic	Five-Hospital System	Community	Rural
Number of hospitals	4	1	3	1

Table 10-4   Number of Years Designated as a Magnet Facility

	< 1 Year	2–4 Years	6–7 Years	10 Years
Number of hospitals	3	3	3	1

the organization at the time. In the initial interviews, only three of the individuals were hired external to the organization, whereas in the most recent interviews only one was an external hire. Initially, 70% of the CNOs were promoted into their CNO roles, whereas 80% of CNOs in recent interviews were promoted from within the organization. Sixty percent of the CNOs were new to their role since 2005. According to Collins (2001), who interviewed CEOs of companies generally regarded for their excellence to identify their differentiating attributes, 10 out of 11 good to great CEOs came from inside the company. This finding is similar to that for the CNO interviewees, where the majority of CNOs were promoted from within their organizations.

In 2004, only two of the organizations had undergone a merger. Three had a change in CEO. Four CNOs described their roles as expanding over the years from operational accountability for nursing only to accountability for many or all clinical departments. One organization transitioned from being a community-based to a tertiary care-based provider, and one organization underwent a significant change in both strategic direction and key leadership owing to financial instability that occurred after its initial designation.

Since 2004, all of the facilities that participated in the initial study had faced challenges such as mergers, acquisitions, and multiple leadership changes. Internal, positive innovations such as technology and capacity had also occurred. While all these events create what the Magnet Commission has termed "controlled destabilization" (Wolf, 2007b), these nursing leaders have adapted to the demands of the ever-changing healthcare landscape.

As part of the study, a convenience sample was used and the interviews were limited to 30 to 45 minutes per CNO. Questions (see **Table 10-5**) were

Table 10-5   Evidence for Nursing Excellence: Magnet CNO Interview Questions

1. If you are new to your CNO at your facility, how long have you been in the role? Did you hold a position in your current organization prior to becoming CNO? If yes, which position did you hold?

2. Have there been any mergers, reorganizations, or changes in organizational strategic direction since 2005?

    a. Have there been changes in key leaders since 2005 (i.e., CEO, CFO, CHRO, CMO, COO)?

3. Which elements, programs, and initiatives contribute to your sustaining the Magnet designation?

    a. Which changes have you made to sustain the Magnet designation?

    b. What are your personal attributes that are critical to your sustaining the Magnet designation?

4. If you are a new CNO (since 2005), what were your initial strategic goals?

    a. Why did you choose those goals?

    b. How did you prioritize your goals?

5. Regarding the 14 Forces of Magnetism (quality of nursing leadership, organizational structure, management style, personnel policies and programs, professional models of care, quality of care, quality improvement, consultation and resources, autonomy, community and hospital, nurses as teachers, image of nursing, collegial nurse–physician relationships, and professional development):

    a. Which, in your experience, are key to your organization's success in sustaining Magnet status?

    b. Please explain and provide examples.

6. Regarding the 8 Essentials of Magnetism (Kramer and Schmalenberg, 2008a: support for education, clinically competent peers, patient-centered culture, supportive nurse–manager relationships, clinical autonomy, control of nursing practice, collegial/collaborative nurse–physician relationships, and perceptions of adequacy of staffing):

    a. Which, in your experience, are key to your organization's success in sustaining Magnet status?

    b. Please explain and provide examples.

7. What are you doing to operationalize Magnet concepts?

8. How are you preparing for redesignation using the five new components and updated requirements?

9. Given that outcomes are a separate component in the 2008 *Manual*, how are you addressing the component to assure that you achieve and sustain the 50th percentile?

10. What are your thoughts about the new model and the redesignation process?

provided in advance of the scheduled telephone interview, so that the nurse leaders could think about them ahead of time. Interviews were conducted during the last months of 2008 during the holiday season. Each one of the original CNOs and even the CNOs being interviewed for the first time agreed to be interviewed without hesitation and found time for the interview despite their demanding schedules and a short scheduling time frame, with the exception of one new CNO. In the remainder of this chapter, the information gleaned from these articulate, knowledgeable leaders is shared throughout the discussion of the FOM and components of the Magnet program.

MAGNET COMPONENTS: EVIDENCE IN PRACTICE

Based on the literature, CNO interviews, and comparing the FOM with Kramer and Schmalenberg's Essentials of Magnetism, the quality of nursing leadership remains the foundation on which to achieve nursing excellence. This finding is consistent with ANCC's new Magnet model (**Figure 10-1**). Each of the five new model components is discussed here and illustrated with CNO examples. **Table 10-6** depicts the relationships of the FOM to the new components; this topic is also addressed here.

In the study of the original Forces of Magnetism, an empirical approach was used to group the original sources of evidence of the Magnet model into succinct, stand-alone clusters. The empirical results were then expanded to reflect the future direction of the nursing profession (Wolf, Triolo, & Reid-Ponte, 2008).

Figure 10-1   New Magnet model.

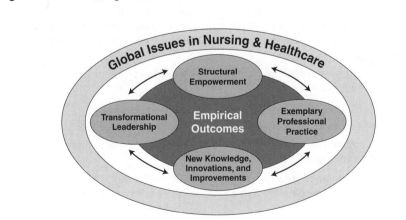

Table 10-6   Derivation of the Magnet Model

Forces of Magnetism	Empirical Domains of Evidence	Magnet Model Components
Quality of Nursing Leadership Management Style	Leadership	Transformational Leadership
Organizational Structure Personnel Policies and Programs Community and the Healthcare Organization Image of Nursing Professional Development	Resource Utilization and Development	Structural Empowerment
Professional Models of Care Consultation and Resources Autonomy Nurses as Teachers Interdisciplinary Relations Quality of Care: Ethics, Patient Safety, and Quality Infrastructure Quality Improvement	Professional Practice Model Safe and Ethical Practice Autonomous Practice Quality Processes	Exemplary Professional Practice
Quality of Care: Research and Evidence-Based Practice Quality Improvement	Research	New Knowledge, Innovations, and Improvements
Quality of Care	Outcomes	Empirical Quality Outcomes

Transformational Leadership

I dream, I test my dreams against my beliefs, I dare to take risks and I execute my vision to make those dreams come true. (Walt Disney)

ANCC (2008a) defines transformational leadership as identifying and communicating the organization's mission, vision, and values in a manner that inspires others to engage in the work to achieve the vision. This kind of leadership transforms the workplace and the healthcare industry. A leader for the future needs to be able to lead people to where they need to be. Such a leader must have strong vision, influence, clinical knowledge, expertise, and professional practice (Wolf, 2007b). This component of the Magnet model encompasses two of the Forces of Magnetism: quality of nursing leadership and management style. The sources of evidence identified by ANCC as demonstrating an organization's transformational leadership aptitude include strategic planning; advocacy, influence, and visibility; accessibility; and communication. The CNOs interviewed were quite articulate in explaining their own paths as transformational leaders. Many examples are included here.

Although none of the CNOs referred to themselves as transformational leaders, their stories, accomplishments, and ability to navigate the turbulent waters of their current healthcare realities while persistently strengthening the work environment were proof of their transformational leadership styles. The CNOs described personal attributes that they believed are critical to their organizations' success in sustaining the Magnet designation. These attributes included resiliency, honest communication, transferring personal beliefs and passions for professional nursing practice to others, servant leadership, developing and fostering relationships with stakeholders, rounding with intention, inspiring and mentoring staff nurses, belief in education, ability to get others excited and committed to their own education, tenacity, trustworthiness, and passion for service and quality, including being a cheerleader for both.

Amidst the chaos of their organizations' states, CNOs set the context for the meaning of work for nursing staff and nurse leaders. Each of the CNOs interviewed is experiencing tremendous change within the organization and spending time recognizing changes in the landscape, informing others of changes to be made, engaging in dialogue with stakeholder groups, and taking action to correct the organization's course. Their astute awareness of their realities, along with their sense-making skills, equip them to make sound decisions that support staff in doing their best work. Assisting others in change is a constant and permanent condition within health care and a key skill and competency needed by CNOs of Magnet organizations.

One CNO who was new to the position of CNO, but not to the organization, described what happens when a new CEO comes into the organization: "The tacit understanding of culture is helpful to confront. It makes one question and really look at what is happening and to truly examine the process and/or the policy" (Wild, 2008). These comments reflect her sense-making skills and openness to exploring the meaning and significance of her work environment.

Another CNO described his personal attribute as passion for service and quality patient care: "I serve as one of the cheerleaders for service and quality" (Luzinski, 2008). He also described himself as always learning and gaining in knowledge to support all staff in their practice.

One CNO described herself as being resilient (Sharkey, 2008). This leader has more than 25 years of tenure in the organization and is adept at managing changes that come her way. Significant organizational leadership changes have occurred in the 2 years she has been in the CNO role, including the hiring of a new CEO without previous Magnet experience; decentralization of nursing departments, such that they reported to four different vice presidents; the lack of a single CNO accountable for nursing practice; and the transition to service lines operating as separate entities. Recently, nursing has resumed reporting to this CNO, who has demonstrated her resiliency and mastery in articulating the value of having a centralized nursing department that reports to a single CNO while also supporting four separate service lines.

Advocacy and Influence

"I stay close to nurses and nurse leaders and talk the talk and provide the business case that supports the forces of Magnetism" (Kerfoot, 2008). This statement illustrates the ability of one CNO to take in information, link it to factors that support and sustain a culture of nursing excellence in a fiscally responsible manner, and be understood by nurses as well as senior leaders in the organization.

Inspiring others through mentoring opportunities was described by one CNO as an attribute that results in staff performing in ways that they did not know were possible. One staff nurse made the following comment: "You make me feel like I can do anything" (Burke, 2008). She also stated, "I am able to inspire people and to get the best of what they have to offer," and described herself as tenacious in her pursuit of excellence. This CNO was recently promoted and now has greater responsibility and more departments. As a result of her change in role, leaders who no longer report to her verbalize their understanding of the need to change reporting relationships. "The Nurse Executive Council is excited about my promotion because they know that I will bring the same standards and expectations to others as I have done in nursing" (Burke, 2008).

The new CNO's first priority at St. Joseph's was to realign nursing as one department following a year of decentralized management. "When the service-line structure was implemented, bedside nurses no longer felt connected to nursing and to the CNO. In the past, staff had a strong relationship and identification to the CNO. I held employee forums and focused on quality indicators and staff satisfaction. Because we were not sustaining these over time, I refocused my energy here. In 2007 I implemented a new initiative, 'Reinvesting in Nursing Excellence'" (Sharkey, 2008).

Visibility, Accessibility, and Communication

Rounding with intention is an effective attribute for another CNO, who gave the following example in which she used an inquiry mode to learn about issues, and then used the information gained in this way to make informed decisions:

> The patient lift equipment was not functioning properly, so during my rounds I would ask questions of the staff: "Tell me about the lift equipment. Does it feel safe to you? What problems are you facing? Do you have any recommendations?" (Bogolin, 2008)

The staff's responses to these questions prepared the CNO to address problems identified efficiently and effectively.

One CNO describes herself as an honest, open communicator who speaks frequently to staff to keep them apprised of decisions that she and her colleagues are making at the executive level:

> In Michigan, it is a tough environment with increasing layoffs and the demise of the auto industry, which is creating personal pressures on families affected. There have also been some layoffs in the hospital, so staff is increasingly nervous. I have promised to keep them informed and to be honest with the communication. (Gokenbach, 2008)

Strategic Planning

Over the course of the past four years, new CEOs were hired in six of the nine hospitals participating in these interviews, while five of the nine CNOs were new to their roles during the same period. Other senior leader changes or additional new roles occurred in each of the hospitals. Growth strategies were evident in six of the hospitals and included the addition of beds to current facilities, acquisition of existing hospitals and building of new hospitals to increase market share, and efforts to strengthen the role of the organization's system in achieving economies of scale and leading healthcare initiatives. Three CNOs discussed changes in their hospitals' strategic direction, which included concerns about patient safety at Miriam following a well-publicized sentinel event (a wrong-side surgery), a service-line approach to care delivery at St. Joseph's, and a greater focus on technology and/or implementing electronic medical records at Beaumont, Aurora, and Poudre Valley.

Despite the changes and their significant impact on the work to be done each day, the nine CNOs were not deterred from staying the Magnet course and achieving redesignation. In fact, from the time of initial designation, five of the nine hospitals have received one redesignation, one has received two redesignations, one achieved a second redesignation in January 2009, one achieved a third redesignation in January 2009, and one has received three redesignations. These achievements emphasize these leaders' mastery of the art of leading through chaos, uncertainty, and tremendous adversity while protecting and fostering healthy work environments for staff within their hospitals. In fact, two CNOs shared the information that the Magnet framework supported their practice during the challenging times. According to one CNO, "Living through Magnet principles has helped me find the 'true north' in times of difficulty (budget struggles, et cetera)" (Wild, 2008). A second CNO stated, "I believe in the tenets of the Magnet program and use them constantly to help guide me and to resolve problems" (Sharkey, 2008).

Each of the five new CNOs clearly identified and executed nursing department strategies once they assumed their new roles. Their emphasis on advocacy for nursing, leadership development, and visibility, accessibility, and communication are evident in their stories. For example, Kerfoot implemented an online nurse manager education program to establish leadership expectations for all managers at Aurora's five Magnet hospitals. Joint practice groups of nurses and physicians were established at the unit level as well as at the hospital and system levels (Aurora Metro Region is designated as a system). Bogolin focused on meeting patients' needs both from a service perspective (examining the implications of the newly implemented HCAHP survey) and from a patient-focused care perspective (implementing the principles of Planetree), which are hallmarks for Delnor; she also emphasized partnering with physicians in new ways to engage them more fully in the hospital and nursing. Bogolin also set expectations for leaders to support, encourage, mentor, and stay close to staff. In fact, "leaders are expected to round on their own units and sister units daily. Sixty percent of their work time is to be devoted to addressing the needs of physicians, patients, visitors, families, and staff" (Bogolin, 2008).

At Southwestern Vermont Medical Center, Riley established the professional model of care and focused on developing clinical competency to support patient-centered care and the care delivery model. The Planetree model (an evidence-based approach to patient care) was the goal, and Lean Six Sigma tools and methods were used to support the journey. The following rationale explains Riley's (2008) decisions:

> The care model had loosened up and, most significantly, there was a change in the nursing population demographics in the last three years. The specialty nurses

have started to age and/or retire. The medical surgical nurses are moving into those areas, and we now are facing an influx of new novice nurses. The isolation of the hospital is a key factor because the culture is that one doesn't drive one hour to work, so recruiting is a challenge.

Wild (2008) described the following situation:

Mostly I figured out the job and to not lose ground, particularly as an "interim," when one can't really do the real thing because it wouldn't be fair to the staff to make too many changes. Since becoming the CNO, my priority was twofold. First, [I want] to reevaluate the model of care and make sure we are where we think we are. Second, recruitment and retention are a focus. Magnet helps get people in the door, but at the two-year mark we are finding they are leaving to be travel nurses and see the world. The experienced nurses aren't moving around—just the new ones after a couple of years. So our new goal is to be creative and look at options: Go travel, but we want you back. We want them to put down roots with UW, and I talk to each new group [about that].

Each of the five new CNOs found her own path based on the unique realities she faced in her market, hospital, and community. Each demonstrated that the path is based on context—that there is no "one right way" and that the Magnet framework can be a beacon of light along the challenging route to sustaining excellence.

Structural Empowerment

To love what you do and feel that it matters—how could anything be more fun? (Katherine Graham, CEO, Washington Post Company)

Structural empowerment: This is where the mission, vision, and values of the organization "come to life" in the structure (Wolf, 2007b). This structure needs to acknowledge value as well as to support and develop strong professional practice. Further strengthening practice are the strong relationships and partnerships developed among all types of community organizations to improve patient outcomes and the health of the communities they serve. This goal is accomplished through the organization's strategic plan, structure, systems, policies, and programs. Staff members need to be developed, directed, and empowered to find the best way to accomplish the organizational goals and achieve desired outcomes. Ultimately, this aim may be accomplished through a variety of structures and programs; one size does not fit all (*http://www.nursecredentialing.org/MagnetNewsArchive2008/NewMagnetModel.aspx*). It also includes several of the FOM: organizational structure, personnel policies and programs, community and the healthcare organization, image of nursing, and professional development.

Key themes of this component are professional engagement, commitment to professional development, teaching and role development, commitment to community involvement, and recognition of nursing. Nurses become engaged through involvement in professional organizations, lifelong learning, autonomy, and empowerment. The following examples provide exceptional evidence that supports the Magnet Commission's premise that structural empowerment is difficult to initially establish, but over time should become hard-wired into the organization (Wolf, 2007b). The examples also illustrate that exceptional outcomes can be obtained through a variety of methods.

Professional Engagement

Lehigh Valley Hospital and Health Network (LVHHN) used a strategic visioning process to determine and define what the future of nursing at LVHHN "should look like and where it should be over the upcoming decade" (Capuano, Durishin, Millard, & Hitchings, 2007). Its key premise was that "engaged nurses create the desired future of nursing" and every nurse—including leaders—should be involved in this process. The nurses had equal voice, which resulted in deepened trust, leveling of the hierarchy and authority, and fully discovering common ground and hope, enthusiasm, and wonder for the future (Capuano et al., 2007). Their extensive research with employee engagement Gallup, Inc. has found that RNs at Magnet hospitals are twice as engaged as RNs at non-Magnet hospitals (Simmons, 2007).

All of the CNOs who participated in the 2008 study discussed strengthening their structures in multiple ways—from revising the nursing structure to more closely reflect the shared governance model (Burke, 2008), to formalizing the Magnet organizational structure to work closely with the professional nurse councils, to creating stronger enculturation of Magnet principles (Gokenbach, 2008).

Katherine Riley (2008), CNO of Southwestern Vermont Medical Center (SVMC), says that her facility has a longstanding culture of empowerment and genuinely looks to the employees to solve problems; according to Riley, it "starts at the top." The CEO at SVMC spends two hours at every employee orientation session talking about the organization's values of quality, empathy, stewardship, teamwork, and safety. Empowerment underscores all of these values, and SVMC even has a policy stating that any employee has the power to solve problems as close to the problem as possible—with up to $200 to use—without prior approval.

Craig Luzinski of Poudre Valley provided an example that shows how powerfully an engaged leader can affect the structure. The clinical coordinators (the traditional head nurse role responsible for daily operations on each unit) meet monthly with Luzinski, which gives him an opportunity to have meaningful "face time" with this key group of leaders. He can easily dispel any rumors that might be circulating, and can listen and guide discussion around the FOM.

In past years, two to three members of the group have been responsible for reviewing and presenting a FOM to the group. Each committee owns one or more FOM and collects data that support the FOM. Two years ago, during the Nursing Day celebration, each nursing unit created a poster on a specific FOM. These posters were all displayed and judged, and prizes were awarded. This presentation has since become an annual event. When the most recent Magnet application was submitted and reviewed by the appraiser team, no additional documentation was requested, which is attributed to the facility's well-developed FOM and to the strong exemplars prepared by various committees and teams and then coordinated by one nurse with expertise in the FOM. The completed application was put in a PDF format and displayed for all staff to view on the organization's intranet site.

Val Gokenbach (2008) of William Beaumont Hospital says, "If the structure isn't in place, it is much harder to move things forward." She now has direct line support, which allows for clearer communication and clearer responsibilities. When first interviewed in 2004, Gokenback described a unique nursing organizational structure in which four CNEs had equal authority and power. One CNE was appointed chairperson by the CEO. This individual was the single voice of nursing and was the CNE who attended the board of directors meetings. All nursing and ancillary departments reported to the CNEs. Communication became very difficult and confusing, resulting in the change in organization structure to have one CNE.

Professional Development

While the commitment to professional development is hard-wired into Magnet organizations as they mature and seek redesignation one or more times, historically the education budget is the one most vulnerable targets during tough financial challenges. Rather than being seen as a "nice to have" item, it should be viewed as an important investment in the people and in the future of the organization (O'Connor, 2008). Magnet hospitals take this notion seriously and have significantly strengthened this commitment further by forming partnerships with local colleges and universities and creating successful coaching, mentoring, graduate nurse residency programs, and strong clinical nurse ladders. The following examples highlight the investment in lifelong learning and wide range of professional development activities pursued by Magnet organizations versus the traditional continuing education program. This dedication to lifelong learning includes recognition of Magnet organizations that support non-nursing staff in pursuing nursing degrees—something that was supported by only anecdotal evidence in the early years of the Magnet Program.

Rebecca Burke (2008) states that "Professional development is important, and we are providing additional educational opportunities for nurses." Miriam

Hospital has a graduate nurse residency program with a waiting list, as the facility has a low turnover rate for RNs. It also initiated a clinical advancement program in 2006.

When first interviewed in 2004, Deb Mals said one of her goals was to have all of the facility's nurses eventually apply for management positions. Currently at Miami Valley Hospital, there are more than 52 nurses who are at some stage of the journey to become an APN, although only a few nurses are pursuing an administration pathway. This skewing may cause difficulties in the future: The hospital is unsure whether it will have enough places for 52 APNs! Mals has instituted a talent mapping process to actually look for nurses with leadership talents. The hospital is reorganizing its nursing department to provide the time for professional and developmental process; so much is experimental that it will take two to three years for the mapping project to see results. Mals believes the "next looming crisis is leadership—this is the number one priority!" She speaks of the need for programs and practices to put leadership into place and create capacity for it, but is nevertheless pleased that Miami Valley Hospital has already created a career specialist role that connects to the schools of nursing; this new role concentrates on career coaching and mentoring (Mals, 2008).

Teaching and Role Development

There are many commonalities and great creativity when it comes to developing and challenging nurses to become leaders in their organization and community. These commonalities include nurses who mentor, teach, and volunteer to share their knowledge in their communities. Nurses have consistently ranked as one of the most trusted professions for nearly a decade by Gallup polls; the only exception was in 2001, when fire fighters claimed the top spot (*http:// www.militaryconnection.com/articles/nursing/gallap-poll-trusted-profession .html*). Magnet hospitals do much to further this trust.

One of the challenges faced by newly designated Magnet facilities is the expectation that they will mentor other facilities on their journey to this status. This expectation has often led to the formation of state and regional consortia and spurred multiple phone calls regarding the new Magnet facility's star status. One of the best places to share best practices on a very large scale is the annual Magnet Conference. One unknown nurse commented during the 2007 Magnet Conference, "I've never witnessed such a great event for nursing...there are no specialty wars, just nurses excited about being nurses." As Rebecca Burke (2008) of Miriam Hospital states, "I believe in education and encourage others to pursue their education and to grow."

Deb Mals of Miami Valley Hospital agrees with Burke, observing that Magnet culture and the Magnet Conference give nurses a chance to recognize their similarities and challenge one another—an important consideration. An example learned from the last conference was a move to create a different clinical ladder. Mals presented the proposal to the MVH board of directors. Although the new clinical ladder represented a huge investment, she felt it was important not to tackle the issue in piecemeal fashion by doing a pilot, but rather to make the full investment and implement it immediately into the system. It is important that CNOs be able to leverage "what Magnet is" as a leveler, because other organizations are following the same course and Magnet brings the very best to the organizations.

Mals did not have to spend a lot of time convincing the executive leadership team that nursing is important. Achieving the best quality is possible only with extraordinary nurses. It also challenges each individual to take the key ideas and implement the best possible variation. "Sharing best practices accelerates our practice!" (Mals, 2008).

Commitment to Community Involvement

Nurses' commitment to their community and the ways in which they are perceived by their patients and colleagues often come to the fore when dress code issues arise. This point was highlighted in 2004 at St. Joseph's and was seen again at Miami Valley Hospital in 2008: The Nurse Executive Council looked at patient satisfaction and did a pilot study related to nurses' attire. Specifically, the hospital created a policy where nurses wore navy and/or white. Although some difficulty arose with acceptance at first, the leaders eventually found that the distinctive attire resulted in increased patient and nurse satisfaction. Other disciplines in the hospital are following the lead of the nursing department and will be wearing a defining color. Adherence to this policy is important because nurses lead the organization and need interdisciplinary support to operate effectively (Mals, 2008).

UWMC is focusing on partnering with its community members by instituting patient/family-centered care. The prior CNO started this trend, but this notion has been a challenge to enculturate within the organization. It means that patient and families have a key place at the decision table, an idea that is difficult for some nurses to accept (Wild, 2008).

Recognition of Nursing

How, why, when and where the hospitals recognize their nurses is an important piece of empowerment and engagement. Magnet CNOs understand this connection and have created strong recognition programs in a variety of areas. The outcome of one such program is described by Lorie Wild of UWMC when she talks about getting control of nursing practice: Evidence supports the idea that nurses run the hospital. For example, physician satisfaction with nurses' performance at UWMC was the most highly ranked item (89%) in a survey of nursing quality of care. This kind of result is very empowering to staff (Wild, 2008).

At St. Joseph's in Atlanta, the Shared Governance Model is a nursing model, not an interdisciplinary model. There are six councils and a steering council (the Nursing Executive Council). A liaison group serves as an interdisciplinary group. In the event that issues requiring an interdisciplinary approach arise, those items are brought to this group. This model empowers nurses to do the work of nursing. Currently 60–75% of all St. Joseph's staff members participate in shared governance; the organization's ultimate goal is 100%. In the 2008 Strategic Plan for Nursing, St. Joseph's set a target of 18 months to achieve 100% full- and part-time staff participation in shared governance. The three-year goal is to have 100% of the per diem staff participating in this program. As an example of what a mature, strong unit-based shared governance council can accomplish, the St. Joseph's staff identified the need to have a peer review process for all staff members (Sharkey, 2008).

Collaborative Nurse–Physician Relationships

Physicians express confidence that nurses have good critical thinking skills, which is an excellent recognition for nursing (Burke, 2008). SVMC, for example, has had shared governance since 1994. The organization continues to revive, strengthen, and evaluate this structure, but considers the councils to be both relevant and active. The councils continually address pertinent issues. For example, if their members get caught up in a discussion of structure, the leaders help to work with them to move forward. In addition, medical staff often bring issues to the councils to address. These shared governance bodies are viewed as having significant input for practice issues at SVMC.

THE ESSENTIALS OF MAGNETISM: EVIDENCE IN SUPPORT OF THE STRUCTURAL EMPOWERMENT COMPONENT

Table 10-7 shows the essentials of clinically competent peers. The ongoing support for education clearly supports the importance of this component. Studies have provided ample evidence that best practices include a variety of forms of professional development support, ranging from annual competency reviews to national certification in specialty areas.

Table 10-7   Essentials of Magnetism

Working with other nurses who are clinically competent	Nurses stated in the study that "recognition and reward for clinical competence" were important, not the clinical ladder programs (p. 30). Clinical competence was one of four value themes identified by CNEs. Also, this is the factor most significantly correlated with perception of adequate staffing, job satisfaction, and perceived ability to give quality care.
Good nurse–physician relationships and communication	These relationships are essential to Magnetism. They are essential to provide quality care and to ensure effective nurse–physician collaborative practice programs. A five-category scale was identified to describe nurse–physician relationships (beginning with the best): collegial, collaborative, student–teacher, neutral, and negative (p. 33).
Nurse autonomy and accountability	The general definition of the concept of autonomy used in the study was the freedom to act on what you know (p. 36). Two additional dimensions were added: scope ("Does practice relate to nursing care only or extend more broadly to patient care?") and sanction ("Is practice organizationally sanctioned?") (p. 36).
Supportive nurse manager or supervisor	The quality and support of the leadership team has been recognized as a central factor in the success of Magnet hospitals, affecting job satisfaction, quality care, and ability to attract nurses to the facility (p. 41). It is also essential for establishing and maintaining both nurse–physician collaborative practice and shared governance or some kind of control over nursing practice structure.
Control over nursing practice and practice environment	This factor was identified by staff nurses as essential to giving quality care. Control over practice also distinguished Magnet organizations in prior research. Domains of control usually include clinical practice, management, quality control of practitioners, and education. One outcome of control over practice cited by many nurses was "increased status, respect, and recognition" (p. 43).
Support for education (in-service, continuing education)	The focus of support for education has changed from the on-site BSN programs once attached to job satisfaction and effectiveness. Over the years, educational support has become more varied, including tuition for short-term courses, internships, externships, and on-site BSN/MSN programs and in-service education that affects attraction and retention as well as job satisfaction and the ability to give quality care (p. 43).

Adequate nurse staffing	In an organization where nurses perceive their co-workers as competent, "staff are able to work with less staff and oftentimes produce more and better-quality nursing care because they are confident in one another's abilities and trust the work of their colleagues" (p. 30). Six indicators are routinely used to measure the nurse shortage: vacancy rate, RN-to-patient ratio, turnover rate, use of supplemental staff, multiple applicants for available positions, and staff nurse perception of adequacy (p. 45).
Concern for the patient is paramount in this organization	A mark of excellence in organizations is the extent to which a system of common and shared core values is in place with values that go beyond the technical requirements of a job. When staff nurses have autonomy and trust management to listen, be responsive to, and have respect for their role and value difference, a dynamic institution exists (p. 51).

Source: Used with permission from Kramer & Schmalenberg, 2002, pp. 25–59.

EXEMPLARY PROFESSIONAL PRACTICE

We are focused on providing world-class care and service, and our goal is to be in the top decile or top 10% of all databases that we are benchmarked against. (Craig Luzinski)

"Exemplary professional practice" describes the processes of how nurses practice, collaborate, and communicate to provide excellent patient care (ANCC, 2008b). Seven of the Forces of Magnetism have been proven to have statistically clustered into this component (see Table 10-6). Nine sources of evidence make up this component: a professional practice model; a care delivery system; staffing, scheduling, and budgeting processes; interdisciplinary care; accountability, competence, and autonomy; ethics, privacy security, and confidentiality; diversity and workplace advocacy; a culture of safety; and quality care monitoring and improvement. Each of the nine CNOs interviewed provided multiple examples of how implementing processes and programs that integrate philosophies and theories of professional practice resulted in demonstrated clinical quality, operational excellence, and desirable financial outcomes.

Professional Practice Model

Staff nurses at Miami Valley Hospital participated in the development of a new clinical ladder. The CNO presented it to the board of directors, as this proposition had significant financial implications. It was important for the CNO to explain the business case for this program. Although expensive to implement, the clinical ladder was also an investment that would achieve high-quality care with extraordinary nurses. It was important that the CNO could articulate the importance of Magnet redesignation as recognizing the very best of organizations. This CNO did not have to spend a lot of time convincing the executive leadership team and board that nursing and the new clinical ladder program were important to sustaining excellence (Mals, 2008).

As part of his work, Luzinski asks his staff, "What makes you want to get out of bed and come to work each day?"(2008). At Poudre Valley Health System, staff own their practice. When a new discharge phone calls program was started in this organization, staff nurses were actively involved. Even then, deployment did not go smoothly. With staff support and process review, however, the new practice eventually became part of nurses' daily work activities.

Poudre Valley Hospital's (PVH) professional practice model also addresses the issue of preventing ventilator-associated pneumonia (VAP). Staff, in partnership with other clinical providers, have eradicated these events. Today, a case of VAP would be treated as a sentinel event and a root-cause analysis (RCA) would be conducted. In addition, each code arrest that occurs on the medical–surgical units is treated as a sentinel event and an RCA is conducted. Problems are identified quickly, resulting in education and/or process improvement. Although no real trends have been identified, respiratory assessment appears to be a common issue involved in most events. For this reason, a few years ago, a respiratory assessment course was developed at PVH and all staff were required to participate in it. Now, upon being hired, every new nurse must complete this course.

Care Delivery System

Redesignation came at a good time at Miami Valley Hospital (Mals, 2008). Over the previous few years, 60% of the hospital's hires were new graduates, so it was important to take a fresh look at what anchored them to practice: Relationship-based care provided the framework, philosophy, and foundation of nursing practice, which included what nurses were doing, how their decision making occurred, how they demonstrated value to the organization, how they cared for themselves, and how they cared for families and patients. During their site visit, the Magnet appraisers learned firsthand from nurses how things are done at the hospital: Staff are clear in their directions. They have implemented handoffs in patient rooms, and patients and families participate in this practice. Nurses keep an open mind about their new process, and they have the perseverance and commitment to sustain the change.

In 2005, Delnor Community Hospital began its patient-centered care journey. The Planetree care delivery philosophy and principles were translated into Delnor's care delivery model by the CNO (Bogolin, 2008). Practices that were implemented in support of the Planetree philosophy included having an open medical record so that patients and family members can view their records during their hospital stay and remain informed about their care, tests, and treatments ordered. Medical staff members initially were hesitant to adopt this philosophy because they did not believe that patients would understand progress notes and consultant notes. However, Bogolin and other senior leaders continually worked with the medical staff to win their support. Today, there are fewer requests for medical records post discharge; anecdotally, the hospital has faced reduced litigation and liability, as reported by Bogolin.

Staffing, Scheduling, and Budgeting Processes

A professional practice model, care delivery model, and staffing plans to support both new models were developed at St. Joseph's (Sharkey, 2008). Although requirements have always been in place for Magnet designation and redesignation, during the few years of nursing decentralization, nursing practice and care delivery became fragmented and were not deemed as exemplary by the CNO. She quickly solicited the support and leadership of the hospital's very strong shared governance councils to develop the new models. Once developed, additional nursing resources were needed to support the new models. Finding financial resources to maintain a budget-neutral proposal was the CNO's next task. Changes in scheduling and pay practices were identified, approved, and implemented to provide funding to support the new needs.

All of these changes were not perceived positively by all staff. For example, the organization had a traditional Baylor plan for the past 20 years, which many staff enjoyed; however, the staffing pattern was no longer supporting patient care needs. Equal distribution of staff was now required each day of the week, whereas when the Baylor plan was initiated, staffing needs were greatest on the weekends during the peak volume periods. In October 2008, the CNO announced that as of March 2009, Baylor plan positions (which required 24 worked hours on weekends for 40 hours of pay) would be eliminated. Ninety staff members are currently in these positions, and they now have the opportunity to find new positions within the organization. The money saved by implementing programs such as this one will be used to fund higher nurse–patient ratios as well as more clinical educator positions.

Interdisciplinary Care

Exemplary professional practice is also evident in the communication process of care delivery at Delnor. Three forms of rounding occur on a regular basis.

First, the change of shift report now takes place at the bedside and includes the patient, the patient's care partner/family member, and oncoming and off-going RNs.

Second, progress rounds are conducted every two days on each medical–surgical and telemetry unit. The patient's RN, patient care coordinator (charge nurse), case manager, social worker, and chaplain visit each patient on the unit to discuss each patient's progress toward discharge. Daily goals are then written on the patient's whiteboard so that all providers and family members know the plan of care.

Third, hourly rounding is performed by the clinical staff on the unit. RNs and technicians round every other hour so that patients have access to a care provider each and every hour of the day. The focus of these rounds is to meet patients' needs (not clinicians' needs). Hanging intravenous medications and doing medical interventions are not tasks that are included in these rounds. Instead, the intent of these rounds is to ask patients what they need (e.g., assistance to the bathroom, water, assistance to a chair or bed). As a result, there are fewer call lights; nurses comment that the night shift is calm and quiet.

As evidence of the Planetree philosophy being acculturated at the unit level, physicians—many of whom are splitters (going to more than one hospital, without loyalty to any one hospital)—often ask the CNO and clinical leaders to go to the other hospitals to teach nurses how to really get to know their patients as nurses do at Delnor. Delnor was awarded the Planetree designation in the fall of 2008.

Accountability, Competence, and Autonomy

There are many programs that exemplify professional practice. Two such programs are at the Miriam Hospital: the on-site clinical nurse leader program and the graduate nurse residency program.

The University of Rhode Island provides the nurse leader program. Burke started this pilot program with 5 nurses, and then took the first cohort of 10 in 2007:

> We now have master's-prepared nurses at the bedside. We now have very low turnover on our medical unit. New grads love working with our clinical nurse leader on the medical unit. In addition to mentoring new grads, she is involved in developing protocols to improve patient care. For example, she was involved in developing an oral care protocol, which is now hospital-wide. She developed a COPD patient protocol, as pulmonary patients are seen on this medical unit. She develops robust plans of care for complex patients. When she is providing patient care, her assignment is typically three patients, all of whom are the most critical patients on the unit. She negotiates for nondirect patient care days to work on

projects. On average, she has a research day each month and is a key driver of change management at the bedside. (Burke, 2008)

The graduate nurse residency program supported the hiring of 80–90 new graduates in 2007 and resulted in a positive impact on retention and turnover. Today, this organization has a waiting list for new nurses in a current environment of nursing shortages and high vacancy rates.

Ethics, Privacy, Security, and Confidentiality

Poudre Valley Health System prides itself on its culture of safety and ability to successfully influence the rate of patient falls (a nurse-sensitive indicator). Balancing the needs for patient privacy with patient safety was a dilemma that the staff addressed. Three years ago, the unassisted falls contributed to two deaths, which led to an extensive review. Bathrooms were identified as a contributor. Today, in addition to the use of bed alarms, any patient at high risk for falling is never left unattended in the bathroom. Someone stays with the patient and explains that his or her safety is the reason for someone remaining in the bathroom and that safety is a higher priority than privacy.

The neurology unit had the highest fall rate, which led to staff actively seeking new ways to provide safe patient care. This unit instituted 24/7 video monitoring of patients at high risk of falls. Again, patients' privacy is trumped by patient safety concerns.

Since inception of these approaches to patient safety, there have been no falls with harm at Poudre Valley Hospital.

Diversity and Workplace Advocacy

None of the interview questions in the study directly asked the CNOs to describe activities under way at their hospitals that support this source of evidence; however, two organizations are implementing the Planetree model of patient-focused care, which includes giving patients the right to read their medical records and actively involving patients and families in developing the patient's plan of care. Delnor Community Hospital, as previously mentioned, has already achieved recognition by the Planetree organization as one of 6 hospitals to successfully incorporate each of the principles into practice.

A second example of addressing this source of evidence is Poudre Valley Health System's implementation of David Marx's (2001) "just culture," which uses a decision matrix to determine culpability for unsafe acts performed by staff. This process differentiates system-induced errors and deficiencies in training from intentional unacceptable actions. The level of discipline is determined by culpability rather than based on the severity of the mishap. Finally, Poudre Valley Health System has developed a culture of appreciation, whereby staff explicitly recognize one another for the work that each person does. Staff have the opportunity to recognize and award their peers with $3 coupons when they do good work. As this example demonstrates, the key to engagement is understanding and living our mission and values.

Culture of Safety

In support of a culture of safety and diversity, Bogolin described another practice at Delnor Community Hospital. Patients' stories of harm that occurred during hospitalization are told by patients at the Quality Committee of the board of directors each meeting. For example, at one board meeting a recently discharged patient who had acquired a methicillin-resistant *Staphylococcus aureus* (MRSA) infection during his hospitalization told the story of his "Lost Summer," in which he had to be taken into the hospital for intravenous administration of antibiotics for several weeks. A second patient who had a community-acquired case of MRSA shared his observations while a patient at Delnor, including the fact that staff and physicians were inconsistent in hand-washing and use of contact precautions. His story was videotaped, and the story has since been shared with all employees during quarterly forums and medical staff committee meetings.

The Project Zero campaign resulted from these cases. All adult patients who are admitted to Delnor Community Hospital are now screened for MRSA upon admission, and hand-washing and use of contact precautions are frequently discussed and monitored.

Quality Care Monitoring and Improvement

Quality care monitoring and improvement was one of the sources of evidence that was repeatedly discussed by the CNOs. "I serve as one of the cheerleaders for service and quality," said Luzinski (2008). "I am responsible for being knowledgeable about quality care and improvement." Poudre Valley Health System's Quality Department reports to this CNO, and he actively works with the department to implement a robust program. Poudre Valley Hospital has also been implementing the principles of David Marx's "just culture," including the use of inquiry as a method to involve staff by asking them questions to help them understand the episode of poor performance rather than using a punitive approach for dealing with poor performance.

"Compared to most organization, we have taken a hard line on employees becoming involved and following safe practices," says Luzinski. For example, bedside medication verification started 1.5 years ago at his organization. Compliance was measured at 50% with use of scanners. New goals were set and, within 9 months, a level of 90% compliance was reached. Along the way, staff members identified a set of process problems and worked with others to improve those processes. Today, because the processes were addressed explicitly and are working smoothly, any further lack of noncompliance results in a focus on the individual; the disciplinary process is invoked if the employee knowingly disregarded the current process and no barrier prevented him or her from being compliant. The use of patient identifiers is a well-known expectation: The first event of noncompliance is occasion for a "final warning"; a second event is terms for termination. However, each event is investigated thoroughly using the "just culture" matrix. Implementation of this process demonstrated the organization's shift to a culture of safety, which is critical to support reduced morbidity and mortality. Staff members are included in reviews of any event that leads to patient harm. Actions to resolve these events are first accepted by staff before they are implemented.

At Aurora Health Care, each facility has a quality dashboard and action plans are developed for indicators not meeting targets. For the Centers for Medicare/Medicaid Services' (CMS) "never events," rates are no longer reported, but each event is counted and examined. Nurses at Delnor Community Hospital now own their own core measures and are responsible for implementing their own interventions to improve performance. Quality management staff support their activities but are not the drivers of the changes. Over the past year, Lean principles have been applied to several projects, including addressing process and system changes to meet obstetrical capacity issues and sterile processing changes to support surgical patient care and smoother operating room throughput.

At Poudre Valley Health System, unit-based committees have been involved in the Baldridge process and staff have attended classes intended to help them develop quality improvement projects, conduct data collection, and develop action plans. All staff members are well versed in the process, although a few patient care units have not achieved greater than a 90th percentile ranking. Transparency is a part of the culture, so staff and leaders learn to discuss their performance openly. Hospital efforts and resources are shifted to underperforming units so that they can develop and implement approaches to move their performance to a higher level. Says Craig Luzinski (2008), "We believe and demonstrate that we are a learning community. We expect all units to be well versed in using run charts and conducting their own data analysis by providing them resources to be successful." During monthly nursing director meetings, score cards are reviewed: World-class performance (top 10% of benchmark) is recognized, while those units not meeting their targets are identified.

CNOs of Magnet hospitals openly admit their passion for nursing excellence in their statements. Says Mals (2008), "Sharing best practices accelerates our practice!" According to Sharkey (2008), "My personal philosophy is that Magnet is not a prize to hold to yourself. Our goal should be to mentor and support as many hospitals as possible to seek and achieve Magnet designation. In Georgia, I have worked with the CNOs of the other three Magnet hospitals to form a consortium to improve patient outcomes and to advance nursing."

When Poudre Valley Hospital was awarded the prestigious Malcolm Baldrige Award in November 2008, Luzinski (2008) commented that he had a responsibility to share the organization's best practices and learnings with colleagues across the country so that they can implement any of the practices that meet their needs. His open, generous approach to help others achieve and sustain excellent patient care demonstrates his commitment to safe, effective nursing care.

THE ESSENTIALS OF MAGNETISM: EVIDENCE IN SUPPORT OF THE EXEMPLARY PROFESSIONAL PRACTICE COMPONENT

Kramer and Schmalenberg have conducted extensive research studies over the past 23 years to first identify and then verify, elucidate, and evaluate the Essentials of Magnetism (EOM)—that is, the elements necessary to support a healthy work environment for clinical nurses. As of June 2009, they will have published 37 studies on the EOM (personal communication). Table 10-7 summarizes their most recent work, which identifies the structures, processes, and outcomes of healthy work environments from the perspective of bedside nurses. Although these studies are not randomized control trials (which are perceived as the gold standard for strength of evidence), they are nevertheless well-designed studies using large samples of practicing nurses from many hospitals from across the United States and involve both qualitative and quantitative methods (DiCenso, Guyatt, & Ciliska, 2005). These studies clearly differentiate staff nurses' perceived work environment needs from those of formal leaders and professional organizations. Staff nurses value competent peers above all else. They also desire autonomous decision making, both independent and interdependent. Control over nursing practice is another dominant concern of bedside nurses. Kramer and Schmalenberg (2008a, 2008b, 2008c, 2008d; Kramer et al., 2008; Schmalenberg et al., 2008) have identified a variety of best practices that contribute to the healthy work environment; these are also apparent in the sources of evidence for each of the five components previously discussed in this chapter.

New Knowledge, Innovations, and Improvements

Magnet organizations are in an ideal position to advance the science of nursing and should be the pioneers of our future. (Gail Wolf)

Magnet organizations conscientiously integrate evidence-based practice and research into their clinical and operational processes. They possess established and evolving programs related to evidence-based practices and research programs. Indeed, innovations in patient care, nursing, and the practice environment are the hallmark of hospitals receiving the Magnet designation (ANCC, 2008a). Magnet organizations that are preparing for redesignation tend to not take risks lest they compromise their redesignation. Creating reformation in health care will cause a bit of controlled destabilization, so this component will reflect that risk, encouraging Magnet facilities to make changes based on the evidence and focus on the future (Wolf, 2007a).

The Forces of Magnetism included in this component focus on quality of care through research, evidence-based practice, and quality improvement (innovation). These terms are sometimes used interchangeably, oftentimes because of confusion about the true meaning of each individual term. Once they are hard-wired into a practice culture, however, they are complementary (Newhouse, 2007).

Dr. Janet Houser, Associate Dean for Research at Regis University, was called upon to assist Poudre Valley Health System with its assessment and development efforts. She conducted a series of education events. Since her involvement, all policies and practice are now evidence based and include levels of evidence; master's-level students conduct their research at the hospital. Today, two PhD-prepared nurse researchers are on the Nursing Research Council. Members of the Nursing Research Council presented the results of their study at Sigma Theta Tau International (STTI) in Vienna, Austria, in 2007, which marked a change in attitude and knowledge regarding pre- and post-EBP education. It took 3 years to fully implement and enculturate EBP. Now Clinical Nurse Specialists (CNSs) lead the committees with involvement from all areas of the hospital (Luzinski, 2008).

Other CNOs report that the focus on research, EBP, and innovation is inspiring members of their organizations:

- "The research project that we are doing in partnership with Cerner and UWM is helping us achieve quality outcomes using an evidence-based approach. This is a three-year project. We just went live in July, and we will begin collecting data and evaluating our impact on patient outcomes over the next year." (Kerfoot, 2008).
- "EBP and research is a current priority. Reducing urinary tract infections and other clinical problems is our focus. The hospital's Risk Management department awarded nursing a grant to conduct a patient falls research project" (Burke, 2008).
- "To remain on the cutting edge, I am forming a new Nursing Innovations Team for 2009 and creating a formal structure with two universities to increase research at the bedside and begin to articulate outcomes in a more profound way" (Gokenbach, 2008).

- "Quality issues are paramount, so we always engage staff to help. When helping or mentoring other hospitals, rather than charging for our time, we ask for a donation to the Magnet Research Fund, which funds the Nurse Scholar program (pays for 80 hours to do the EBP or research project). Dr. Tuttle of the University of Iowa is now working with us on a research project. We asked for research champions to collect data and had lots of interest and volunteers to do it on their own time—not part of the scholar program" (Riley, 2008).

- "I believe that one attribute that is critical for us to sustain Magnet [designation] is the belief in what we can achieve despite being a small rural hospital. I look at what larger facilities are doing, and find a way to accomplish similar here. I don't like hearing that we can't do something, I like the approach of 'how can we do this?'" (Riley, 2008).

- "The nurses at the bedside are engaged with research! SVMC has Evidence-Based Competency Validation day that celebrates this; the title also makes the link to practice obvious to newer nurses. Nurses need to understand science as well as technology" (Riley, 2008).

- "To address resource allocation, we use Lean management tools. We must look at efficiency of the system to manage the numbers and types of people we need. We are constantly searching for better ways and trying to convert those into business cases to support our innovation. For example, we examined the staffing model to address nurse managers' span of control. We completed an analysis of what they were currently doing. We looked at tools that would improve efficiency. We know from the research that once span of control is greater than 40–45 people, relationships suffer. We were able to quantify this by a question on the staff satisfaction survey that addresses loyalty" (Kerfoot, 2008).

- "There have to be strong leaders at every level throughout the facility. That is how you innovate! One of UW's core values is innovation, which allows us to constantly improve. Leaders cultivate that kind of environment" (Wild, 2008)

- "We have a clinical nurse scholar program funded to have selected nurses develop EBP or a research project; we get 10–12 applications per year. We also have an EBP/Research week and get 30–40 posters. As a Magnet facility, the nurses understand the importance [of research] and are engaged" (Riley, 2008).

- "Quality is number one: Everything else feeds into quality. From the board of directors and senior leaders to staff at the bedside, the focus is quality first. Leaders provide the resources for staff to do their jobs, and we have created an environment and provided tools so that we have quality outcomes" (Luzinski, 2008).

Empirical Quality Outcomes

The 50th percentile of today is the 75th percentile of tomorrow. (Deb Mals)

The assumption is that Magnet organizations should be leading the way in terms of outcomes. These outcomes are dynamic and measurable and may be reported at an individual unit, department, population, or organizational level. They define areas of improved performance and areas requiring additional effort to achieve improvement. These outcomes focus on the results and differences that can be demonstrated based on application of sound structure and process in the healthcare team and other external and internal factors. The dynamic nature of outcomes allows for the "controlled destabilization" in a transformational environment and answers the question, "So what?" (ANCC, 2008b; Wolf & Greenhouse, 2007). The CNOs who participated in the 2008 study unanimously supported the notion of Magnet moving more toward outcomes and the goal of reaching or sustaining achievement in the 50th percentile.

An additional item addressed in the area of excellence was the awards that each facility had received. **Table 10-8** illustrates the types and numbers of awards the facilities in this chapter have earned in addition to Magnet recognition. This demonstrates the ongoing quest of Magnet organizations to not just meet excellence but to exceed the standard. The theme in this component is quality of care.

Currently we are at the 50th percentile for all indicators. Our NDNQI results are good as are our Core Measures. For example, we have a nurse-driven protocol for the pneumonia vaccine and we are doing well. Also, our pressure ulcer rate is very good. (Burke, 2008)

We have done a good job focusing on outcomes and achieving and sustaining the 50th percentile. One difficulty might be employee satisfaction. The organization is facing some economic struggles (like everyone else) and had to implement a change to healthcare benefits for employees, from an HMO to a consumer-directed plan. Even though [the change] is being implemented in stages, at some point keeping both plans will be too expensive and there will be a tipping point—not too popular with employees. We will continue to address concerns. (Riley, 2008)

Our system president uses the metaphor of a *work-horse philosophy*, which is to keep enough energy over time to maintain the heavy burden in today's challenging healthcare industry. Too many organizations today have a *race-horse mentality*, which is focused on achieving the goal but are unable to sustain over time, which leads others to believe that the organization has a "flavor of the month" philosophy. (Luzinski, 2008).

Table 10-8   Chief Nursing Officer, Hospital Affiliation, and State and National Recognition Awards

CNO and Hospital	State and National Recognition Awards for Excellence (2004–2008)
Rebecca Burke, MS, RN Miriam Hospital Providence, Rhode Island	2008: Blue Distinction Centers for Complex and Rare Cancer, from Blue Cross and Blue Shield 2008: Number 1 Diagnostic Imaging Residency, from Brown University 2007, 2006: Top 100 Cardiovascular Hospitals, from Solucient 2006: Primary Stroke Designation
Lore Bogolin, MSN, RN Delnor Community Hospital Geneva, Illinois	2008: Best Place to Work in Illinois (#4) 2008, 2007, 2006, 2005, 2004: National List of Companies That Care, from the Center for Companies That Care 2007: Planetree Designated Hospital (one of 6 hospitals as of 2007)
Karlene Kerfoot, PhD, RN, CNAA, FAAN Aurora Health Care Metro Region: St. Luke's Medical Center, St. Luke's South Shore, Aurora Sinai Medical Center, West Allis Memorial Hospital, and Aurora Medical Center Washington County, Wisconsin	2008: World Wide Web Health Award, Bronze Medal for Health Promotion/Disease and Injury Prevention 2007, 2006, 2005, 2004: One of the Most Wired Healthcare Providers, from *Hospital and Health Network* magazine 2006 (Aurora Sinai): One of the top 59 hospitals recognized nationally by Leapfrog Group for Patient Safety 2006, 2005 (Aurora Sinai): Premier Award for Quality for Community-Acquired Pneumonia and Maternal, Neonatal Care
Val Gokenbach, DM, RN, RWJF William Beaumont Hospital Royal Oak, Michigan	2008: *U.S. News and World Report* Best Hospitals (ranked for 14 years) Governor Award for Family Medicine Center (5 years) 2008: National Research Corporation Consumer Choice Award 2008: Most Preferred Hospital in Southeastern Michigan (awarded for 13 consecutive years) 2005: Automation Alley's "Nonprofit of the Year"

Lorie Wild, PhD, RN, NEA-BC
University of Washington
   Medical Center
Seattle, Washington
	U.S. News and World Report Best Hospitals
	   (2007, ranked #11; 2008, ranked #10)
	2008: Practice Green Health Environmental
	   Leadership Award
	Washington State Quality Award, Leadership
	   Level

Craig Luzinski, MS, RN
Poudre Valley Health System
Fort Collins, Colorado
	2008: Malcolm Baldrige National Quality Award
	2008, 2007, 2006, 2005, 2004: Thompson Top 100
	   Hospitals
	2008: One of America's 100 Best Places to Work,
	   from *Modern Healthcare*
	2008: Highest Award for Sustained Overall
	   Excellence in Nursing Quality, from the
	   American Nurses Association
	2008, 2007, 2006, 2005: Top 100 Hospitals, from
	   Solucient

Deb Mals, MS, RN, NEA-BC
Miami Valley Hospital
Dayton, Ohio
	2008–2009: Consumer's Choice Award for
	   Dayton Area (13 consecutive years)
	Health Grade's Distinguished Hospital Award
	   for Clinical Excellence™
	June 2007: Top One Percent in United States for
	   Cardiac Care, from CMS
	2007: *U.S. News and World Report* Best
	   Hospital

Kim Sharkey, RN, MBA,
   NEA-BC
St. Joseph's Hospital
Atlanta, Georgia
	2006: Distinguished Hospital Award for Patient
	   Safety, from HealthGrades
	2004: A+ Employer, from *Atlanta Business
	   Chronicle*

Katherine Riley, MSN, RN,
   CAN, BC
Southwestern Vermont
   Medical Center
Bennington, Vermont
	2007: VHA Leadership Award for Clinical
	   Excellence
	2007: Press Ganey Summit Award
	Three Vermont State Quality Awards, from the
	   Center for Living and Rehabilitation

Over the last three years, our organization has changed significantly, which has created uncertainty among those who work here. We have been able to sustain our outcomes. We are recognized as one of the top 100 hospitals, and our NDNQI nurse-sensitive indicators remain strong overall. (Sharkey, 2008)

[We use a] balanced score card; goals are adjusted annually. For example, in our bedside medication verification process, our year 1 goal was 50% compliance to achieve green [status]; our second-year goal was 50% compliance (red); and the new green target was 75% compliance. Another example of different goals for different areas is the Emergency Department (ED), where we have lower, realistic goals for patient satisfaction because it is more difficult for the ED to achieve similar patient satisfaction results due to wait times [and other factors that lead to] significant patient [dissatisfaction]. (Luzinski, 2008)

[We] feel good about the new directions. The need to challenge MVH is there; there is no real hurdle, but the challenge for us is whether the 50th [percentile] is good enough. (Mals, 2008)

We have a very robust system for collecting and reporting data and outcomes. There is a great deal of evidence-based processes and research at the bedside. I also thought that it would be valuable for all nurse managers and PNC members to become "yellow belts" in Six Sigma, which we completed this year. Many of the building blocks are already in place. (Gokenbach, 2008)

Since the HCAHP's survey was newly implemented, it was important for everyone to understand the new rating scale. The Likert rating scale uses "always," and it was important to understand what it means to patients and to staff. What do staff need to do to meet patients' needs consistently? Also the ED had been at the 99th percentile using the Press Ganey survey, and now their scores went down on the item "Likelihood to recommend the ED to others." The staff created a video that is played in the waiting room to explain to patients and families what to expect while in the ED. (Bogolin, 2008)

Nurses now own their own core measures and are responsible for implementing their own interventions to improve performance. Quality Management staff support their activities but are not the drivers of the changes. Over the past year, lead principles have been applied to several projects, including addressing process and system changes to meet OB capacity issues and sterile processing changes to support surgical patient care and smoother OR throughput. (Bogolin, 2008).

SUMMARY

Maggie McClure and Ada Sue Hinshaw, authors of the chapter "The Future of Magnet Hospitals" in *Magnet Hospitals Revisited*, stated that "Magnet status is not a permanent institutional characteristic, but rather one that requires constant nurturing" (2002, p. 119). All of the CNOs of the Magnet hospitals interviewed for this chapter related many personal struggles and institutional challenges in preparing for redesignation and keeping the momentum and excitement fresh. Our discussions in 2008 with the CNO group revealed a maturing of the role of Magnet CNO, including greater willingness to take risks and try other directions should one not be initially successful. The new Magnet model has been embraced by the interviewed CNOs despite the challenges of learning a new manual each time they seek redesignation of the organization. Realizing that hospitals have life cycles and changing the way redesignated hospitals are evaluated have also been welcome trends.

The Magnet Program reached a tipping point in 2003, and it continues to gain prestige as the number of facilities achieving this designation grows. Magnet hospitals now account for 5% of the nation's 5,708 hospitals (AHA, 2008). In addition, Magnet hospitals continue to dominate *U.S. News and World Report*'s list of 100 Best Hospitals.

The economic challenges facing health care today are enormous. Nevertheless, according to Tom Mason, founding head of Rose-Hulman Institute of Technology and founding Vice President of Entrepreneurship and Business Planning of Rose-Hulman Ventures (2008), "Economic history has taught us that new waves of technology and innovation bring higher and higher levels of prosperity and that great problems can be viewed as great opportunities."

The Magnet Commission has published a dynamic model for the Forces of Magnetism that creates an environment in which leadership, innovation, quality, and safety are rewarded and celebrated. "Successful transformation must be led by the nurse executive with an unrelenting passion" (Wolf & Greenhouse, 2007). After her institution's recent redesignation, Karen Haller, Vice President of Nursing and Patient Care Services at Johns Hopkins Hospital, stated, "Magnet allows us to think about what is right, good, excellent" (2008, p. 25). These are the words of the pioneers of our future.

REFERENCES

American Hospital Association (AHA). (2008). *Fast facts on US hospitals.* Retrieved May 12, 2009, from http://www.aha.org/aha/resource-center/Statistics-and-Studies/fast-facts.html

American Nurses Association (ANA). (1991). *Standards for organized nursing services and responsibilities of nurse administrators across all settings.* Washington, DC: Author.

American Nurses Credentialing Center (ANCC). (2004). *Nursing: Scope and standards of practice.* Washington, DC: American Nurses Association.

American Nurses Credentialing Center (ANCC). (2008a). *Announcing a new model for ANCC's Magnet Recognition Program.* Retrieved December 1, 2008, from http://www.nursecredentialing.org/MagnetNewsArchive2008/NewMagnetModel.aspx

American Nurses Credentialing Center (ANCC). (2008b). *Application manual: Magnet Recognition Program, 2008 edition.* Silver Spring, MD: American Nurses Association.

Bogolin, L. (2008). Personal communication, Delnor Community Hospital, Geneva, IL.

Burke, R. (2008). Personal communication, The Miriam Hospital, Providence, RI.

Capuano, T., Durishin, L., Millard, J., & Hitchings, K. (2007). The desired future of nursing doesn't just happen: Engaged nurses create it. *Journal of Nursing Administration, 37*(2), 61–63.

Collins, J. (2001). *Good to great: Why some companies make the leap and others don't.* New York: HarperCollins.

DiCenso, A., Guyatt, G., & Ciliska, D. (2005). *Evidence-based nursing: A guide to clinical practice.* St. Louis, MO: Elsevier Mosby.

Gokenbach, V. (2008). Personal communication, William Beaumont Hospital, Royal Oak, MI.

Haller, K. (2008, Fall). Patient safety heroes save the day. *Johns Hopkins Nursing, 6*(3), 25.

Havens, D. S., Thompson, P. A., & Jones, C. B. (2008). Chief nursing officer turnover. *Journal of Nursing Administration, 38*(12), 516–525.

Kerfoot, K. (2008). Personal communication, Aurora Health Care System, Washington County, WI.

Kleinman, D. M. (2008, October 25–26). Critical questions: Helping patients make informed choices. *Wall Street Journal,* pp. A8A–A8C.

Kramer, M., & Schmalenberg, C. (2002). Staff nurses identify essentials of magnetism. In M. McClure & A. S. Hinshaw (Eds.), *Magnet hospitals revisited: Attraction and retention of professional nurses* (pp. 25–59). Washington, DC: American Nurses Association.

Kramer, M., & Schmalenberg, C. (2008a). Confirmation of a healthy work environment. *Critical Care Nurse, 28*(2), 56–63.

Kramer, M., & Schmalenberg, C. (2008b). The practice of clinical autonomy in hospitals: 20,000 nurses tell their story. *Critical Care Nurse, 28*(6), 1–13.

Kramer, M., & Schmalenberg, C. (2008c). Nine structures and leadership practices essential to a magnetic work environment. NAQ accepted for publication.

Kramer, M., & Schmalenberg, C. (2008d). Clinical unit with the healthiest work environments. *Critical Care Nurse, 28*(3), 65–77.

Kramer, M., Schmalenberg, C., Maguire, P., Brewer, B., Burke, R., Chmielewski, L., et al. (2008). Structures and practices enabling staff nurses to control their practice. *Western Journal of Nursing Research, 30*(5), 539–559.

Luzinski, C. (2008). Personal communication, Poudre Valley Health System, Fort Collins, CO.

Mals, D. (2008). Personal communication, Miami Valley Hospital, Dayton, OH.

Marquez, L. (2006, January 21). Nursing shortage: How it may affect you. *ABC News.* Retrieved May 8, 2009, from http://abcnews.go.com/WNT/Health/story?id=1529546

Marx, D. (2001, April 17). Medical event reporting system—transfusion medicine (MERS-TM). In *Patient safety and the "Just Culture:" A Primer for Health Care Executives* (pp. 1–28). Funded by a grant from the National Heart, Lung, and Blood Institute, National Institutes of Health. Retrieved May 3, 2009, from http://dodpatientsafety.usuhs.mil/index.php?name=Downloads&req=getit&lid=724

Mason, T. (2008). Flashpoint: Surviving the financial crisis. *TribStar.com.* Retrieved June 18, 2009, from http://www.tribstar.com/opinion/local_story_348112050.html/resources_printstory

McClure, M. L., & Hinshaw, A. S. (2002). The future of hospitals. In *Magnet hospitals revisited: Attraction and retention of professional nurses* (pp. 116–128). Washington, DC: American Nurses Association.

Newhouse, R. P. (2007). Evidence and the executive: Diffusing confusion among evidence-based practice, quality improvement and research. *Journal of Nursing Administration, 37*(10), 432–435.

Nurse Retention and Quality of Care Act of 2001 (Introduced in Senate) S 1594 IS (2001). Retrieved June 18, 2009, from http://thomas.loc.gov/cgi-bin/query/z?c107:S.1594:

O'Connor, M. (2008). The dimensions of leadership: A foundation for caring competency. *Nursing Administration Quarterly, 32*(1), 21–26.

Pekkanen, J. (2003, September). Condition: Critical. *Reader's Digest,* 84–93.

Porter-O'Grady, T, & Malloch, K. (2008). Beyond myth and magic: The future of evidence-based leadership. *Nursing Administration Quarterly, 32*(3), 176–187.

Riley, K. (2008). Personal communication, Southwestern Vermont Medical Center, Bennington, VT.

Schmalenberg, C., Kramer, M., Brewer, B. B., Burke, R., Chmielewski, L., Cox, K., et al. (2008). Clinically competent peers and support for education: Structures and practices that work. *Critical Care Nurse, 28*(4), 54–65.

Sharkey, K. (2008). Personal communication, St. Joseph's Hospital, Atlanta, GA.

Simmons, S. (2007). Personal communication, The Gallup Organization, Washington, DC.

Triolo, P. K., Scherer, E. M., & Floyd, J. M. (2006). Evaluation of the Magnet Recognition Program. *Journal of Nursing Administration, 36*(1), 42–48.

Trofino, J. (2007, May). *Magnet recognition: The Nobel Prize for nursing practice.* Retrieved May 12, 2009, from http://www.entrepreneur.com/tradejournals/article/168512990.html

Wild, L. (2008). Personal communication, University of Washington Medical Center, Seattle, WA.

Wolf, G. (2007a). Introduction of the New Magnet Model, presentation at Magnet Conference, October.

Wolf, G. (2007b). The New Magnet Model [Webinar]. October.

Wolf, G. A., & Greenhouse, P. K. (2007). Blueprint for design: Creating models that direct change. *Journal of Nursing Administration, 37*(9), 381–387.

Wolf, G., Triolo, P., & Reid-Ponte, P. (2008). Magnet Recognition Program: The next generation. *Journal of Nursing Administration, 38*(4), 200–204.

CHAPTER 11

Evidence-Based Regulation: Emerging Knowledge Management to Inform Policy

Joey Ridenour

Crucial to finding the way is this: there is no beginning or end. You must make your own map. (Joy Hargo, "A Map to the Next World")

INTRODUCTION

This chapter has three aims. First, it addresses the emergence and importance of evidence-based regulation (EBR) as the means to inform policy. Second, it explores the challenges related to EBR as well as lessons learned in the implementation of evidence-informed regulation. Third, it concludes with suggestions for future research in EBR as the means to support higher levels of performance in regulatory agencies.

THE EMERGENCE OF EVIDENCE-BASED REGULATION

Effective policy must be informed by valid knowledge regarding the correlates of performance and provide input for policy makers' deliberations. (Smith, 2004)

According to Keehley and Abercrombie (2008), most government and non-profit agencies are using a wide array of performance measures to manage their resources and demonstrate to the public or their constituents that they are meeting their regulatory mandates.

Evidence-based or -informed policy and practice is complex and creates a diverse literature of its own, which ranges widely across issues from primary research as a source of evidence to its implementation in policy and practice ("Lessons from the Literature," 2008). Much of the literature on evidence-based policy has been produced in the United Kingdom, where researchers have focused on identification and synthesis of academic and research evidence that relates to the central government's support of the national healthcare system. The emphasis of the United Kingdom is on raising basic awareness of the importance of information and is generally interpreted as a call for data to support better decision making.

Chalmers argues that "practitioners in all fields sometimes do things which are not beneficial, and occasionally do harm" (quoted in Hammeresley, 2005). Furthermore, research has an important role to play in providing information for policy making and practice. There is a strong tendency for all manner of ideas to be presented as if they were high-level research evidence when, in fact, they are not the product of research and are not reliable. Even in the realm of research, some over-claiming occurs. This stems, in part, from the demands that researchers demonstrate the practical value and interest of their work. Reviews are, therefore, an essential bridge between the worlds of research and those of policy making and practice (Hammeresley, 2005).

In the United States, the passage of the Government Performance and Results Act (GPRA) in 1993 demonstrated that elected officials wanted the government's services to improve (Keehley & Abercrombie, 2008). This act marked the first time public officials had legislated a strategic approach to administering government. Departments and agencies were allowed several years to align their performance measures with their strategic plan. In 2003, the U.S. Office of Management and Budget (OMB) required all federal agencies to report on their performance measures as a way to enhance their performance based on evidence. Boyne, Meier, O'Toole, and Walker (2006) and Petch (2008) assert that public management and organizational performance rapidly developed from a non-issue to big issue as part of this requirement. According to a study done by Howard and Kilmartin (2006), 73% of government executives reported asking, "How do we compare to neighboring jurisdictions?" or "Have we improved service delivery in the last year?"

To develop pragmatic plans to produce evidence-based regulation, regulatory leaders should rigorously address several independent questions as a framework to increase their impact for change:

- What are the results for which will we hold ourselves accountable?
- How will we achieve those results?
- What will those results really cost?
- How do we build the organization we need to deliver the results?

NURSING REGULATION

Boards of Nursing have a legal mandate to protect the public from unsafe nurses, improve the outcomes of nursing education, and remove regulatory barriers in the licensing of practitioners. In the past ten years, the public and state legislatures have also formulated expectations for board staff and members to be more explicit about the evidence that provides a linkage to their public protection mandate.

In 1998, National Council of State Boards of Nursing (NCSBN), which is a nonprofit agency comprising member boards of the 50 states plus U.S. territories, embarked on a ground-breaking project to further the evidence-based regulation model. NCSBN began the development of a performance measurement system for state and territorial Boards of Nursing that incorporated data collected from internal and external sources. A key element of this system was defining and measuring performance based on outcome-oriented indicators to assist nursing regulatory boards in managing and improving program outcomes for their customers and to assist them in providing accountability to the citizens of their state (Smith, 2004). The project is called Commitment to Ongoing Regulatory Excellence (CORE).

TERMINOLOGY AND BASIC CONCEPTS

While there is not agreement on the definition of evidence-based regulation or evidence-informed policy, three global definitions to define the basic concepts of EBR have been proposed. The first definition comes from the United Kingdom. The U.K. Government Policy Hub's definition of evidence has been modified to describe evidence-based regulation:

> The raw ingredient of evidence-based regulation is information. Good-quality policy making depends on high-quality information, derived from a variety of sources—expert knowledge; existing domestic and international research; existing statistics; stakeholder consultation; evaluation of previous policies; new research, if appropriate; or secondary sources, including the Internet. Evidence-based regulation can also include analysis of the outcomes of board functions and cost of policy options (International Conference on Evidence-Based Best Practice Guideline, 2007).

The second definition was developed by the Center for Health System Research and Analysis (CHSRF, 2006) and has also been adapted to define evidence-based regulation:

> Evidence-based regulation is information that comes closest to the facts of the matter. The form it takes depends on context. The findings of high-quality, methodologically appropriate regulatory research are the most accurate evidence. Because research is often incomplete and sometimes contradictory or unavailable, other kinds of regulatory information are necessary supplements to or stand in for research. The evidence base for decision is the multiple forms of

evidence combined with rigor with expedience—while privileging the former over the latter.

The third description is from the World Health Organization of Europe (2004):

> Findings from research and other knowledge that may serve as a useful basis for decision making in public health and health care.

Interestingly, Petch (2008) prefers to reframe the terminology as "evidence informed" rather than "evidence based" because "evidence does not make decisions, people do." Evidence-based regulation is based on outcome measures associated with the organization's purpose and long-term strategic goals, and is intended to ensure the safety of citizens and identify regulated parties that place the public at risk for harm. According to Keehley and Abercrombie (2008), measures place performance in context by providing comparisons and are important because they can change the way people view performance. Measures also reveal where the agency needs to improve. *Outputs* are those services delivered to the citizens of the state. Public organizations such as boards of nursing are learning to link their outputs and outcomes, and should be held accountable for doing so. A *link* is described as a logical, intuitive, or empirical direct connection between producing outputs and ultimate outcomes. **Figure 11-1** illustrates the relationships among inputs, processes, and outcomes.

Figure 11-1   Links between producing outputs and ultimate outcomes.

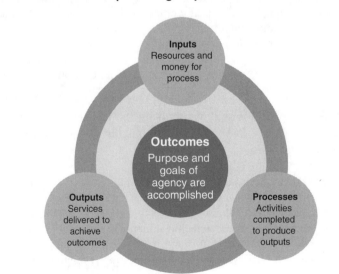

Other relevant concepts in an evidence-based regulatory model include measurement, promising practices, benchmarking, and knowledge management. Steven Medlin from the iKon Group has defined *measurement* as the process of assigning numbers to something according to a defined set of rules (Keehley & Abercrombie, 2008). *Inputs* are resources such as money spent on staff compensation, overhead, and other items to ensure that the processes are completed. A *process is a* series of work steps that results in the delivery of an output.

Specific outcomes and outputs are measured for each of the four areas of nursing regulatory board function:

- Investigating and disciplining nurses who violate the Nurse Practice Act
- Licensing of qualified applicants
- Approving nursing education programs
- Educating and responding to scope of practice inquiries (Smith, 2004)

Promising practices are described as ideas, practices, process steps, or policies that will improve performance in the organization that adopts them (Keehley & Abercrombie, 2008). Identification of promising practices relates to identifying boards with consistently high ratings in terms of outputs and effectiveness.

Benchmarking is a methodology used to improve performance by finding high-performing organizations and importing their practices to the home organization (Keehley & Abercrombie, 2008).

Productivity in regulation is often difficult to define and describe beyond the basic definition of "the ratio of outputs to inputs or efficiency." However, the need to more effectively and clearly define productivity has never been greater, and use of an evidence-based model is an important step in this process. Productivity analysis includes determination of unit costs or the ratio of inputs to outputs as well as consideration of quality. Quality is the error rate or the degree to which the outcome meets with customer satisfaction (Bradach, Tierney, & Stone, 2008).

Knowledge management is the "creation and subsequent management of an environment which encourages knowledge to be created, shared, learned, enhanced, organized, and utilized for the benefit of the organization and its customers" (Petch, 2008).

MAJOR BENEFITS OF EVIDENCE-BASED REGULATION

Apart from global economic competitiveness, the rhetoric and practice of evidence-based policy and practice within the United Kingdom and elsewhere has placed enormous emphasis on the generation, identification, and use of robust and reliable evidence. (Sin, 2008)

The challenge that many stakeholders and regulators face is the need to define the benefits or outcomes of effective regulation—namely, the benefits to and protection of the public. Several other benefits also emerge from evidence-based regulation, including the provision of data, linking of data points to inform resource allocations, improved decision making, and better accountability (Poister, 2003). The evidence-based regulation model requires regulators to engage in continuous quality improvement activities by asking challenging questions about practices and the manner in which the agency is currently operating. Examples of questions that should be asked regularly include these:

- Why are we conducting licensing and investigative programs this way?
- Why have we not solved problems and complaints from the public that we have known about for a period of time?
- Which regulatory barriers are perceived to be not in the public's best interest in the twenty-first century?
- How do regulatory leaders align the limited resources with the regulatory activities to create the greatest impact?
- Is the problem under my control?
- If I don't fix the issue, is the public or the board at risk?

Recently, state and government executives were surveyed by Howard and Kilmartin (2006), who sought to determine the major benefits of evidence-based regulation. As part of their study, these researchers identified several compelling reasons to collect data or evidence:

- Improve productivity or efficiency (identified by 79% of respondents)
- Increase constituent satisfaction (70%)
- Improve accountability and transparency (59%)
- Increase employee satisfaction, loyalty, and motivation (52%)
- Improve technology utilization (47%)
- Complete transformation of functions (36%)

Another benefit derived from an evidence-based regulatory model is the framework it creates for responsible and accountable behaviors. Keehley and Abercrombie (2008) assert that many of the services provided by governments operate very much like private-sector businesses. Managers in top-performing state agencies insist on accountability from subordinates and expect to be held to the same standard of accountability by their superiors.

Theodore Poister (2003, p. 250) states that "comparative data may be useful in a number of ways, not the least of which is to provide an incentive for less efficient and effective programs to improve their performance. Indeed, just participating in efforts to define and report common measurements on a uniform basis may spur some agencies to upgrade their own measurement systems and use them more productively." Poister also believes that more gains are achieved through the sharing of leading-edge practices than by penalizing under-performing programs. Conversely, managing regulatory programs or agencies without performance measures has been likened to flying blind, with no instruments to indicate where the enterprise is heading (Poister, 2003).

EVIDENCE-BASED REGULATION EXEMPLARS

Different questions need different types of evidence. (Petch, 2008)

This section outlines a step-by-step process for developing a foundation for evidence-based regulation to inform policy based on two projects: the Arizona Medication Technician Pilot Study, which was completed in 2008, and the evidence of public protection based on "A Regulatory Performance Measurement System" developed by the National Council of State Boards of Nursing. While some overlap may exist, the steps to design and implement the Medication Technician Pilot Study processes are described here deliberately and systematically, as well as those steps responsible for each of the various tasks to better illustrate the processes.

Exemplar 1: Evidence-Based Policy: Arizona Medication Technician Pilot Project Study

In 2002, a report to explore the regulation and establishment of a new medication technician role was filed by the Arizona Association of Homes and Housing for the Aging and the Arizona Health Care Association requesting regulatory oversight of a medication technician pilot study. The legislature approved the pilot study concept outlined in the sunrise report, leading to the introduction and passage of legislation enacted for the pilot to be overseen by the Board of Nursing (Arizona House Bill 2256, 2004). This law authorized the Board of Nursing to establish a pilot program to provide the evidence "to determine the impact to patient health and safety of allowing nursing assistants [to act] as pilot study medication technicians to administer medications under educational requirements and conditions prescribed by the board" (Arizona House Bill 2256, 2004, Section A). With funding secured from nongovernmental sources, the pilot study involved six long-term care facilities throughout the state. Although the study included only a small number of participants, the evidence-informed policy supports the idea that when facilities have properly integrated medication technicians into the care delivery system, resident care improves because the work of the medication technicians frees up nurses to perform higher-level tasks.

Arizona House Bill 2256 (2004) made the Board of Nursing responsible for developing protocols, prescribing the education, overseeing the project and preparing a report to the legislature by December 2008. It also incorporated patient safety-related measures including the following:

- Prohibitions to keep facilities from requiring a nurse to delegate medication administration to medication technicians
- Prohibitions against medication technicians administering medications to unstable or sub-acute residents
- Prohibitions against a medication technician administering any medication by needle
- Other measures incorporated within the study

The Board of Nursing formed a steering committee to oversee the project. The committee developed protocols regarding which medications' administration could be delegated to a medication assistant. The Board approved the recommendations that certain medications and tasks associated with medications could not be delegated to a medication technician. It based this decision on whether the task would require the skill of a licensed nurse and whether the task had an increased potential for harm to residents. Tasks that could not be delegated included the following duties:

- The first dose of a medication
- Administration of a medication requiring a complex mathematical conversion
- Administration of inhalant medications
- Emplacement of skin patches
- Administration of vaginal medications
- Administration of sublingual medications
- Administration of PRN ("as needed") medications, with some exceptions for low-risk medications

The Steering Committee then formed three subcommittees to focus on research, education, and funding. The research subcommittee determined the research priorities and design of the pilot study. The funding subcommittee worked to secure funding to conduct the research. Finally, the education subcommittee developed relevant course guidelines and curriculum, and contributed to a legally defensible competency exam.

The research subcommittee reviewed various indicators and approaches to study the safety of using medication technicians, with the goal of comparing patterns of medication errors before and six months after the use of medication technicians began in selected facilities. The original sunrise legislation identified safety of medication administration by medication technicians as the central public policy to be explored by the Board of Nursing. The Board also believed that participant satisfaction would be an important indicator of acceptance of the medication technician role. Therefore the pilot study was limited to these two indicators.

The subcommittee reviewed various methods to measure medication errors and ultimately recommended use of the Flynn and Barker Naive Observation Method (Barker, Flynn, & Pepper, 2002). This method is widely recognized as the most valid and reliable for measuring medication error rates in healthcare settings. In this methodology, an observer watches and records each medication pass and then compares what the resident received to the medication ordered in the resident's chart, without having any knowledge of the resident's prescribed medications and without reviewing the administration record (MAR) during the observation. The Board of Nursing decided to measure satisfaction levels by using structured interviews of pilot program participants, including medication technicians, delegating nurses, and directors of nursing.

The education subcommittee reviewed course requirements in 19 states that allow for the delivery of medications by unlicensed persons under a licensed nurse's delegation and supervision. The setting options considered by the subcommittee included community colleges or facilities participating in the pilot study. Given the small number of participating facilities and the possibility of diverse geographic locations, facility-based training proved to be the most feasible model for adoption.

A 100-hour medication technician course consisting of 45 hours of didactic instruction, 15 hours of skill lab, and 40 hours of supervised medication administration to residents was approved by the Board. The course guidelines and a curriculum included basic pharmacology information and safe medication administration principles. Approximately 300 multiple-choice items were developed for the state-administered competency exam. A training program for all instructors was also developed.

After the establishment of the curriculum, research, and funding mechanisms, the Board of Nursing and the Arizona Health Care Association issued a "Scope of Work" call for a researcher to determine the impact to patient health and safety of allowing medication technician to administer medications. The Board hired D&S Diversified Technologies (D&SDT), the current vendor for Arizona's certified nursing assistant exam, to conduct the research. In turn, D&SDT hired Dr. Jill Scott-Cawiezell, a nationally recognized expert on medication delivery and errors in long-term care facilities, to serve as a consultant. D&SDT also developed a standardized competency exam with both written and manual-skills portions based on the approved curriculum.

The Board of Nursing conducted its first training session with instructors in March 2006; additional training sessions were conducted in 2007. Board staff visited all facilities during training, which included a specific education program directed at all delegating nursing staff of the facility.

Working with Board staff and the education subcommittee, D&SDT developed an item pool for a written competency medication technician exam consisting of more than 1,200 items. The test pool contained 761 total active items, with each exam consisting of 50 items distributed according to a Board-approved test plan. The subcommittee designed the test plan based on the time allotted in the curriculum for each topic and the importance of each topic in terms of patient safety. Other states that draw from the same item pool include Arkansas, Montana, Ohio, and Oklahoma. D&SDT also developed a skills competency exam, using check-off lists developed by the education subcommittee.

Students in the pilot study had a limited number of chances to pass the test before being required to retake the course. In total, 21 persons passed both the written and manual skills tests out of 32 total exam administrations. The skills exam proved less challenging than the written exam, with 78% of applicants passing the skills exam on their first attempt and only 41% passing the written exam on their first attempt. All but one student passed the skills exam on the second attempt, and 59% of test takers passed the written exam on the second attempt.

All six participating facilities sent representatives to a two-day "train the trainer" session. The training sessions provided opportunities for participants in the pilot study to discuss the unique features of the project; reinforce teaching–learning principles, including test construction; and augment the textbook adopted by the Board of Nursing for training the technicians.

The Steering Committee invited all pilot study participants to attend all steering committee meetings and offer their perspective. Some common themes arose in these sessions:

- *Difficulty recruiting CNAs for the role.* Many facilities found that attracting CNAs to the program presented more challenges than anticipated and that they needed to increase hourly wages and offer other incentives to gain participation.
- *CNA shortages.* Even with an adequate number of CNAs trained and qualified for the role, shortages of CNAs in the facility necessitated that these personnel work primarily as CNAs rather than as medication technicians.
- *Positive acceptance of delegation to medication technicians.* Nurses who delegated medication administration to CNAs reported very positive results and experiences. In some facilities, additional CNAs became attracted to the role after observing their colleagues functioning as medication technicians.

- *Positive impact on medication administration by nurses.* The medication technicians discovered and reported unsafe medication practices and RN/LPN medication errors. One facility changed its medication administration schedule in response to a medication technician's concern that residents' medications were inappropriately scheduled.

As of November 2008, 21 qualified medication technicians were continuing to administer medications under the delegation of a licensed nurse in five long-term care facilities in Arizona. Participating facilities want to continue to use medication technicians, but face the ongoing challenges of CNA shortages, high staff turnover, and other fiscal constraints. Rollout of a state-wide program may eventually lead recognized educational institutions to participate in training, with a resultant increase in training opportunities, higher passing rates on the competency exam, and less reliance on facility staff for training.

Research Results

Research analysis was completed by D&SDT (2008), an agency external to the Board of Nursing, to further assure validity and reliability of the data. Information specific to medication errors and staff satisfaction is discussed here.

Medication Error Rates   The pre-implementation mean medication error rate was found to be 10.4% (LPNs, 10.12%; RNs, 11.54%). These rates were not statistically or clinically different for RN and LPN levels of licensure.

Post-implementation observation revealed a mean medication error rate of 6.6% (LPNs, 7.25%; RNs, 2.75%; medication technicians, 6.06%). Again, no statistical or clinically significant differences were noted among the medication administrators based on credential. Likewise, no statistically significant differences in either rate or pattern of error were found before or after the utilization of medication technicians. While it appears that there was an actual lowering of the medication error rate, due to the limited power of the study, the result is not considered significant.

Staff Satisfaction   Interviews of study participants from the five nursing homes after the post pilot study intervention data collection period provided insight into staff perceptions and acceptance of the project. Persons interviewed included directors of nursing (DONs), registered nurses (RNs), licensed practical nurses (LPNs), and pilot study medication technicians (PSMTs). All nurses indicated that, despite some early misgivings about the new medication technician role, when they were able to partner with a PSMT, they had more time to work directly with the residents. As a consequence, nurses reported feeling better about their resident care and assessments. These findings closely aligned with those from another study that provided empirical evidence supporting the medication technician role in reducing job stress and increasing satisfaction among licensed nurses.

Nurses had the following comments related to staff satisfaction:

- "The concept is fabulous; I now have more time to assess my residents and work with other staff. In the past, I felt stuck behind the med cart."
- "Nurses are now more available."
- "It is hard when the techs aren't here; they are good partners."

The medication technicians reported that it was their perception that nurses were spending more time with residents. However, medication technicians were affected by the delegating nurse's acceptance of the role:

I had a very difficult time in my new role at first. My nurse was constantly looking over my shoulder and making me very nervous. I could not get the pass done. Now, I have a new partner and I love what I am doing. We work really well together. (D&SDT, 2008, pp. 4–5)

All informants, except one nurse who felt she pampered her residents, reported the residents were very happy with the addition of the medication technician role (D&SDT, 2008, p. 5):

- "They miss her when she is gone. The resident keeps asking me where [she] is today."
- "Residents are glad for the change; they don't have to wait for their meds."

Informants reported minimal changes to the medication administration procedure. Many informants reported they believed there were fewer medication errors and a noticeable improvement in timely delivery of medications.

Informants provided recommendations and lessons learned during the pilot medication technician project. The recommendations include:

- The time frame for the training was too condensed. The training needed to be more spread out to allow time to study the critical concepts.
- More medication technicians are needed, and they need to be consistently assigned to the role to improve and build systems.
- Licensed staff would like to review the training so there can be consistent reinforcements for the medication technicians.

The lessons learned include:

- Speed comes with time. The key is being very careful.
- There is an increase in understanding of the importance of vital signs and their relationships to medications.
- The role of the PSMT adds flexibility to staffing.

Medications Technician Pilot Study Conclusions

Findings suggest that the introduction of medication technicians to the medication team in a long-term care facility will not negatively alter the rate or pattern of medication error. Significantly, an Agency for Healthcare Research and Quality (AHRQ)-funded medication safety study (Scott-Cawiezell, Pepper, Madsen, Petroski, Vogelsmeir, & Zellmer, 2007a, 2007b) reached similar conclusions. In addition to the safety data presented, healthcare personnel consistently reported positive results with the addition of the medication technician to the healthcare team. The study found no evidence that facilities replaced licensed nurses with medication technicians; likewise, there were no incidents of drug diversion by medication technicians.

The Arizona pilot study confirms the results of earlier studies, which indicated that medication technicians can provide safe medication delivery. Nevertheless, nursing home residents have many illnesses and take many medications; these characteristics render them vulnerable to even subtle alterations in their medication regimens. Many of the drugs delivered via routine medication administration do require assessment for potential adverse effects. CNAs and medication technicians lack the assessment skills and knowledge required to make adjustments or watch for many potential changes that a resident may undergo, including adverse drug effects. Thus, as recognized in the sunrise report and the enactment of HB 2256, the role of the licensed nurse remains critical to the management of nursing home residents' health and medications.

As D&SDT stated in its report, nursing homes face many challenges as they seek to provide safe care in a milieu characterized by very fiscally constrained budgets. Innovation and evidence must be critical parts of how care is delivered to this ever-growing and very frail population. In an ideal world, the frail and vulnerable residents would have RNs providing all aspects of their care. In a fiscally constrained world, however, the skills of staff representing many levels of credentialing must be maximized to assure that adequate care is given. The Arizona study provides some initial evidence to suggest that medication technicians can be effectively used for routine medication administration. Understanding the limitations of the medication technicians and creating medication systems that include the RN and the CMT/A as partners could ensure a system of safe medication administration whereby residents get the right medication, at the right time, in the right dose, through the right route, and prepared in the right method, to assure the best therapeutic result (Scott-Cawiezell et al., 2007a; D&SDT, 2008).

Based on the experience with this project and the results of the pilot study, the Steering Committee made the following recommendations to the Arizona Board of Nursing:

- Legislation be pursued to extend the role of the medication technician state-wide.
- All features of the pilot study remain in place, including protocols, education, setting, and testing.
- The time frame for the training be paced so students can better comprehend the material.
- The role of the RN in delegation and medication management be specifically addressed.
- The Board of Nursing collaborate with the Department of Health Services and other licensing boards in crafting legislation related to the medication technician role.

Exemplar 2: Evidence of Public Protection Based on Performance Measurement

Evidence-based regulation is also a journey of measuring outcomes and being accountable to the public.

The second exemplar to illustrate the processes of evidence-based regulation is the Commitment to Ongoing Regulatory Excellence (CORE) project. This work began approximately ten years ago. In 1998, the board of directors of the National Council of State Boards of Nursing (NCSBN) of Directors appointed a project advisory group to partner with the Urban Institute to provide oversight and guide development of an ongoing performance measurement and benchmarking system (CORE). The collection of data, research, and analysis of quantitative and empirical data has assisted Boards of Nursing in carrying out their public mandate to protect the public by isolating weaknesses and identifying strengths. The 2005 evidence (i.e., data) assisted the 42 participating Boards of Nursing to make connections between performance differences and best practices.

Examples of metrics deemed essential to understand the operational health of the board of nursing in fulfilling its public protection mission included the following items:

- Staff productivity (i.e., number of applicants licensed, investigative cases processed, or educational programs approved)
- Cost-effectiveness (i.e., expense calculations per licensee; see **Figure 11-2**)
- Cycle times (i.e., processing of licensure applications and investigations; see **Figure 11-3**)

Stakeholder satisfaction and perceptions are also critical to understanding the *operational health* of the regulatory board. The CORE ratings and open-ended questions were intended to provide information to direct efforts in gaps in service.

Figure 11-2   Dashboard processing licensure applications from receipt of required information.

FY 2005	n	Aggregate Average	Arizona	Variance
APRN	19	9 days	3.31 days	<5.69> days less than aggregate
RN	27	18	0.78	<17.22> days less than aggregate
LPN	23	16	1.98	<14.02> days less than aggregate
Licensure Verification to Another Board of Nursing	15	8	14	+6 days greater than aggregate

Figure 11-3   Dashboard estimated days to resolve cases, FY 2005.

FY 2005	n	Aggregate Average	Arizona	Variance
Number of days	31	274 9.13 months	218 7.3 months	<1.87 months> below aggregate

FY 2008 data to resolve cases is ranging 6.8–7.2 months.

The CORE measurement categories are reported every two years in the *Arizona State Board of Nursing Regulatory Journal* as a "dashboard of measures" for the evidence-based regulation framework. Similar to a dashboard in an airplane, which provides the pilot with an overview of the critical functions of the airplane, a Board of Nursing dashboard provides a high level of understanding of how the Board is performing. In addition to these performance measures, the Board wants to know how to improve outcomes in better protecting the public. The Arizona State Board of Nursing finds that the connection between the numbers and regulatory practices that drive performance is a way to achieve this goal.

Researchers at the NCSBN, in conjunction with the Commitment to Ongoing Regulatory Excellence Committee, have provided the necessary connections between the performance differences and identified best practices. Discipline, licensure, educational program approval, practice, and governance best practices were based on interviews with those Boards receiving the highest ratings in the CORE research.

CHALLENGES IN DELIVERING EVIDENCE-BASED REGULATION

In terms of political and managerial contexts, the prospects of evidence-based regulation are associated with both challenges and opportunities. Comparing the performance of individual agencies or programs based on a set of common measures is a sensitive issue, as some organizations may look bad in comparison with others whether or not the indicators have been adjusted for contextual factors (Poister, 2003).

One of the more significant challenges in regulation is the difficulty in attaching a dollar value to public protection. The daily routine of executive directors of regulatory boards is filled with constant *scatterization*—that is, the quest to serve multiple constituencies ranging from nursing applicants to members of the legislature. In the business world, market forces serve as feedback on company performance. According to Bradach, Tierney, and Stone (2008), performance is relatively easy to quantify through quarterly earnings, return on investment, customer loyalty scores, and the like. In contrast, in the regulatory world, the mission to protect the public—not markets—is the magnet that attracts essential resources (Bradach et al., 2008). Regulators struggle with competing priorities in systems and infrastructures needed to provide the operating data; the challenge lies in keeping everyone focused on the evidence needed to achieve the ultimate goals. Typically organizational capacity needs to assure achievement of performance targets are not considered chief priorities. Similarly, technology is often under-compensated when funding decisions are finalized by entities external to the agency.

Public-Sector Challenges and Barriers

While the need for evidence-based regulation is compelling, it remains under-developed in much of the public sector (Sin, 2008). Sin further asserts that the following structures and cultures within public agencies present a set of barriers to the progress of the evidence-based movement:

- The existence of a rule-based culture that encourages compliance
- Typical hierarchical and bureaucratic structures, which slow down communication and decision making

- Resistance to taking on the movements as a shared responsibility
- High turnover and transfers among staff
- The tendency toward "change fatigue" as a result of the constant introduction of initiatives
- The confidential nature of some types of information and knowledge, which inhibits sharing and access

Measurement Challenges and Conflicting Views

Another challenge is the conflicting perspectives on measurement. Measures, performance, and benchmarking are inextricably linked in providing the foundation for evidence-based regulation (Keehley & Abercrombie, 2008). Measures are important for many reasons in benchmarking in the public sector according to Keehley and Abercrombie, who have been studying benchmarking in the public sector for more than 35 years. Keehley and Abercrombie further assert that leaders need performance measures in both government and nonprofit organizations for managing on a daily, weekly, monthly, and even yearly basis. If government is to operate efficiently and effectively, each agency must have an ongoing gauge or dashboard to guide its actions (Keehley & Abercrombie, 2008).

In essence, performance measures are foundational components for evidence-based regulation because they facilitate the following tasks (Keehley & Abercrombie, 2008):

- Allow comparisons among performance of outputs and outcomes
- Change the way performance is viewed based on evidence
- Reveal where improvements are needed
- Demonstrate when improvement is accomplished
- Overall better direct programs and operations to ensure increased efficiency and effectiveness

Given the diversity of the regulatory programs, there is little agreement on standard outcome metrics with which to measure performance. Translating the public protection mission into goals needs to result in specific enough items to inform resource allocations (Bradach et al., 2008). Audit processes assess and compare performance subjectively and are typically value driven by the philosophy of the state auditor legislative committee.

To facilitate comparisons, organizations must collect "apples to apples" comparative data from like agencies or jurisdictions. They must also ensure that participating jurisdictions use a consistent set of data definitions (Keehley & Abercrombie, 2008). The implementation of a rigorous data collection process will also help to ensure the integrity of the data and other information through internal and external review and oversight.

Rethinking Assumptions

Even without formally gathering evidence or data, regulators can advance the work of evidence-based regulation by rethinking the assumptions that underlie the laws and rules of the agency. As noted by Pfeffer and Sutton (2006), consideration of the assumptions that underpin interventions is often sufficient to reproduce insights gained from empirical research.

Overcoming Resistance

Delivering on the basis of defined set of regulatory outcomes appears straightforward. Nevertheless, the approach is often considered revolutionary in regulation, even though the concept was embraced by business leaders more than three decades ago. Many Boards of Nursing resist data collection on two grounds: (1) that data collection is time-consuming and costly, and (2) that extrapolation of data is exceptionally difficult if the agency resides within an umbrella structure participating in the project. The question of proof also arises. The formal evaluation process of CORE documents the link between a program and a set of outputs or outcomes. Many unseasoned regulators may require reference data and benchmarks as proof before they will adopt the evidentiary mindset and model. The CORE model is especially helpful in closing this gap.

Another source of potential resistance is the perceived cost of an evidence-based approach. Regulatory leaders critical of evidence-based regulation typically do not have enough money to cover existing programs, let alone support activities related to collecting data. Others may be caught in a self-deception trap and have a sense of false security when they state, "We are far better than most others—so why do we need to improve?"

Overcoming resistance to evidence-based regulation is an evolving process—a journey of many years that will ultimately improve the use of resources and improve protection of the public. To make decisions based on evidence, regulatory leaders need to be immersed in a culture where everyone in the organization is committed to getting and using the best facts (Pfeffer & Sutton, 2006).

Transferability of findings is another area that spurs resistance from some regulators. Pawson (2003) argues that, on the whole, evidence from evaluation has a good record in illuminating whether a program has worked and is even often able to say why the program succeeded or failed. He further states that we are not so good at "fortune telling"—that is, estimating whether the same program will work in another place on another occasion. Finally, he asserts that the biggest "bug-bear" is the complexity of programs, which is an elusive limitation associated with evidence-based policy.

To be sure, there is no fairy godmother who will magically wave a wand and enact an evidentiary model (even some regulators would surely welcome such magic). Weiss et al. also note that evaluators sometimes wish for a fairy god-mother who would make decision makers pay attention to evaluation findings on what works; these authors argue that giving the evaluation evidence more clout may, in fact, be a worthwhile way of increasing the rationality of decision making for public policy creation ("Lessons from the Literature," 2008). B. W. Head asserts that, "In reality, policy decisions emerge from politics, judgment, and debate rather than empirical analysis; the 'evidence' is diverse and con-testable" ("Lessons from the Literature," 2008). The social nature of the policy culture, which often results in policy makers choosing, abusing, or ignoring evidence in response to more pressing and arguably important factors such as public opinion or financial restraints, is regretted by many academics ("Lessons from the Literature," 2008).

CAVEATS FOR THE EVIDENCE-BASED REGULATION JOURNEY

Several caveats require consideration for the future. The evidence-based regu-lation journey is an important step for the reasons discussed previously in this chapter and necessarily requires sensitivity to the current culture and a set of interactions that are dynamic and continually evolving.

The first caveat is specific to building leadership capacity and expertise. Senior organizational leaders and board members need to become the stron-gest advocates for working in an evidence-informed way. The executive team is expected to set expectations, in conjunction with staff, that policy and prac-tice will be evidence informed. Without an organizational culture that values learning, evidence-based regulations will seem to be almost a counterculture movement (Best Practice Summary, 2008).

The second caveat is specific to the challenges involved in moving from data collection to action. Although data collection is essential to evidence-based regulation, it is not the end result. Obtaining a lot of comparative data for other jurisdictions or on a national level does not move the agency any closer to pro-viding evidence about improved performance. The public is better served when evidence is used to create a learning organization in which executives are constantly searching for better ways to deliver improved outcomes (Keehley & Abercrombie, 2008). Personal opinions must yield to data.

The third caveat is specific to performance measurement. Selecting the most critical program services to begin evidence-based regulation is often a challenge. It is important to focus on gathering measurement evidence on criti-cal program services that most significantly affect the quality and costs of regu-latory services. In addition, focusing on the desired results rather than volumes of data collected is essential, yet often proves to be a challenge (Poister, 2003). Criteria for selecting measures also need to be based on usefulness in making decisions rather than the fact the data is already available. If full-time equivalent (FTE) measures are used for determining input resources expended, then actual FTEs should be used (not the budgeted number).

The fourth caveat is a consideration related to clarifying the value and importance of process versus outcome measures. While these issues are closely linked and processes are certainly important, the outcomes are the area warranting the greatest attention. Focusing primarily on process work renders the evidence model irrelevant and distracting. For example, the board may consider and measure the cycle time to process a licensure application. What is more important is the accuracy of the process—namely, were the individuals who were licensed prepared to practice safely? Fast processing that results in licensure of unsafe individuals negatively impacts public safety.

Technology is another area deserving of caution in an evidence-based model. The more information technology systems are used to manage access to operations data, the easier it is to conduct consistent and meaningful performance measurement. If the desired performance metrics are not embedded into the software application system, however, the administrative team must spend more time and resources to carry out the work manually. To be sure, there is no such thing as a free outcome. Measuring performance requires an investment (Cole & Parston, 2006). For this reason, the work of evidence-based regulation requires an executive-level position who is committed to be the process owner of evidence-based regulation and budget resources to collect outcome data.

Delivering and sustaining results requires the right people in the right positions. No matter how eloquent the agency's strategy might be or how ready the availability of funds, success is still directly linked to effective people doing their work effectively (Bradach et al., 2008). Boyne (2003) asserts that in reviewing evidence on public service improvement, the two variables that emerge as the most consistent influences on agency performance are resources and management. While some boards are strongly led, some are under-managed. Effective management is always essential for success.

Another caveat is the need to distinguish outputs and outcomes. Outputs represent what the program actually does, whereas outcomes are the results produced by the program (Howard & Kilmartin, 2006).

THE RIGHT METRICS

More metrics are not necessarily better. Instead, organizations should focus on a relatively small number of important measures of success (Poister, 2003). The right questions are actually related to the outcomes for which the agency is to be held accountable. *Metrics mania* or metrics overload should be addressed by narrowing the analysis to only those items that actually gauge whether performance is improving (Cole & Parston, 2006).

Traditionally, public agencies within state government have found it easier to measure inputs, processes, and outputs than to focus on outcomes. Over the past few decades, the search for similar performance measures for public service organizations and the desire to improve performance have driven a great deal of public-sector research around the world (Cole & Parston, 2006). Adopting a methodology and adhering to the defined set of rules can be both helpful and instructive for agency staff. Performance evidence needs to be monitored and tracked to ensure that the higher level of performance is sustained. The search for improvement is a journey, not a destination.

The importance of considering context cannot be overstated. It is important to avoid casual benchmarking in searching for promising practices. The erroneous assumption that what works for one agency will automatically work for another agency deserves scrutiny. Paying close attention to why the process works and whether it will work elsewhere is clearly important. Searching for promising practices is done through asking questions of colleagues or accessing information on the Internet. To prevent engaging in regulatory "tourism syndrome" (i.e., carrying out a site visit without the right preparation), prepare questions such as the following (Keehley & Abercrombie, 2008):

- Have you experienced a challenge similar to long cycle times in completing investigations or licensing?
- How did you solve the problem?
- Which processes did you change, and do you have information on the sequential steps?
- What evidence is available that links the promising practice with improvement?
- What is unique about your organization or your circumstances?

Traditional regulatory performance measures are analogous to monitoring a car that is driving down a freeway to determine how the car is running. To measure inputs (i.e., the resources needed to deliver products or services), gallons of gasoline consumed are tallied. Such a measurement may provide a good view of the car's performance but it does not provide much about the context of the journey. For instance, the car may be high performing but "if it is on the wrong freeway heading in the wrong direction, the best-performing car will not arrive at the desired destination. Plus, whatever the fuel efficiency, the driver will have needlessly used gas getting to a destination he was not trying to reach" (Cole & Parston, 2006).

It is important to realize that everything related to evidence-based regulation takes longer than planned and is often similar to turning a large battleship.

Invest in basic infrastructure and leadership development by providing new tools and skills in creating a balanced approached emphasizing evidence and feasibility. Be patient but persistent as the ship experiences navigating new waters and occasional rough seas. Evidence-based regulation is only useful when it is coupled with a willingness to take action. Even when the evidence is relevant, it will not automatically be used. Having spent months collecting data and having the information marginalized or ignored by superiors in state government is frustrating.

MOVING FORWARD WITH THREE LENSES

According to B. W. Head, three types of evidence or perspectives are important for informing policy (**Figure 11-4**): systematic or scientific research, program or practice experience, and political judgment. The practical craft of policy development involves interweaving strands of information and values from all these disparate bodies of knowledge ("Lessons from the Literature," 2008).

On the first day of class, many deans of medical schools greet their first-year medical students with a sobering fact: Half of what we know is wrong; the problem is, we don't know which half (Pfeffer & Sutton, 2006). Physicians continue with their education even though something more is gained over time that is more important than any single benefit of evidence: wisdom.

> Wisdom means acting with knowledge while doubting what you know. It entails striking a balance between arrogance (assuming you know more than you do) and insecurity (believing that you know too little to act). It requires asking for help and asking questions, as well as giving help and answering questions. With an attitude of wisdom one can do things now, but still keep learning along the way. That is why creating a culture that fosters an evidence-based approach and problem solving is one of a leader's most crucial tasks, regardless of whether they are in charge of a business, nonprofit, or government agency. (Pfeffer & Sutton, 2006, p. 4)

THE FUTURE OF EVIDENCE-BASED REGULATION

Pawson (2003) argues that the latest big shift in the methodology of evidence-based policy is the move to systematic review. In other words, less effort and money are now being spent on "live" evaluations of programs for evidence, and much more attention is being paid to reviewing the existing evidence. Pawson further asserts there is a major role for theory-driven approach in systematically reviewing research evidence.

Figure 11-4   Three lenses of evidence-based informed policy.

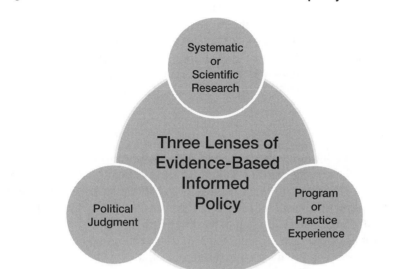

Source: Head, 2008.

Although regulatory agencies have begun to develop evidence to inform policy, embedding new processes needs to be institutionalized and become the standard way of doing things. Compilation of evidence and synthesis of the research findings need to be integrated systematically into the existing processes.

A central clearinghouse needs to be developed to catalog the research completed as well as to collect information on efforts that did not produce the anticipated evidence. "The literature on systematic reviewing tends to promote a single conception of the review process: that it is concerned with pooling the data or findings from multiple studies in order to maximize the accuracy and precision of conclusions about which polices and practice work" (Hammeresley, 2005). The establishment of the proposed clearing house would also add value to the body of knowledge by identifying relationships within the regulatory body of knowledge.

Leaders need to hold a clear vision of EBR and develop networks to build on the best of "what works," while still learning lessons along the way. Leaders need to know each agency's strengths and develop new skills and competencies in building an evidence-based infrastructure that might inform policy and regulation, with which "change management is intertwined." Hammeresley (2005) further asserts that while research can provide evidence about the consequences of various policies, on its own it "cannot tell the best thing to do, either in general terms or in particular cases."

Evidence encompasses more than just research within evidence-informed policy; it is sustained even though skepticism and misperceptions might still prevail in some sectors of the regulatory milieu. We can expect to see efforts continue to improve outcomes and performance as well as to provide accountability to legislatures through a common-sense, yet data-driven approach.

CONCLUSION

The time has come for an evidence-based, regulation-informed policy movement. Evidence-based regulation can help leaders in health care determine what works and what doesn't, "identify dangerous half truths that constitute so much of what passes for wisdom, and reject the nonsense that too often passes for sound advice" in the development of health policy (Pfeffer & Sutton, 2006).

Evidence-based regulation is complex and multidimensional. Although such regulation can aid greatly in informing policy, it is by no means a panacea to all that ails the current regulatory system. Nevertheless, good evidence can provide regulatory leaders and policy makers with valid and timely information about how well or poorly specific programs or research projects performed. It is then up to the collective to respond deliberately and effectively in improving the protection of the public. Clearly, the time for evidence-based regulation has arrived, and regulatory agencies have a key role to play in developing new systems that will provide policy makers with valuable information that truly makes a difference.

REFERENCES

AZ H. B. 2256, Arizona Session Laws 36–121.02 (2004).

Barker, K., Flynn, E., & Pepper, G. (2002, December 1). Observation method of detecting medication errors. *American Journal of Health-System Pharmacy, 59*(23), 2314–2316.

Best Practices, LLC Online. (1998, November 28). *Developing the benchmarking function: Lessons learned.* Available at: http://www3.best-in-class.com

Boyne, G. (2003). Sources of public service improvement: A critical review and research agenda. *Journal of Public Administration Research and Theory, 13*(3), 367–394.

Boyne, G., Meier, K., O'Toole, L. Jr., & Walker, E. (2006). *Public service performance: Perspectives on measurement and management.* Cambridge, UK: Cambridge University Press.

Bradach, J. L., Tierney, T. J., & Stone, N. (2008, December). Delivering on the promise of nonprofits. *Harvard Business Review, 86*(12), 88–97.

Canadian Health Services Research Foundation (CHSRF). (2006). *The foundation's definition of evidence.* Retrieved June 19, 2009, from http://www.chsrf.ca/other_documents_e.php

Cole, M., & Parston, G. (2006). *Unlocking public value: A new model for achieving high performance in public service.* Hoboken, NJ: John Wiley & Sons.

D & S Diversified Technologies (D&SDT). (2008). *Arizona pilot study medication technician final report.* Submitted to the Arizona State Board of Nursing on June 13, 2008.

Hammeresley, M. (2005). Is the evidence-based practice movement doing more good than harm? Reflections on Iain Chalmers' case for research-based policy making and practice. *Evidence & Policy, 1*(1), 85–100.

Head, B. W. (2008). Three lenses of evidence-based policy. *Australian Journal of Public Administration, 67*(1), 1–11.

Howard, M., & Kilmartin, B. (2006, May). *Assessment of benchmarking within government organizations.* Retrieved May 12, 2009, from http://www.nasact.org/nasact/benchmarking/downloads/AssessBenchmarkGovOrg.pdf

International Conference on Evidence-Based Best Practice Guidelines. (2007, June 7). Evidence-informed management decision making: Is it a possibility in healthcare? Markham, Ontario.

Keehley, P., & Abercrombie, N. (2008). *Benchmarking in the public and nonprofit sectors: Best practices for achieving performance breakthroughs.* San Francisco: Jossey-Bass.

Lessons from the literature. (2008, August). *Evidence & Policy, 4*(3), 263–288.

Pawson, R. (2003). Nothing as practical as a good theory. *Evaluation, 9*(4), 471–490.

Petch, A. (2008, April 8). Presentation: What do we mean by evidence-informed practice? *Research in Practice for Adults*, London, UK.

Pfeffer, J., & Sutton, R. (2006, April). Act on facts, not faith: How management can follow medicine's lead and rely on evidence, not on half truths. *Stanford Social Innovation Review.* Retrieved May 12, 2009, from http://www.ssireview.org/images/articles/2006SP_feature_Pfeffer_Sutton.pdf

Poister, T. (2003). *Measuring performance in public and nonprofit organizations.* San Francisco: Jossey-Bass.

Scott-Cawiezell, J., Pepper, G., Madsen, R., Petroski, G., Vogelsmeir, A., & Zellmer, D. (2007a). Nursing home error and level of staff credentials. *Clinical Nursing Research, 16*(1), 72–78.

Scott-Cawiezell, J., Pepper, G., Madsen, R., Petroski, G., Vogelsmeir, A., & Zellmer, D. (2007b). *Final report: Technology to improve medication safety in nursing homes.* Submitted to the Agency for Healthcare Research and Quality.

Sin, C., (2008). Developments within knowledge management and their relevance for the evidence-based movement. *Evidence & Policy, 4*(3), 227–249.

Smith, J. (2004, April). Executive summary: Evidence-based regulation: A regulatory performance measurement system. *National Council State Boards of Nursing Research Brief, 8*, 1–3.

Weiss, C. H., Murphy-Graham, E., Petrosino, A., & Gandhi, A. G. (2008). The fairy godmother—and her warts: Making the dream of evidence-based policy come true. *American Journal of Evaluation, 29*(1), 29–47.

World Health Organization (WHO). (2004). *Health Evidence Network (HEN).* Retrieved June 19, 2009, from http://www.euro.who.int/HEN/20030610_10

CHAPTER 12

Evidence-Based Leadership: Solid Foundations for Management Practices

Tim Porter-O'Grady and Kathy Malloch

INTRODUCTION

As we move more inexorably and confidently deeper into the twenty-first century, it is clear that the rules of engagement are significantly changing the emergence of an informational and technological foundation for human experiences and practices (Trompenaars & Hampden-Turner, 2002). These emerging realities are calling organizations and leaders into a different contextual framework for leadership and the management of work (Wolper, 2004). The information age is changing all the rules affecting structure and the processes associated with doing work, achieving outcomes, or producing products (Watkins, 2004). In particular, the information infrastructure is now able to aggregate huge volumes of data, correlate that information, integrate it, and report it clearly and efficiently. This ability to aggregate and manage data changes the foundation of decision making and action in a major way (Janecka, 2008).

This chapter presents an overview of accountability, knowledge work, the relationship between emerging leadership and manager accountabilities, the importance of values alignment, decision making and data, the challenges of overcoming dogma, and complexity as key considerations in the new work of evidence-based leadership. The chapter concludes with an application of an evidentiary model using a zero-based or *wilderness* approach to assist leaders in actualizing an effective and closely interrelated evidence-driven leadership-management model.

A GROWING DEMAND FOR ACCOUNTABILITY

In the past decade, much has been made of the high level of judgment and assumptions-based clinical practices that characterize all of the healthcare disciplines (Freshwater & Rolfe, 2004). The attempt to build evidence-based practice has raised a number of significant concerns regarding the foundations of judgment of clinical practitioners (McNamara, 2002). The evidence indicates that much weight has been applied to past practices, individual experiences, and traditional foundations of learning used in the formation of the body of knowledge upon which most practitioners base their own clinical judgments and actions (Smith, 2004). Of course, this foundation for behavior is quite unstable and unreliable—the inadequacies inherent in the dependence on past practice and individual assumptions cannot be understated (McSherry, Simmons, & Abbott, 2002). Even so, for most practitioners, even in contemporary clinical situations, the past remains the foundation of the vast majority of practice decisions and actions in the present.

This reality of uninformed and evidence-lacking decision making and action, which is readily apparent in clinical practice, is only extended and broadened when we consider leadership and management practices in health care. Indeed, much of management practice is based on an unbounded and wide variation of myth, whim, fancy, fad, and fashion (Tourish & Hargie, 2004; Malloch & Porter-O'Grady, 1999). In no area of human endeavor are there as many nonvalidated assumptions of practice and the management of human behavior as in the arena of management and leadership (Albrecht, 2003). Almost weekly, self-proclaimed management gurus announce new insights regarding leadership and management practice based solely on the expression of their own thinking and fantasy regarding what works and does not work in the leadership of people and organizations. Management and leadership is most bereft of any continuous aggregated and related body of knowledge that would in any way validate the foundations upon which many of the practices of leadership and management are based (Drucker, 2001; Drucker & Stone, 1998; Mintzberg, 1990).

Contemporary notions of accountability would require the resolution of such a difficulty. Yet, still new tomes appear weekly on the bookshelves attesting to emerging personal insights with regard to judgments of what makes effective leaders and what produces sustainable outcomes in business and service. At the same time, broad-based evidence of the lack of accountability and ownership with regard to personal decisions and actions in almost every arena is rife both in the United States and on the global stage, demonstrating the paucity of real and effective leadership (Gitlow, 2005; Goodpaster, Nash, & Bettignies, 2006; Jackson & Nelson, 2004; McDaniel, 2004). This lack of accountability, and the corresponding lack of understanding regarding what accountability means, underpins much of the problem associated with building an evidentiary foundation to leadership decisions and practices (McDaniel, 2004; Oliver, 2004; Price, 2006).

While often used in the same sentences, the terms "responsibility" and "accountability" describe fundamentally different performances. Responsibility relates to how well the work is done, a notion that encompasses issues of knowledge, competence, and efficiency of the effort. Responsibility focuses on the work, how well it is done and how competent and capable the worker is in performing it. Thus it is a fundamental focus on process (Porter-O'Grady & Malloch, 2007). Accountability, by comparison, focuses on the product of work; it is a measure of value. It focuses on the results of work—the outcome, the impact, the actual difference that work makes (**Figure 12-1**). Accountability relates to the viability, value, and impact of the products of work and can be articulated by measures of outcome, meaning, and financial value.

One is accountable to the extent that the anticipated outcome is actually achieved or advanced by the combined and integrated efforts of people. Individuals can work conscientiously, with determination, commitment, and high levels of responsibility, yet still not demonstrate accountability. Working responsibly means doing the work well—in short, doing it right. Accountability, by comparison, means doing the right work—that is, work that achieves defined purposes, outcomes, and value (Hickman, Smith, & Conners, 2004; Malloch & Porter-O'Grady, 2005). One can be working responsibly with great diligence, yet still perform an action that does not necessarily achieve desirable outcomes or value. In fact, many people do work that may not relate to outcome or value. Nurses, for example, are commonly involved in rituals and routines to which no definitive outcome is attached and from which no purposeful value is achieved (Berwick, Nolan, & Whittington, 2008; Osborne, 2002; Tilley, 2008). These nurses may act very responsibly as demonstrated

---

Figure 12-1   Leadership and accountability.

Responsibility (20th Century)	Accountability (21st Century)
Process	Product
Action	Result
Work	Outcome
Do	Accomplish
Task	Difference
Function	Fit
Job	Role
Incremental	Sustainable
Externally generated	Internally generated

by the depth of their commitment and the quality of their work processes, yet still fail to demonstrate accountability in tying those work processes to any measurable or meaningful value or outcome. If no difference is made, the sustainable value of the work is missed and, therefore, accountability is not demonstrated (Barry, Murcko, & Brubaker, 2002; Berwick et al., 2008; Fottler, Ford, & Heaton, 2002).

Work is not inherently valuable. Rather, work is valuable only to the extent that it is informed by purpose and achieves the ends to which it is directed (Bossidy, Charan, & Burck, 2002). Failing to accomplish these two elements, work has no value. This notion is significant in light of the foundations related to constructing an evidentiary baseline to which the value trajectory of work can be related. This intersection between process and impact is a fundamental component found in evidence-based processes. Evidence of the value of a particular work is demonstrated by the goodness of fit between the desired outcomes or value of the work and the effective processes associated with obtaining them (Barry et al., 2002). The strength of this connection is the centerpiece of evidence-driven processes and represents the essential relationship between the processes of work and the achievement of the values to which they are directed.

In knowledge work environments such as hospitals and healthcare systems, the notion of accountability takes on special meaning. Knowledge workers own the means of their own capital, and this means is now as significant as any other sources of capital- and human-intensive organizations (Sveiby, 1997). Knowledge workers have an individually driven sense of ownership with regard to their knowledge and its demonstration in the applications of work (Hooker & Csikszentmihalvi, 2003). Embedded in this understanding of knowledge work ownership are the mobility and portability of that knowledge, as the knowledge worker carries the knowledge wherever he or she operates in the system. This flexibility is another important consideration with regard to accountability. Knowledge workers' ownership of the knowledge tools and capacities necessary to do the work of practice creates an additional burden of understanding in relationship to the expression of accountability: Knowledge workers do not transfer the locus of control for their accountability to institutions, organizations, or others outside of their knowledge work community.

Nurses and physicians are especially notable examples of this phenomenon (Apker, Ford, & Fox, 2003). Nurses and physicians, like other professionals, demonstrate the ownership of the body of knowledge and the translation and application of that knowledge into clinical practice and patient impact. These professionals own both the knowledge and the activities associated with expressing it. Employment does not transfer the locus of control for that knowledge to the employing entities. Accountability for the performance and achievement of clinical outcomes rests exclusively and solely with the competent practitioners. It is expected that these practitioners will fully own their accountability, and that such accountability will be evidenced in the positive clinical outcomes achieved through its expression (Malloch & Porter-O'Grady, 2006).

This notion of ownership in relationship to accountability is critical to the professional knowledge worker; it also informs the management of these workers (**Figure 12-2**). As such, ownership for the work of practice does not transfer to the management role, and managers cannot be held accountable for the outcomes of practice owned by the knowledge workers whose capacity and competence are essential to both achieving and sustaining outcomes (Porter-O'Grady, 2000). Because ownership is invested in the practitioner, if the desired outcomes are to be achieved, the role of management is to create an organization and systems context that facilitates, supports, and encourages the ownership and expression of accountability on the part of knowledge workers (Albrecht, 2003).

In short, the accountability of management differs in important ways from the accountability of the knowledge worker staff. The effectiveness of work and the achievement of outcomes belongs to the knowledge work staff; the creation of context that frames and supports the work and accountability of staff is the source of accountability for management (Dotlich & Cairo, 2002). The outcome of the management role is the same as that of the knowledge worker staff: effective patient care, leading to positive clinical outcomes (**Figure 12-3**). However, accountability for achieving those ends is significantly different in a management role as compared to the knowledge worker staff role. The activities associated with one are differentiated from the activities associated with the other. Yet, both roles are necessary to create the dynamic—the intersection—necessary to sustain performance outcomes.

Figure 12-2   Evidence-based leadership: Foundations.

Foundations

- Hard facts and culture of truth
- Fact-based decisions
- Work as unfinished prototype
- Always look behind the line
- Have no strongly held beliefs
- All work is a learning journey

Figure 12-3   Evidence-based leadership: Performance.

Performance

- Clear accountability
- Clear expectations
- Staff drive performance
- Performance demonstration
- Contract for outcomes

The definitive delineation of the management role is articulated in the five accountabilities of management: human, fiscal, material, support, and systems resources (Drucker, 1977). Management accountability relates to the quality and integrity of the direction and infrastructure of systems and the degree of integrity of their relationship with the work and performance outcomes of the knowledge worker stakeholders. In partnership with knowledge workers, the leaders of the organization aggregate the efforts of systems and people in a mosaic of intersection and performance that networks strategy, infrastructure, resources, and knowledge work in the configuration (a dance, if you will) of consonance and contribution that advances both the clinical outcomes for patients and the organizational viability of the system (Pidd, 2004).

These five management accountabilities provide the contextual framework for the functional role of the management leader. They not only define the content of leadership, but also clarify the boundaries of leadership practice essential to the effectiveness of the role of the manager (Mintzberg, 2004). It is the failure of organizations to clearly articulate this bounded role for managers, yet still expect high levels of competence in its expression, that is most problematic for health institutions. In fact, because most managers are drawn from the ranks of clinical practitioners, their affiliation and association with the role of clinical practice frequently remain stronger in them than their understanding, attachment, and commitment to the exercise of the role of manager. In addition, the organization's commitment to high levels of leadership and management development has been limited in the past. As a result, the competencies, effectiveness, and skills necessary to demonstrate high levels of management application and accountability have historically been missing. Much of the learning in the role comprises on-the-job training, which is hardly a firm foundation for developing appropriate and effective management and leadership capacity (Gandossy & Sonnenfeld, 2004; Leach, 2005).

Further creating challenges to the accountability of management is the dramatic shift in performance expectations between the clinical and management roles (**Figure 12-4**). Clinical excellence is a poor predictor of management success. The knowledge, translational, and applications competencies required for clinical excellence operate in an entirely different frame of reference than do the skills necessary for management excellence (Bass, 1990; Force, 2005; Kleinman, 2003). Unless this point is made clear, excellent clinical practitioners may continue to be promoted to roles in management without adequate acknowledgment of their management incapacity with the expectation that, because they are excellent practitioners, they will obtain the necessary management skills through osmosis or through their own efforts (Mathena, 2002). Of course, neither is true. As a result, exchanging clinical competence for management expertise rarely occurs with any measure of effectiveness, and the lack of leadership excellence is the price paid for not changing this circumstance (Badawy, 2003; Traynor, 1999).

This is the contextual framework leading to the paucity of accountability evidenced in healthcare management and leadership today. Both now and in the future, this endeavor desperately needs to be informed through the development of an evidence-based frame for the five management accountabilities in the effective exercise of the leadership role.

KNOWING WHAT YOU KNOW

Perhaps a key element of evidence-based management and leadership is understanding what a manager knows and doesn't know. As mentioned previously, much of management today is based on previous parental experiences, individuals' own organizational history, and whatever beliefs individuals have constructed as a part of their own personal approach to leadership. Dissecting this set of variables is a critical place for beginning to understand what is certain and what is myth. A good starting point is the understanding that much of which we identify as certain in management is actually myth (Hatch, Kostera, & Kozminski, 2005).

Figure 12-4 Evidence-based leadership: Value.

Value

- Focus on product of work
- What makes a difference
- Unbundle attachment to process
- Change is the work
- Shift patient expectation

Organizational leaders and individual managers begin the process of clarifying and applying evidence-based mechanics to leadership behavior by identifying practices and processes that have existed over the long term but have no foundation in fact (Kanter, 2004; Keating, 2004; Useem, 2004). A classic example is managers' general impression that they have an obligation to motivate their staff. While there is no evidence that managers can motivate staff to do anything (indeed, the evidence runs counter to that belief), many—if not most—managers still talk as though motivating staff is one of their role obligations (Herzberg, 1991; Miner, 2005). From the classic research of Hertzberg to contemporary data, studies have consistently shown that motivating others to sustainable action is the one thing managers cannot do (Herzberg, 2008). Yet myriad books on the topic, course content related to it, and major organizational efforts at staff motivation are the signposts of contemporary efforts to apply this myth. Instead of seeking to understand the psychodynamics of motivation and the necessity of its originating from within individuals, management efforts continue to focus on creating motivation as a management capacity—and continue to miss the mark (Christiansen, 2003).

MOTIVATION VERSUS VALUES ALIGNMENT

If the forces of motivation were understood and the research related to those forces were incorporated into management capacity, managers might spend more of their resources and energy on creating the conditions of alignment (Barry et al., 2002; Fottler et al., 2002). (See **Figure 12-5**.) Aligning individual motivations with organizational goals has a much longer history of well-researched validation than do efforts at employee motivation (Gottlieb, 2003; Lencioni, 2002). Creating both the infrastructure and the expectation of alignment of individual behaviors with organizational goals requires a particular set of skills, including ownership, engagement, investment, and strong linked and integrated efforts at performance evaluation and course correction (Malloch & Porter-O'Grady, 2006). Good evidence suggests that efforts in this arena have a direct payoff in terms of accomplishment and outcomes. No such body of evidence has been uncovered for organizational efforts at employee motivation.

Figure 12-5   Evidence-based motivation.

Truth

- You can't motivate anyone to do anything! People are already motivated. However, their motivation may not be aligned with group goals. The role of the leader is to create this alignment, not to motivate people.

The critical point here is the call for leadership staff to begin to build both structures and processes that reflect the laying of an evidentiary foundation for making decisions and taking action. This endeavor requires a series of steps that begin with personal and organizational reflection and call to the table the most senior leaders as they begin work on prescriptives that generate both a framework and set of expectations with regard to evidence-based decision making and action taking (Giacco, 2003; Wager, Wickham, & Glaser, 2005). Reflection at the highest levels of the organization and the construction of evidentiary foundations upon which strategy, tactics, performance, and outcome measures can be based create a basis from which data building of evidence-driven practices can emerge and their relationship to positive impacts and outcomes can be established.

DECISION MAKING AND ANALYSIS

All organizations are awash with data. It isn't so much the collection of data that is important in today's contemporary organization, but rather the ability to use those data, analyze them, and make decisions and take action based on what the analysis reveals (Chakravarthy, 2003; Garvin & Roberto, 2001; Porter-O'Grady & Afable, 2003). Without question, in today's information-driven business world, the ability to manage data and use it appropriately is a fundamental management skill set. This love for and attachment to data, including the management of data and the analysis of data's impacts, is a central prerequisite and an essential tool in the armamentarium of the good leader (Davenport, 2006). Attachment to data means having a facility for its gathering, aggregation, translation, interpretation, and application in a way that is meaningful and makes a difference in the lives of those who will use the data (**Figure 12-6**). Data-driven decision making means more than simply relating to the data:

Figure 12-6   Data-driven skill sets.

Knowledge Worker (New)	Employee (Old)
• Conceptual synthesis	• Manual dexterity
• Use of analytics	• Functional proficiency
• Multiple "intelligences"	• Fixed skill set
• Outcome driven	• Process (volume) value
• Value "fit"	• Unilateral performance
• Data driven decisions	

It means establishing an intense relationship with data processes so that the structure of data becomes both a facilitating factor and a seamless integration. The data-driven process supports real-time communication and information, and the application of data entails real-time informing, guidance, and solution seeking at the point of decision and action (Ball, 2000; Oostendorp, 2003).

Of real importance to managers is the ability to make this strong attachment to data and analysis a part of the fundamental work experience of the knowledge worker. Translating data management into a real attachment to the use of data by knowledge workers is a formidable undertaking. Nevertheless, if the connection can be made between the value of work and the extent to which it is informed by data-driven decision making and evaluated by data-clarified measures, then leaders can begin to establish attachment between the use of data and evidence and the clinical decisions made and actions taken at the point of service. To accomplish this goal, such processes must be seamlessly integrated into the recording, collection, and assessment of information and directly connected to the decision processes whose value and accuracy depend on both the veracity and the utility of the knowledge produced in real time by such data processes (Goad, 2002). The fluidity, portability, and mobility of data systems and processes as they are incorporated into knowledge worker activity are the keys to accelerating their viability as tools for both informing decisions and evaluating actions. Competent managers now view this approach not as a new way of doing business, but rather as the *only* way to think and do the work effectively.

To create a meaningful attachment to data and the analytics related to creating relevance from it will require that both practitioners and information systems experts and developers focus on the utility of such systems from the users' perspective (Hildreth & Kimble, 2004). To date, much data have been collected in health care, yet much of those data are neither relevant nor valuable to individuals at the point of service, where the ability to establish the evidence of clinical viability is compromised without this input. The "heavy," complex, and overwhelming systems for collecting and managing data simply make them untenable in the work life of the knowledge worker, especially given the myriad clinical pressures constraining her or his time. Continuing emphasis on the development of portability through the use of mobile data devices, remote data access, and other hand-held devices is essential to creating ease-of-use conditions that satisfy the point-of-service user who needs ready access to critical and real-time data. It is the obligation of managers, in their role of creating and enabling context for evidentiary practices, to make sure that such data processes are both available and useful. If the point-of-service utility of data management systems does not advance, the currently great distance between truly effective evidence-based processes and clinical practices will be sustained over a long period of time (Geisler, Krabbendam, & Schuring, 2003).

Building effective analytics calls for organizations to recalibrate the way in which they collect and integrate data. In hospitals, for example, financial, flow, patient, and clinical performance data should not be looked at as separable elements. Instead, they should be viewed as representing distinct components of essentially the same data set. Each of these elements of data affects the others, thereby providing multiple sources of related information for guiding decision making and action (Locsin, 2001). From a purely business perspective, clinical requirements generated from patient assessment have a direct and immediate impact on financial considerations: They influence how hospitals will get paid for those activities, as they invariably fall both under and outside of the auspices of third-party payers. This, in turn, has a direct impact on both the patient and the organization—one that can be ignored only at the peril of both. Evidence-based management requires knowing the value of these interfaces, recognizing how the implications of the data may affect both the business and the practices of the organization, and subsequently taking the requisite actions necessary to positively problem solve (Jurewicz & Cutler, 2003). Laying the foundation for analytics as a process for linking and integrating the business of care with the practice of care is essential to generate practitioner-centered values that directly relate to the patients they serve, the decisions they make, and the positive outcomes they attempt to achieve.

OVERCOMING DOGMA AND BELIEF

Past practice, historical precedent, dogma, belief, and ideology all serve to create a contextual framework that informs action. Professions—most notably, nursing and medicine—have long historical attachments to process in the memories, mythologies, fantasies, and stories that create an idealization of practice and a disconnect from fact and reality (Anderson & Willson, 2008). For example, the traditional attachment to policy and procedure now represents a significant impediment to building evidence-based systems and infrastructure (**Figure 12-7**). In fact, policy and procedure are anathema to evidentiary processes representing a mental model and organizational framework that operate with constructs demonstrating a polar difference from the ones that now represent the fluidity of information management and clinical decision making (Birch, 2007; Oostendorp, 2003).

Attachment to policy and procedural constructs represents an understanding of practice as being part of a "fixed" operational and clinical system. Policy and procedural constructs demonstrate a belief that change is external, incremental, and situational—none of which, as we now know, holds true. In quantum thinking and within complexity-defined systems, change is a constant, a fundamental dynamic of existence. In this circumstance, change is

Figure 12-7   From process to synthesis.

Critical Process

- Newtonian
- Reductionistic
- Policy and procedure
- Provider driven
- Process centric
- Interventional

Critical Synthesis

- Quantum
- Multilateral
- Evidentiary
- Value/goal centric
- Referent (continuous)

an existential condition, uncontrolled, beyond human manipulation; it is also a fundamental characteristic and operation of the universe (Blum, 2006). The belief that it can be bounded, defined, and controlled as represented in fixed policy and procedural frameworks is simply no longer reasonable. Yet, 4165 acute care hospitals across the United States still write policies and procedures and depend on them to inform appropriate action. Besides the gross idiocy of time wasted in redundancy and duplication in policy content and work processes as each hospital writes the same policy for itself, the format itself is no longer relevant.

Evidentiary systems reflect quantum understanding in the digital reality. The partnership inherent in these two elements redefines process and action. The capacity of the technology of information management and documentation now makes it possible for evidentiary data to be "real time" in nature, with a continuous feed of input, throughput, and output creating a truly effective and useful cybernetic loop (Malloch & Porter-O'Grady, 2006). Now clinical data can be collected, integrated, and synthesized in the input and throughput stages. Those data can then prove useful in the output phase when they are used to constructively challenge past practices, change current practice, and advise future practice, all in real time (Melnyk & Fineout-Overholt, 2004). Thanks to the availability of contemporary portable hardware and truly effective data management and application software, the user may now use "just-in-time" information as the basis upon which to make decisions and to take action. Validation, improvement, and transformation of practice can now occur in an instant in time, aided by the veracity, accuracy, and timeliness of the clinical data management system and the responsiveness of the human interface with it. No longer is there a six- to nine-month policy development–definition–approval turnaround time, which robs the patient of the immediate benefit from a new clinical product, process, or action. Now clinical action is itself the product of the confluence between demonstrated experience with data inputs, up-to-date contemporary research, aggregated inputs informing best practice, and actual clinical practices representing the most current standards or protocols guiding clinical action (Straus, Richardson, Glasziou, & Haynes, 2005.

The role of leadership in this movement is self-evident. Because leaders have the predominant role in creating the context and providing the supports necessary to ensure that appropriate decisions and actions are undertaken, resourcing and applying structure to these new models are obligations of the leader role. Performing this role effectively requires clarity of the conceptual role, personal knowledge, leadership principles, collaboration, synthesis, knowledge management, and mentoring. Aware and informed healthcare leaders stay abreast of the changing conditions and context for the application of clinical service. Through deliberation and dialogue at the strategic and tactical levels of the organization (where managers should be spending their leadership capital), these managers facilitate the planning and construction of designs for creating infrastructure and processes that would support point-of-service, evidence-based data integration and translation of its utility into clinical practice (**Figure 12-8**). The manager's requisite abilities related to scanning, predictive capacity, and adaptation now come to bear as a critical skill set in the creation of the structures and processes in support of contemporary evidence-based initiatives (Hesselbein, 2002). Indeed, managers represent in their own practice and performance the use of evidentiary strategies and tactics in advising decisions and taking actions related to resource use, demonstrated in their own management of human, fiscal, material, support, and systems accountabilities. The role played by strong, evidence-committed management leaders is enhanced by their willingness to both model and mentor evidentiary dynamics as the appropriate contemporary framework within which all work relationships and clinical performance unfold.

Figure 12-8   Principles of sustainable leadership.

Critical Process	New Models for Leaders
Directing	Clearinghouse
Organizing	Enrolling
Leading	Investing
Controlling	Conflicting
Informing	Challenging
Parenting	Moderating
Telling	Inquiring
Managing	Facilitating
Evaluating	Stretching

LEADERSHIP AND COMPLEXITY

Complexity and complex systems thinking and research have provided a strong contemporary foundation for rethinking and reconfiguring the role of management in complex organizations (Murphy, Ruch, Pepicello, & Murph, 1997; Shan & Ang, 2008; Suh, 2005; Zimmerman, Lindberg, & Plsek, 1998). Much of the complex-systems literature has demonstrated the power and influence of system self-organization and emergent system behaviors (Miller & Scott, 2007). This new research is revising the foundations for understanding leadership practices and behavior and even reconceptualizing the role and application of leadership in organization decisions and actions (Morrison, 2007).

Much of the work on complex-systems sciences emerged from the biological, social, and physical sciences. The convergence of those data revealed patterns of behavior that emerged from examples of interacting and intersecting human societies, e-systems, ecosystems, the human brain, and bee colonies, among others (Rouse, 2007). These various exemplars of system now serve to inform our understanding of the role of the leader in the interactions of leaders with and within the systems of which they are a part (Stacey, 2007). (See **Figure 12-9**.)

A larger question related to complex systems is how much control should be exercised by the agent of control (the manager) within systems—in this case,

---

Figure 12-9   Complexity is a network of interdependent relationships and intersections, interacting together for a common purpose advancing mutual goals.

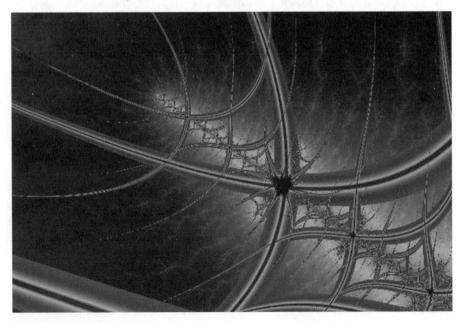

within the healthcare system. We know that varying levels of agency control are evident in a variety of systems. For example, on the Internet, almost no central control is exerted. In contrast, in the military and the solar system, high levels of control are exhibited. In the human body, intermediate interacting levels of control are evidenced.

Degrees of criticalness also influence level of agent control. In highly critical circumstances, where the life of an organism or system is directly and dramatically threatened, high levels of control are necessary to stabilize the system and bring it back into balance. By comparison, in systems with a high level of equilibrium and good responsive interface between external environmental challenges and demands and internal mechanisms of response, low levels of critical condition exist and, therefore, there is a reduced need for levels of agent control (Solow & Szmerekovsky, 2006).

Within the frame of complexity, there is the understanding that complex adaptive systems represent a highly complex dynamic of interacting and intersecting forces operating externally and internally, constantly affecting the life of the system (Yin & Ang, 2008). (See **Figure 12-10**.) For example, the management of a patient in a critical care unit requires much more agent intervention surveillance and intensity than does the management of a patient in

Figure 12-10   Complexity frame for evidence-driven synthesis/adaptative realities.

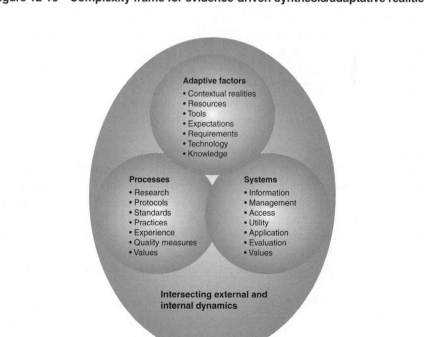

a long-term care facility or hospice setting. The degree of agent control and manipulation of circumstance and relational variables leads to different agent roles and relationship with control. Evidence-based management perceives this relationship in terms of the complex network of intersections and interactions and the degree of internally generated locus of control or the degree of external management of control. In broad terms, the incidence of emergent leadership and its influence on decision making and action may be directly related to the level of agent control, ranging from highly critical (greatest agent control) to highly self-managed (least agent control).

In an evidence-based framework, engagement and involvement inside the innovation process would reflect the least intensity of agent control, allowing the greatest freedom in an environment that fosters successful innovation. Ready access to all of the supports, resources, tools, and processes that facilitate the energetic and free-flowing activities of creativity would be essential to innovation. The manager in this case would create conditions and circumstances that permit this more "open" dynamic to thrive. By contrast, emergence of this type of control would be less likely in a situation where the variables need to be tightly manipulated and managed with narrowly defined but clearly applied manager (agent) control, such as in situations involving employee discipline, critical interventions, system control (such as in a prison), or terrorism.

The effective evidence-based manager recognizes the action of complexity and the value of establishing the evolving role factors, including new roles responding to the current circumstances and the activities unfolding within them. Also, the evidence-driven leader is aware of the confluence and consonance of interaction between external environmental forces and internal relational, operational, and behavioral responses to an ever-changing set of circumstances (Frandkov, 1999). (See **Figure 12-11**.) For this reason, managers need to raise their level of awareness with regard to the conflicting competencies learned as a part of traditional management development from those more contemporary competencies reflected in factors of agency and the role of the manager in a complex adaptive system. The most important element to shift to an evidentiary framework for the leader is the recognition that past leadership practices have been guided by linear, cognitive, and rational processes that reflect rather predictable changes in process and outputs. In the new environment, decision making and action must reflect more nonlinear and quantum influences in human dynamics and behavior. The evidence-based leader understands that human (and, therefore, health) behavior, such that change is better conceptualized, understood, and addressed through the lens of complex adaptive/responsive processes (Ang & Yin, 2008).

Research findings related to fractal patterns, which are central to the understanding of chaos theory, demonstrate that recurring patterns are present in

Figure 12-11   Complexity frames for the 21st century.

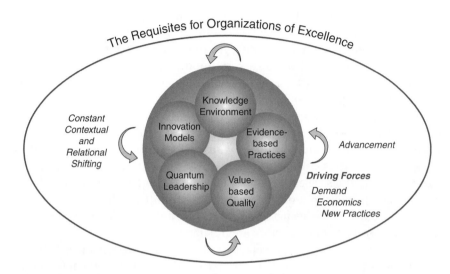

larger systems that are self-similar at all stages of magnification (Ang & Yin, 2008). When that concept is applied to behavioral change that can be expressed in infinite permutations, it implies that there are deeply embedded, recurrent patterns of change within groups, within individuals, and between individuals. The evidence-driven leader constantly looks for patterns in the system—that is, networks of intersections and relationships that recur in a wide variety of situations and circumstances (Janecka, 2008). By harnessing those definitive patterns, cross-referencing them, and looking for common elements, themes, and behaviors, the leader sees the emergence of the necessary insights, vehicles, resources, and actions that can be used and applied in related systems, networks, relationships, intersections, decisions, and actions (Hildreth & Kimble, 2004).

For the manager, then, evidence-based leadership represents the contemporary application of the theory and research of the action of complex systems and the translation and use of that understanding in decisions and actions in the workplace. For the manager, just as for the clinician, the development of the infrastructure—that is, a framework for good evidence-based leadership—reflects the application of complexity theory and complex adaptive systems to the work relationships, behaviors, and structures constantly operating to influence clinical practice and outcomes. If the leaders seek to uncover evidence-based practice in the lives of the knowledge work professionals, it is critical that the lens used in this endeavor be the leader's own evidence-driven behaviors and practices (Bennet & Bennet, 2004).

LEADERSHIP AND SOCIAL CONSTRUCTION: BUILDING COMMUNITIES OF PRACTICE

Managing environments where the preponderance of players are professional knowledge workers raises a unique set of circumstances with regard to knowledge creation, generation, and utility. All of these are key factors in knowledge work communities with regard to building a culture of evidence that drives professional thinking, relationship, and action. Communities of practice comprise groups of people informally bound together by shared expertise and enterprise related specifically to particular field of practice (Hildreth & Kimble, 2004). These communities share knowledge, insight, and experiences with others who have similar content and goals. Through their relationships and interactions, these groups typically form foundations for best practice, protocols, and actions. These groups of knowledge workers base their value on their common frame of reference, seeking opportunities to find best practices, strengthen their knowledge networks, and contribute directly to realizing the value of the products of their work and its impact.

The concept of knowledge is central to the work of professional practice. In communities of practice, knowledge transfer is the product of the interactions between knowledge workers (agents) who are working to comprehend, define, and apply knowledge (Higgs, Richardson, & Dahlgren, 2004). In this set of circumstances, the leader is constantly observing the group's construction, needs, and work requisites; attempting to blend their actions with the prevailing reality; and trying to integrate external realities with emerging responses so as to assure a tighter goodness of fit between them. In essence, the manager is constantly creating a context of reality orientation, including an understanding of the overriding reality of constant change. The manager brings to the table the reality that systems exist in the context of specific goals. Indeed, adaptive systems simply reflect or denote the essential requisite of systems—namely, their ability to support adaptation as a way of better achieving goals (Bradford & Burke, 2005).

From the perspective of the leader, the fundamental of the role of knowledge worker is as "agent of change," where change *is* the work of the knowledge worker. In short, knowledge workers exist to make change (their sole purpose). The manager as system agent makes sure that there is congruence between the external demands for change and the internal mechanisms and response to change, such that the changes undertaken by the agents of change (knowledge workers) are relevant, timely, and appropriate.

By creating this environment or context for communities of practice or accountability groups, the leader creates a level of engagement and ownership on the part of the knowledge worker with regard to the stakes and purposes of the community. This level of mutuality serves as a common frame of reference for ownership. It increases the obligation of accountability and creates a circumstance in which accountability becomes the driving force for the alignment of effective decisions and actions. In short, the leader creates an evidence-oriented environment in which all activities of the stakeholders reinforce their participation and investment in activities built on an evidentiary frame, a feat that requires full engagement on the part of the organization's members in advancing that work. The value of evidence-based management, in this scenario, is reflected in the effectiveness and success of evidence-based practice. In short, the manager works to create a culture of evidence-based practice (Anderson & Willson, 2008).

Furthermore, when the leader creates a culture of evidence-based practice and a medium supporting communities of practice, the system's clinical intellectual and creative capital—that is, the clinical practitioners—perceive themselves as the central medium of decision and action; in essence, the life of the system depends on them (Chrispeels, 2004). Through this evidentiary membership community, research, experience, best practice, social and technological shifts, and new knowledge become normative elements of relationship and practice. These social networks become the brokers of best practices reflected in their affinity and absorptive capacity for information that informs, challenges, and changes practice (Hamaaskorpi & Niukkanen, 2007). Members of this community see change as the normative context for practice and, with the manager, build the context that facilitates their being fluid, flexible, focused, portable, and mobile. Within this context, then, the knowledge worker stakeholders can create an environment characterized by critical thinking, embracing change, and building multiple feedback loops and monitoring mechanisms that facilitate their ability to adapt new knowledge, translate it, and change practice accordingly. In this scenario, the evidence-based manager orchestrates the cultural dynamics that create the urge to succeed in these networks, translates the conditions and circumstances of reality, and makes it possible for the practitioners to continually adapt and succeed.

BUILDING THE CONTEXTUAL FRAMEWORK FOR EVIDENCE-BASED LEADERSHIP

For evidence-based leadership and management to exist as a way of doing business in organizations, certain organizational and role capacities must be established. Evidence-based leadership does not occur by osmosis or by accident. Instead, intentional design and construction are critical processes necessary to create the context and constructs that ultimately lead to an evidentiary framework within which both the business and the action of clinical practice can successfully unfold.

The following components must be incorporated in the construction of evidentiary environments to assure an appropriate environment for evidence-based leadership:

1. Commitment to data- and information-driven decision making at the very senior levels of the organization in a way that assures the decisions will be generated from within a data framework.

2. Investment in the resources needed to build the data and informational infrastructure, including appropriation of sufficient hardware and software to assure the utility and effectiveness of information-driven decision making and determination of fixed-process approaches to operational and clinical decision making.

3. Engagement of and investment in point-of-service knowledge workers at the outset in the design of management and clinical information infrastructure, software, processes and effectiveness evaluation, as a way of assuring a goodness of fit between the proposed data tools and the utility of their application.

4. Reconceptualization and retraining of managers and leaders in the new concepts of complex adaptive/responsive systems, role agency, and emergent leadership, and in the manager behaviors necessary to facilitate a framework for innovation and creativity as a way of doing business in the organization.

5. Conception of healthcare organizations and hospitals as complex systems and networked relationships that demonstrate high levels of multifocal interaction and interdependence in a way that eliminates vertical decision models, operating silos, and nonaligned departmental configurations.

6. Elimination of discipline-specific locus of control in favor of interdisciplinary processes, teams, and decision making, resulting in an integrated model of evidence-driven decision making, practice, and impact evaluation. This step includes recognizing that sustainable outcome-oriented, evidence-driven practice represents the synthesis of the effort of all stakeholders influencing clinical outcomes, rather than being a unilateral measure of incremental impact (isolated, nonaligned disciplinary outcome).

7. Construction and development of a strategic plan and timeline for transforming the system environment from a fixed operational model to a fluid, data-driven organizational framework supporting evidentiary systems, structures, processes, applications, and evaluation. This step includes consonance between the evidence-driven strategic trajectory, resource capitalization for it, management and operational reconfiguration for leading it, and clinical facility in doing it.

This series of steps provides governance and senior leadership with a framework for constructing the foundation of an evidence-driven organization and all that is necessary to initiate and sustain that philosophy. It certainly calls for major commitment to transforming the healthcare organization. The requisite for doing so, however, is clearly evidenced by the emerging and maturing synthesis between technology and human action. Indeed, technology and human experience are, in the twenty-first century, no longer separate entities. Effective leadership in health care focuses diligently not on establishing this relationship (its establishment has already occurred), but rather on facilitating and refining its positive development in a way that yields net accelerated value within the healing community. As clearly indicated by all authors in this text, evidence-based practice cannot unfold without the discussion and inclusion of technological factors and forces influencing advancing clinical practice and the evidence upon which such advances will be founded.

The next section presents an application of these theoretical principles in a transformational model intended to guide leaders on this important journey.

IMAGINE THIS...

Today's healthcare professionals now have the opportunity to turn the evidence-based leadership and management model into reality—especially given the economic downturns and work force shortages that characterize the current environment. A better and more effective way to work is desperately needed. The "monkey wrench" thrown into the healthcare industry by the current economic hardships may, in fact, be the best thing that could happen to health care, as it offers healthcare organization the chance to create an evidence-driven healthcare model that includes both clinical practices and leadership and management practices. Put simply, the current marketplace is the ideal milieu for healthcare professionals to create new models for health care.

One strategy involves the application of these principles as the guiding force in the transformation to an evidence-based leadership and management model. To be sure, health care has always had its share of great ideas and innovators, especially in technology and pharmaceuticals. What has been lacking, however, is the contemporary infrastructure to support and sustain these new ideas. New ideas and innovations require a disciplined approach toward their evaluation, implementation, and sustainability. The following model provides this structure and support for sustainability. Six steps are included in the *Imagine this...* approach, as shown in **Figure 12-12**.

Step 1

Step 1 begins with the vision—that is, envisioning the new reality or dreaming the big dream. This step sets the stage for the work to be done and develops rules of engagement for this work. The principles of evidence-based leadership and management are foundational for this work to occur. The principles include the following expectations:

- Processes are best understood using complex adaptive and responsive frameworks. Complexity tenets specific to self-organization, emergent behaviors, uncertainty, lack of central control, nonlinear activities, dynamic interacting and intersecting, and evolving roles guide the work of evidence-based leadership and management. Similarly, work relationships among individuals reflect the reality of complexity and complex adaptive systems.

- Uncertainty is normative. Reality evolves as actions and individuals interact and intersect. There is no template or algorithm for determining how the future will unfold.

- Accountability is based on outcomes and results rather than processes and outputs. In addition, accountability for performance and achievement based on knowledge rather than opinion is the norm. The elimination of non-value-added work is expected.

- The value equation is continually evaluated; namely, the relationship among resources, outcomes, and value is summarily positive.

- The processes are knowledge driven. Doing the right work, which is itself based on knowledge or evidence, is essential. The locus of control for knowledge and knowledge management lies within the individual rather than with the organization. At the same time, knowledge is owned and managed by communities of knowledge workers who are bound together by shared expertise. Thus knowledge management goes well beyond traditional organizational boundaries.

- Teamwork, values alignment, and community building are the essential relationship skills needed to support the evidence-based model. The work focuses on facilitating the understanding and engagement of common values and goals by team members; it is not geared toward externally motivating individuals to participate for a stipend reward. The work of creating *fire in the bellies* of all team members is deemed far more important and sustainable than enlisting a group of followers.

- The paradox of time is recognized: Timing is everything. Change takes time, but we don't have time to over-process new ideas. Failing to move and to take rational and strategic risks will be detrimental to organizational survival.

Figure 12-12 Imagine this...

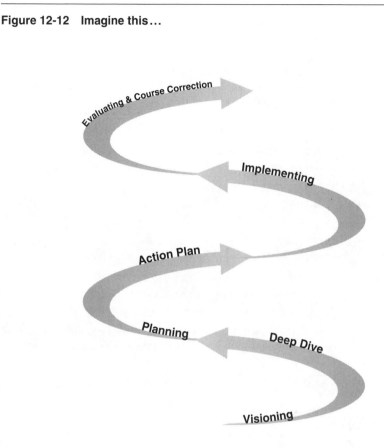

The visioning process can be similar to the process used in the design of the Fable Hospital, a composite of recently built or redesigned healthcare facilities that has implemented facets of evidence-based design. Fable Hospital doesn't yet exist; however, its authors believe it will be built (Berry, Parker, Coile, Hamilton, O'Neill, & Sadler, 2004). Fable Hospital serves as an idealized template to illustrate how evidence-based design can improve outcomes from many perspectives. **Table 12-1** lists the elements within the healthcare environment that might potentially be linked to evidentiary resources within this structure.

This model and approach can serve as a guide for the evolution of the evidence-based leadership model. Similarly, a model for evidence-based leadership could and should do the same. Information specific to patient and staff satisfaction, clinical outcomes, safety, organizational effectiveness, cost-efficiency, resource allocations, and financial performance should be examined as part of this step.

Table 12-1   Fable Hospital: The Evidence-Based Design Dream

Fable Hospital's core values include superior quality, safety, patient-focused care, family friendliness, staff support, cost sensitivity, eco-sustainability and community responsibility. Management engaged a philosophically aligned design team based on the premise that the building should reflect the organization's core values and strategic aspirations. The designers responded with an array of design innovations and upgrades for the new facility, including the following:

OVERSIZED SINGLE ROOMS with dedicated space for patient, family and staff activities and sufficient capacity for in-room procedures. The design maximizes daylight exposure to patient rooms and work spaces.

VARIABLE ACUITY ROOMS standardized in shape, size and headwall to eliminate the need to move patients as their condition changes.

DOUBLE-DOOR BATHROOM ACCESS enabling caregivers to more easily assist patients to and from the bathroom on foot, in wheelchairs, or in their beds.

DECENTRALIZED, BARRIERFREE NURSING STATIONS that place nurses in close proximity to their patients and supplies, most of which are stored in or near patient rooms.

ADDITIONAL HAND-WASHING FACILITIES located conveniently to encourage staff to use them to reduce transmission of infections and enabling patients to see them being used.

HEPA FILTERS to improve the filtration of incoming outside air and eliminate re-circulated air.

FLEXIBLE SPACES for advanced technologies including operating rooms sized for robotic surgery, endovascular suites for minimally invasive surgery with sophisticated imaging, and imaging rooms designed to support continuous equipment advances.

PEACEFUL SETTINGS including artwork displays, space to listen to piano music, and gardens with fountains and benches to moderate the stress of building occupants.

NOISE-REDUCING MEASURES including sound-absorbing ceilings and a wireless communications system that eliminates overhead paging, to moderate the stress of building occupants.

CONSULTATION SPACES conveniently located to facilitate private communication between caregivers and families.

PATIENT EDUCATION CENTERS on each floor offering brochures, books, videotapes and Internet access to disease-specific information and online support groups that improve patient and family understanding of illness.

STAFF SUPPORT FACILITIES including a staff-only cafeteria, windowed break rooms with outside access, a day-care facility, and an exercise club.

Source: Berry, Parker, Coile, Hamilton, O'Neill, & Sadler, 2004.

Step 2

The second step is the "deep dive" into the healthcare environment. The deep dive, similar to the approach advocated by Kelley (2001), is an experiential observation process that provides a systematic methodology for teams to be both innovative and creative in finding solutions to improve, eliminate, or add new practices. In a deep dive, teams observe processes, interview those involved in the process, take pictures, write notes, and generate new ideas from their observations (Kelley, 2001). Participant observations emphasize opportunities to strengthen the value of work, opportunities to eliminate non-essential or non-value-added work, and the potential for increasing or adding experiences that exceed value expectations.

In the deep dive experience, the assignment of roles or faces of innovation can assist in the explication of a rich array of information. According to Kelley (2005), there are ten faces of innovation:

- *Anthropologist:* This role observes behaviors and seeks to understand how people interact in certain settings. In the leadership deep dive, individuals would be observing the interactions between team members, the communication styles, and the equipment and technology used, among other things.

- *Experimenter:* This perspective focuses on prototyping new ideas; it deals with proposing and testing new methods or models. For the leader, an experimenter might propose new ideas using the "What if we..." approach.

- *Cross-pollinator:* A cross-pollinator looks from one industry or culture to another to see how different ideas or products exist in different areas. For example, a clinical leader might propose nonclinical approaches in the clinical setting to test responses and effect.

- *Hurdler:* The hurdler thrives on overcoming obstacles and escaping seemingly impossible situations. For the leader seeking to advance the evidence-driven model, the hurdler persona would propose new and different ways to gain support for an unpopular but needed change.

- *Collaborator:* This persona brings eclectic individuals together to find common ground. To be sure, collaboration and dialogue will be needed in an evidence-driven model as individuals learn about one another, including their different values and different needs. Coming to consensus without eliminating distinctions is the hallmark of success for the collaborator.

- *Director:* The director persona is an orchestra leader-type individual; he or she can work with multiple individuals and inspire their creative spirits. Often times in healthcare organizations, the director is essential to getting individuals together to begin meaningful dialogue and then move to collaboration.

- *Experience Architect:* For this persona, participation in a special event is essential. Experiencing a particular feeling is believed to be an approach to inspiring creativity. For the healthcare professional, experiencing or facilitating a high level of patient satisfaction is especially motivating.

- *Set Designer:* The set designer organizes the environment so that the best work can occur. For the healthcare experience, a set designer might be the person who selected a great, quiet retreat place for thinking and brainstorming.

- *Caregiver:* In Kelley's model (2005), the caregiver persona is the individual who goes beyond basic service and works to anticipate needs and be ready to assist. Similarly, in the leadership model, the caregiver could be the person making sure everyone is happy with staffing schedules or lunch breaks. What is often a challenge for this role is the tendency to go beyond caregiving to mothering and assuming accountability for another person or entity.

- *Storyteller:* This persona represents a very high level of understanding of a situation. The storyteller is able to use situations and events to make a point or engage others in meaningful ways. Often the storyteller is able to distill very complex issues into a story for illustration purposes and is able to assist others in understanding the issues quickly.

When individuals assume these different personas in the work of assessing an environment, the resulting richness of information is incredible. The results are far superior to those possible when individuals view a situation from their typical persona. Once this information is gained, the team can aggregate it into a wilderness infrastructure table (**Table 12-2**) to identify specific strengths, work to be done, work to be eliminated, and metrics for measurement.

Step 3

The third step is planning for the future is both specific and personal. For a leader steeped in uncertainty and the realities of a complex system, constant and unrelenting change can be either transformational or debilitating. Necessarily, the sometimes intimidating and unsettling activities must serve as inspiration for transformation—even in the toughest of times. According to Rosen (2008), three capabilities are needed: self-awareness, a commitment to lifelong learning, and nonattachment. Self-awareness means knowing what you know and what you don't know. A commitment to lifelong learning entails continually feeding both the mind and the soul with new resources to solve problems

Table 12-2 Wilderness Infrastructure Table: Moving from the Unknown to the Known

		Wilderness: If we had it all/ dreaming the big dream	Reality: What we have today	Gaps between the wilderness and the reality	Strategy to close gaps: What can be done? When can it be done? What will it cost?	Work to give up: What work is redundant or not adding value to patient outcomes?	Measures of success: What value was created for the patient? How will we measure it?
1	Data and information driven decision making						
2	Hardware and software resources						
3	Engagement of point-of-service knowledge workers						
4	Support for skill and competence transition						
5	Complexity knowledge						
6	Interdisciplinary processes						
7	Strategic organizational transitioning						

and grow. Nonattachment is probably the most challenging of the three capabilities: It is about letting go of negative habits and limiting behaviors, and focusing on what needs to occur to achieve goals rather than worrying about one's personal feelings.

Step 4

Step 4 involves developing an action plan based on the information collected in the wilderness infrastructure template. Creating an action plan for an uncertain future requires a somewhat rigorous process. The wilderness template can be used to guide and document this process through the steps of visioning, assessment, gap analysis, action planning, work modifications, and evaluation metrics. Using this approach, team members are able to more clearly review, distill, and prioritize the ideas into a strategic action plan.

The action plan should include not only action items for additional work, but also identification of redundant or non-value-added work that can be eliminated. Too often efforts focus only on the additional work without consideration being given to elimination of outmoded work.

Within the action plan, the business case or rationale for new work must be included in an evidentiary model. The business case is an important component to advance the evidence journey. The specific resources, risks, and anticipated outcomes are essential inputs to the model from which to propose new and different strategies. Failing to consider all of the options and potential outcomes hinders both progress and the possible improvements.

As the organization's roles evolve into the evidentiary model, it is important to assure that transition between roles relies on adding new and different skills rather than increasing the depth to current skills. For example, to advance from a knowledge worker to an evidence-driven manager, new skills and competencies are needed (**Table 12-3**). Rather than learning more about

---

Table 12-3   Role Accountabilities

Leader accountable for creating the conditions for excellence in clinical care optimal outcomes in a way that is sustainable and valued.

Manager accountable for creating a context that facilitates and supports ownership and expression of accountability on the part of the knowledge workers.

Knowledge worker accountable for effective patient care work and the achievement outcomes.

---

pharmaceuticals, the aspiring manager needs to learn how to create the conditions for others to own the accountability for knowledge management needed to safely and effectively administer medications. Under the evidentiary model, roles for leaders, managers, and knowledge workers are clear and outcome driven. The leader is accountable for creating the conditions for excellence in clinical care work and optimal outcomes in a way that is both sustainable and valued. The manager is accountable for creating a context that facilitates, supports, and encourages the ownership and expression of accountability on the part of knowledge workers. The knowledge workers are accountable for effective patient care work and the achievement of outcomes.

To assess the evidentiary nature of leaders, manager, and knowledge workers and the supporting culture, use of the wilderness role template is recommended (**Table 12-4**). The teamwork required to complete the template—which includes desired and actual behaviors, gaps between desired and actual plans, metrics, and work to eliminate—can be both enlightening and instructive in this regard.

As the team considers the action plan, specific measures need to be selected for implementation. The data and analytics for measurement of outcomes include those metrics and qualitative summaries that reflect endpoint results directly related to value for the community, organization, providers, and patients. Necessarily, multiple metrics need to be evaluated simultaneously and within the context of the service. For example, numerous variables affect rates of patient falls, nosocomial infection rates, drug costs, and nursing turnover. Thus, not only are these metrics important to examine on their own, but they should also be addressed within the context of the available staff, their skill levels, technology resources, and the physical environment. Multivariate analyses are essential to portray the system results both accurately and comprehensively.

As the action plan is developed, efforts to overcome dogma should be considered. For example, the extant clinical policy and procedure manuals can be rethought from the evidentiary model. The evaluation should begin by considering the desired value-based outcome—namely, information is needed by caregivers to provide safe and effective patient care.

Step 5

Implementing the plan is Step 5 in the evidence-based model and necessarily requires significant time and rollout considerations. No matter how clear and definitive the action plan is, unforeseen events and challenges will inevitably arise; to be sure, plan implementation is an exercise in living with complexity and learning to respect and value the reality of the healthcare environment. Traditional project management concepts are helpful to stage the implementation.

Table 12-4   Wilderness Role Table: Moving from the Unknown to the Known

	Wilderness: If we had it all/ dreaming the big dream	Reality: What we have today	Gaps between the wilderness and the reality	Strategy to close gaps: What can be done? When can it be done? What will it cost?	Work to give up: What work is redundant or not adding value to patient outcomes?	Measures of success: What value was created for the patient? How will we measure it?
1	Leadership role clarity					
2	Manager role clarity					
3	Knowledge worker role clarity					
4	Resources: People and dollars					
5	Culture					

Complexity principles and sensitivity to uncertainty and the chaos resulting from the evolution are best supported through teamwork and collaboration.

Step 6

The sixth step includes evaluating the plan and course correction. Given the complex, interactive, and intersecting work that is being analyzed, a mind map (**Figure 12-13**) is often a very useful tool to document this iterative and evolving work. This tool provides an excellent way to gather multiple documents, Web sites, and video files into a single site. The resulting mind map best demonstrates the aggregation and synthesis of the complexities of the current healthcare system and the breadth and depth of the work of transforming leadership behaviors.

Next Steps

As leaders emerge into the evidentiary leadership world, there is both work to do and much to be gained. Thinking and behaving in ways that are better defined based on evidence and enhanced by digital innovations are essential for not only success, but also for survival. The desired foundation will

---

Figure 12-13   Mind Map Example

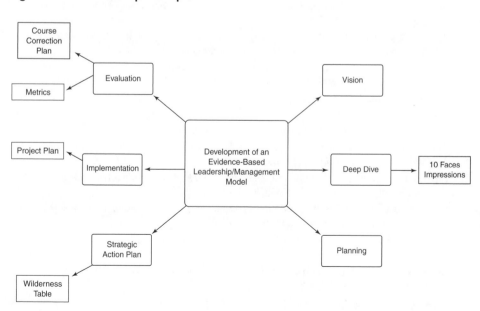

support ongoing commitment to role accountability, evidence, effective relationships, and core values of respect, integrity, and caring. Three distinct and clearly defined roles are essential for the future; the leader, the manager and the knowledge worker in order to assure work that is outcome driven and recognized for its value to the patient.

REFERENCES

Albrecht, K. (2003). *The power of minds at work: Organizational intelligence in action.* New York: AMACOM.

Anderson, J., & Willson, P. (2008). Clinical decision support systems in nursing: Synthesis of the science for evidence-based practice. *CIN: Computers, Informatics, Nursing, 26*(3), 151–158.

Ang, Y., & Yin, S. (2008). *Intelligent complex adaptive systems.* Chicago: IGI.

Apker, J., Ford, S., & Fox, D. (2003). Predicting nurses organizational and professional identification: The effect of nursing roles, professional economy, and supportive communication. *Nursing Economics, 21*(5), 226–232.

Badawy, M. (2003). Why managers fail. In R. Katz (Ed.), *The human side of managing technological innovation* (pp. 34–46). New York: Oxford University Press.

Ball, M.J. (2000). *Nursing informatics: Where caring and technology meet* (3rd ed.). New York: Springer.

Barry, R., Murcko, A., & Brubaker, C. (2002). *The Six Sigma book for healthcare.* Chicago: Health Administration Press.

Bass, B. (1990). *Bass & Stogdill's handbook of leadership: Theory, research, and managerial applications.* New York: Free Press.

Bennet, A., & Bennet, D. (2004). *Organizational survival in the New World: The intelligent complex adaptive system.* New York: Butterworth-Heinemann.

Berry, L. L., Parker, D., Coile, R. C., Jr., Hamilton, D. K., O'Neill, D. D., & Sadler, J. D. (2004). The business case for better buildings. *Frontiers of Health Services Management, 21*(1), 3–24.

Berwick, D., Nolan, T., & Whittington, J. (2008). The triple aim: Care, health, and cost. *Health Affairs, 27*(3), 759–769.

Birch, D. (2007). *Digital identity management.* Los Angeles: Gower.

Blum, M. (2006). *Continuity, quantum, continuum, and dialectic: The foundational logics of Western historical thinking.* Chicago: Peter Lang.

Bossidy, L., Charan, R., & Burck, C. (2002). *Execution: The discipline of getting things done.* New York: Crown Business.

Bradford, D. L., & Burke, W. W. (2005). *Reinventing organization development: New approaches to change in organizations.* San Francisco: Pfeiffer.

Chakravarthy, B. (2003). *Strategy process: Shaping the contours of the field.* Malden, MA: Blackwell.

Chrispeels, J.H. (2004). *Learning to lead together: The promise and challenge of sharing leadership.* Thousand Oaks, CA: Sage.

Christiansen, C. (2003). *The innovator's dilemma: The revolutionary book that will change the way you do business.* New York: HarperCollins.

Davenport, T. (2006). Competing on analytics. *Harvard Business Review, 82*(1), 24–36.

Dotlich, D. L., & Cairo, P. C. (2002). *Unnatural leadership: Going against intuition and experience to develop ten new leadership instincts.* San Francisco: Jossey-Bass.

Drucker, P. (1977). *Management.* New York: Harper & Row.

Drucker, P. F. (2001). *The essential Drucker: Selections from the management works of Peter F. Drucker.* New York: HarperBusiness.

Drucker, P., & Stone, N. (1998). *On the profession of management.* Boston: Harvard Business School Publishing.

Force, M. (2005). The relationship between effective nurse managers and nursing retention. *Journal of Nursing Administration, 35*(7–8), 336–341.

Fottler, M., Ford, R., & Heaton, C. (2002). *Achieving service excellence.* Chicago: Health Administration Press.

Frandkov, A. (1999). *Nonlinear and adaptive control of complex systems.* New York: Springer.

Freshwater, D., & Rolfe, G. (2004). *Deconstructing evidence based practice.* New York: Routledge.

Gandossy, R. P., & Sonnenfeld, J. A. (2004). I see nothing, I hear nothing: Culture, corruption, and apathy. In R. P. Gandossy & J. A. Sonnenfeld (Eds.), *Leadership and governance from the inside out* (pp. 3–26). New York: John Wiley & Sons.

Garvin, D., & Roberto, M. (2001). What you don't know about making decisions. *Harvard Business Review, 79*(9), 108–118.

Geisler, E., Krabbendam, K., & Schuring, R. (2003). *Technology, health care, and management in the hospital of the future.* Westport, CT: Praeger.

Giacco, A. F. (2003). *Maverick management: Strategies for success.* Newark, NJ: University of Delaware Press.

Gitlow, A. L. (2005). *Corruption in corporate America: Who is responsible? Who will protect the public interest?* Lanham, MD: University Press of America.

Goad, T. W. (2002). *Information literacy and workplace performance.* Westport, CT: Quorum Books.

Goodpaster, K., Nash, L. L., & Bettignies, H. (2006). *Business ethics: Policies and persons* (4th ed.). Boston: McGraw-Hill/Irwin.

Gottlieb, M. R. (2003). *Managing group process.* Westport, CT: Praeger.

Hamaaskorpi, V., & Niukkanen, H. (2007). Leadership in different kinds of regional development networks. *Baltic Journal of Management, 2*(1), 80–96.

Hatch, M. J., Kostera, M., & Kozminski, A. (2005). *The three faces of leadership: Manager, artist, priest.* Malden, MA: Blackwell.

Herzberg, F. (1991). *Motivation to work.* Cleveland, OH: Penton Media.

Herzberg, F. (2008). *One more time: How do you motivate employees?* Boston: Harvard Business School Press.

Hesselbein, F. (2002). *Hesselbein on leadership.* San Francisco: Jossey-Bass.

Hickman, C., Smith, T., & Conners, R. (2004). *The Oz principle: Getting results through individual and organizational accountability.* New York: Portfolio Hardcover.

Higgs, J., Richardson, B., & Dahlgren, M. A. (2004). *Developing practice knowledge for health professionals.* New York: Butterworth-Heinemann.

Hildreth, P. M., & Kimble, C. (2004). *Knowledge networks: Innovation through communities of practice.* Hershey, PA: Idea Group.

Hooker, C., & Csikszentmihalvi, M. (2003). Rethinking the motivation and structuring of knowledge work. In C. Pearce & J. Conger (Eds.), *Shared leadership: Reframing the hows and whys of leadership* (pp. 217–233). Thousand Oaks, CA: Sage.

Jackson, I. A., & Nelson, J. (2004). *Profits with principles: Seven strategies for delivering value with values.* New York: Currency/Doubleday.

Janecka, I. (2008). A review of managing information in complex organizations: Semiotics and signals, complexity and chaos. *Emergence: Complexity and Organization, 10*(1), 91–96.

Jurewicz, L., & Cutler, T. (2003). *High tech, high touch: Library customer service through technology.* Chicago: American Library Association.

Kanter, R. (2004). How leaders restore confidence. In R. P. Gandossy & J. A. Sonnenfeld (Eds.), *Leadership and governance from the inside out* (pp. 39–50). New York: John Wiley & Sons.

Keating, S. (2004). If I only knew then what I know now. In R. P. Gandossy & J. A. Sonnenfeld (Eds.), *Leadership and governance from the inside and out* (pp. 271–276). New York: John Wiley & Sons.

Kelley, T. (2001). *The art of innovation: Lessons in creativity from IDEO America's leading design firm.* New York: Doubleday.

Kelley, T. (2005). *The ten faces of innovation.* New York: Doubleday.

Kleinman, C. (2003). Leadership roles, competencies, and education: How prepared are nurse managers. *Journal of Nursing Administration, 33*(9), 451–455.

Leach, L. (2005). Nurse executive transformational leadership and organizational commitment. *Journal of Nursing Administration, 35*(5), 228–237.

Lencioni, P. (2002). *The five dysfunctions of a team.* San Francisco: Jossey-Bass.

Locsin, R. C. (2001). *Advancing technology, caring, and nursing.* Westport, CT: Auburn House.

Malloch, K., & Porter-O'Grady, T. (1999). Partnership economics: Nursing's challenge in a quantum age. *Nursing Economics, 17*(6), 299–307.

Malloch, K., & Porter-O'Grady, T. (2005). *The quantum leader: Applications for the new world of work.* Sudbury, MA: Jones and Bartlett Publishers.

Malloch, K., & Porter-O'Grady, T. (2006). *Introduction to evidence-based practice in nursing and health care.* Sudbury, MA: Jones and Bartlett Publishers.

Mathena, K. (2002). Nursing manager leadership skills. *Journal of Nursing Administration, 32*(3), 136–142.

McDaniel, C. (2004). *Organizational ethics: Research and ethical environments.* Burlington, VT: Ashgate.

McNamara, O. (2002). *Becoming an evidence-based practitioner: A framework for teacher–researchers.* New York: Routledge/Falmer.

McSherry, R., Simmons, M., & Abbott, P. (2002). *Evidence-informed nursing: A guide for clinical nurses.* New York: Routledge.

Melnyk, B., & Fineout-Overholt, E. (2004). *Evidence-based practice in nursing and healthcare: A guide to best practice.* St. Louis, MO: Lippincott Williams & Wilkins.

Miller, J., & Scott, P. (2007). *Complex adaptive systems: An introduction to computational models of social life.* Princeton, NJ: Princeton University Press.

Miner, J. B. (2005). *Organizational behavior.* Armonk, NY: M. E. Sharpe.

Mintzberg, H. (1990). The manager's job: Folklore and fact. *Harvard Business Review, 48*(2), 163–176.

Mintzberg, H. (2004). *Managers, not MBAs: A hard look at the soft practice of managing and management development.* San Francisco: Barrett Koehler.

Morrison, K. (2007). *Complexity leadership.* Charlotte, NC: Information Age Publishing.

Murphy, E., Ruch, S., Pepicello, J., & Murphy, M. (1997). Managing an increasingly complex system. *Nursing Management, 28*(10), 33–38.

Oliver, R. W. (2004). *What is transparency?* New York: McGraw-Hill.

Oostendorp, H. V. (2003). *Cognition in a digital world.* Mahwah, NJ: Lawrence Erlbaum Associates.

Osborne, H. (2002). *Partnering with patients to improve health outcomes.* Gaithersburg, MD: Aspen.

Pidd, M. (2004). *Systems modeling: Theory and practice.* Hoboken, NJ: John Wiley & Sons.

Porter-O'Grady, T. (2000). Interdisciplinary shared governance: A partnership model for high performance in a managed care environment. *Seminars for Nurse Managers, 8*(3), 158–169.

Porter-O'Grady, T., & Afable, R. (2003). The technology of partnership. *Health Progress, 84*(3), 41–52.

Porter-O'Grady, T., & Malloch, K. (2007). *Quantum leadership: A resource for healthcare innovation.* Sudbury, MA: Jones and Bartlett Publishers.

Price, T. L. (2006). *Understanding ethical failures in leadership.* New York: Cambridge University Press.

Rosen, R. H. (2008, Fall). Embracing uncertainty and anxiety. *Leader to Leader, 2008*(50), 34–38.

Rouse, W. (2007). Complex engineered, organizational and natural systems: Issues underlying the complexity of systems and fundamental research needed to address these issues. *Systems Engineering, 10*(3), 260–271.

Shan, Y., & Ang, Y. (2008). *Applications of complex adaptive systems.* Hershey, PA: IGI.

Smith, P. (2004). *Shaping the facts: Evidence-based nursing and health care.* New York: Churchill Livingstone.

Solow, D., & Szmerekovsky, J. (2006). The role of leadership: What management science can give back to the study of complex systems. *Emergence: Complexity and Organizations, 8*(4), 52–60.

Stacey, R. (2007). *Complexity and the experience of leading organizations.* New York: Routledge.

Straus, S., Richardson, W., Glasziou, P., & Haynes, R. (2005). *Evidence-based medicine.* London: Churchill Livingstone.

Suh, N. P. (2005). *Complexity: Theory and applications.* New York: Oxford University Press.

Sveiby, K. (1997). *The new organizational wealth.* San Francisco: Berrett-Koehler.

Tilley, D. (2008). Competency in nursing: A concept analysis. *Journal of Continuing Education in Nursing, 39*(2), 58–65.

Tourish, D., & Hargie, O. (2004). *Key issues in organizational communication.* New York: Routledge.

Traynor, M. (1999). *Managerialism and nursing: Beyond oppression and profession.* London: Rutledge.

Trompenaars, A., & Hampden-Turner, C. (2002). *21 leaders for the 21st century: How innovative leaders manage in the digital age.* New York: McGraw-Hill.

Useem, M. (2004). The essence of leading and governing is deciding. In R. P. Gandossy & J. A. Sonnenfeld (Eds.), *Leadership and governance from the inside out* (pp. 63–74). New York: John Wiley & Sons.

Wager, K., Wickham, F., & Glaser, J. (2005). *Managing healthcare information systems: A practical approach for healthcare executives.* San Francisco: Jossey-Bass.

Watkins, S. (2004). 21st-century corporate governance: The growing pressure on the board toward a corporate solution. In R. P. Gandossy & J. A. Sonnenfeld (Eds.), *Leadership and governance from the inside out* (pp. 27–36). New York: John Wiley & Sons.

Wolper, L. F. (2004). *Health care administration: Planning, implementing, and managing organized delivery systems* (4th ed.). Sudbury, MA: Jones and Bartlett Publishers.

Yin, S., & Ang, Y. (2008). *Applications of complex adaptive systems.* Chicago: IGI.

Zimmerman, B., Lindberg, C., & Plsek, P. (1998). *Edgeware.* Irving, TX: VHA.

Index